Addiction Psychiatry: Challenges and Recent Advances

Editors

SUNIL KHUSHALANI
GEORGE KOLODNER
CHRISTOPHER WELSH

PSYCHIATRIC CLINICS OF NORTH AMERICA

www.psych.theclinics.com

Consulting Editor
HARSH K. TRIVEDI

September 2022 • Volume 45 • Number 3

ELSEVIER

1600 John F. Kennedy Boulevard ● Suite 1800 ● Philadelphia, Pennsylvania, 19103-2899

http://www.theclinics.com

PSYCHIATRIC CLINICS OF NORTH AMERICA Volume 45, Number 3
September 2022 ISSN 0193-953X, ISBN-13: 978-0-323-93961-4

Editor: Megan Ashdown
Developmental Editor: Diana Grace Ang

Psychiatric Clinics of North America (ISSN 0193-953X) is published quarterly by Elsevier Inc., 360 Park Avenue South, New York, NY 10010-1710. Months of issue are March, June, September, and December. Business and Editorial Offices: 1600 John F. Kennedy Blvd., Suite 1800, Philadelphia, PA 19103-2899. Periodicals postage paid at New York, NY and additional mailing offices. Subscription prices are $345.00 per year (US individuals), $985.00 per year (US institutions), $100.00 per year (US students/residents), $414.00 per year (Canadian individuals), $509.00 per year (international individuals), $1005.00 per year (Canadian & international institutions), and $220.00 per year (international students/residents), $100.00 per year (Canadian & students/residents). Foreign air speed delivery is included in all *Clinics'* subscription prices. All prices are subject to change without notice. **POSTMASTER:** Send address changes to *Psychiatric Clinics of North America*, Elsevier Health Sciences Division, Subscription Customer Service, 3251 Riverport Lane, Maryland Heights, MO 63043. **Customer Service: 1-800-654-2452 (US). From outside the United States, call 1-314-447-8871. Fax: 1-314-447-8029. E-mail: journalscustomerservice-usa@elsevier.com (for print support) and journalsonlinesupport-usa@elsevier.com (for online support).**

Reprints. For copies of 100 or more, of articles in this publication, please contact the Commercial Reprints Department, Elsevier Inc., 360 Park Avenue South, New York, New York 10010-1710. Tel.: 212-633-3874, Fax: 212-633-3820, E-mail: reprints@elsevier.com.

Psychiatric Clinics of North America is covered in *MEDLINE/PubMed (Index Medicus), Current Contents/Social and Behavioral Sciences, Social Science Citation Index, Embase/Excerpta Medica,* and PsycINFO.

Printed in the United States of America.

Contributors

CONSULTING EDITOR

HARSH K. TRIVEDI, MD, MBA
President and Chief Executive Officer, Sheppard Pratt, Clinical Professor of Psychiatry, University of Maryland School of Medicine, Baltimore, Maryland, USA

EDITORS

SUNIL KHUSHALANI, MD, DLFAPA, FASAM
System Medical Director, Behavioral Health, Atlantic Health System, Adjunct Assistant Professor, Department of Psychiatry, University of Maryland School of Medicine, Morristown, New Jersey, USA

GEORGE KOLODNER, MD, DLFAPA, FASAM
Medical Director, Triple Track, Clinical Professor of Psychiatry, Georgetown University School of Medicine, Washington, DC, USA

CHRISTOPHER WELSH, MD
Associate Professor, Division of Addiction Research and Treatment, Department of Psychiatry, University of Maryland School of Medicine, Baltimore, Maryland, USA

AUTHORS

ANNABELLE M. BELCHER, PhD
Division of Addiction Research and Treatment, Assistant Professor, Department of Psychiatry, University of Maryland School of Medicine, Baltimore, Maryland, USA

DAVID BEST, PhD
Professor of Criminology, Business, Law and Social Sciences, University of Derby, Derby, Derbyshire, United Kingdom

MEGAN BURESH, MD
Department of Medicine, Division of Addiction Medicine, Johns Hopkins School of Medicine, Baltimore, Maryland, USA

GREGORY MALIK BURNETT, MD, MBA, MPH
Adjunct Assistant Professor, Center for Addiction Medicine, University of Maryland Midtown Campus, Baltimore, Maryland, USA

WILSON M. COMPTON, MD, MPE
Deputy Director, National Institute on Drug Abuse, Bethesda, Maryland, USA

ABHILASH DESAI, MD
Adjunct Associate Professor, Division of Geriatric Psychiatry, Department of Psychiatry and Behavioral Neuroscience, Saint Louis University School of Medicine, St Louis,

Missouri, USA; Adjunct Associate Professor, Department of Psychiatry and Behavioral Sciences, University of Washington School of Medicine

CARLO C. DICLEMENTE, PhD, ABPP
Emeritus Professor of Psychology, University of Maryland Baltimore County, Baltimore, Maryland, USA

MICHAEL FINGERHOOD, MD
Department of Medicine, Division of Addiction Medicine, Johns Hopkins School of Medicine, Baltimore, Maryland, USA

DAVID R. GASTFRIEND, MD, DFASAM
Chief Architect, CONTINUUM – The ASAM Criteria Decision Engine, Chief Medical Officer and Co-Founder, DynamiCare Health, Inc, Wareham, Massachusetts, USA; DynamiCare Health, Boston, Massachusetts, USA

DAVID A. GORELICK, MD, PhD, DLFAPA, FASAM
Professor of Psychiatry, University of Maryland School of Medicine, Baltimore, Maryland, USA

GEORGE GROSSBERG, MD
Samuel W. Fordyce Professor, Division of Geriatric Psychiatry, Department of Psychiatry and Behavioral Neuroscience, Saint Louis University School of Medicine, St Louis, Missouri, USA

MARIELY HERNANDEZ, PhD
Postdoctoral Fellow in Child and Adolescent Psychiatry, Columbia University Medical Center, New York State Psychiatric Institute, New York, New York, USA

KEVIN P. HILL, MD, MHS
Associate Professor, Department of Psychiatry, Harvard Medical School, Division of Addiction Psychiatry, Beth Israel Deaconess Medical Center, Boston, Massachusetts, USA

AUGUST F. HOLTYN, PhD
Assistant Professor, Department of Psychiatry and Behavioral Sciences, Behavioral Pharmacology Research Unit, Johns Hopkins School of Medicine, Baltimore, Maryland, USA

BENJAMIN ISRAEL, MD
Division of Consultation-Liaison Psychiatry, Assistant Professor, Department of Psychiatry, University of Maryland School of Medicine, Private Consultant in Psychiatry, Psychotherapy, Trauma-Based Care

JOHN F. KELLY, PhD
MGH Recovery Research Institute, Massachusetts General Hospital, Harvard Medical School, Boston, Massachusetts, USA

MARY B. KLEINMAN, MS, MPH
Doctoral Candidate, Department of Psychology, University of Maryland at College Park, College Park, Maryland, USA

GEORGE KOLODNER, MD, DLFAPA, FASAM
Medical Director, Triple Track, Clinical Professor of Psychiatry, Georgetown University School of Medicine, Washington, DC, USA

FRANCES R. LEVIN, MD
Kennedy-Leavy Professor of Psychiatry, Chief, Division on Substance Use Disorders, Director NIDA T32 Substance Abuse Research Fellowship, Columbia University Vagelos College of Physicians and Surgeons, New York State Psychiatric Institute, New York, New York, USA

PETROS LEVOUNIS, MD, MA
Chair, Department of Psychiatry, Rutgers New Jersey Medical School, New York, New York, USA

DAVID MEE-LEE, MD, DFASAM
President, DML Training and Consulting, Davis, California, USA

MICHAEL M. MILLER, MD, DLFAPA, DFASAM
Clinical Adjunct Professor, University of Wisconsin-Madison School of Medicine and Public Health, Madison, Wisconsin, USA; Clinical Associate Professor, Medical College of Wisconsin, Wauwatosa, Wisconsin, USA

MULKA NISIC, MSc
PhD Student, Business, Law and Social Sciences, University of Derby, Derby, Derbyshire, United Kingdom

MARC N. POTENZA, MD, PhD
Department of Neuroscience, Wu Tsai Institute, Yale University, Director, Division on Addictions Research at Yale, Director, Yale Impulsivity Research Program, Yale Center of Excellence in Gambling Research, Director, Women and Addictions Core of Women's Health Research at Yale, Professor of Psychiatry, Neuroscience and Child Study, Department of Psychiatry, Yale School of Medicine, Yale Child Study Center, Connecticut Mental Health Center, New Haven, Connecticut, USA; Connecticut Council on Problem Gambling, Wethersfield, Connecticut, USA

SAVITHA RACHA, MD
Department of Medicine, Division of Addiction Medicine, Johns Hopkins School of Medicine, Baltimore, Maryland, USA

AVINASH RAMPRASHAD, MD
Assistant Professor, Division of Addiction Research and Treatment, Department of Psychiatry, University of Maryland School of Medicine, Baltimore, Maryland, USA

NEIL SANDSON, MD
Clinical Associate Professor, Department of Psychiatry, University of Maryland School of Medicine, Timonium, Maryland, USA; Director of Hospital-Based Services, Director of Psychiatry at the Perry Point site, Deputy Chief of Psychiatry, VA Maryland Health Care System, Baltimore, Maryland, USA

JAMES SHERER, MD
Addiction Psychiatry Fellow, NYU Grossman School of Medicine, New York, New York, USA

MAX SPADERNA, MD
Assistant Professor, Division of Addiction Research and Treatment, University of Maryland School of Medicine, Baltimore, Maryland, USA

ELINA A. STEFANOVICS, PhD
Department of Psychiatry, Yale School of Medicine, New Haven, Connecticut, USA; US Department of Veterans Affairs New England Mental Illness Research and Education Clinical Center (MIRECC), West Haven, Connecticut, USA

MAXINE L. STITZER, PhD
Emeritus Professor, Department of Psychiatry and Behavioral Sciences, Behavioral Pharmacology Research Unit, Johns Hopkins School of Medicine, Friends Research Institute, Baltimore, Maryland, USA

MARY M. SWEENEY, PhD
Assistant Professor, Department of Psychiatry and Behavioral Sciences, Behavioral Pharmacology Research Unit, Johns Hopkins School of Medicine, Baltimore, Maryland, USA

NORA D. VOLKOW, MD
National Institute on Drug Abuse, Bethesda, Maryland, USA

ERIC M. WARGO, PhD
National Institute on Drug Abuse, Bethesda, Maryland, USA

ERIC WEINTRAUB, MD
Professor of Psychiatry, Division of Addiction Research and Treatment, University of Maryland School of Medicine, Baltimore, Maryland, USA

CHRISTOPHER WELSH, MD
Associate Professor, Division of Addiction Research and Treatment, Department of Psychiatry, University of Maryland School of Medicine, Baltimore, Maryland, USA

ALICIA E. WIPROVNICK, PhD
Division of Addiction Research and Treatment, Assistant Professor, Department of Psychiatry, University of Maryland School of Medicine, Baltimore, Maryland, USA

Contents

Preface: Challenges and Advances in the Field of Addiction Psychiatry   xiii

Sunil Khushalani, George Kolodner and Christopher Welsh

Neuropsychiatric Model of Addiction Simplified   321

Wilson M. Compton, Eric M. Wargo, and Nora D. Volkow

> While substance experimentation typically begins in adolescence, sub-
> stance use disorders (SUDs) usually develop in late teens or early adult-
> hood, often in individuals who are vulnerable because of biological and
> socioeconomic risk factors. Severe SUDs—synonymous with addic-
> tion—involve changes in limbic and prefrontal brain areas after chronic
> drug exposure. These changes involve learned associations between
> drug reward and cues that trigger the anticipation of that reward (known
> as incentive salience), as well as heightened dysphoria during withdrawal
> and weakened prefrontal circuits needed for inhibiting habitual responses.

Pharmacotherapy of Opioid Use Disorder—Update and Current Challenges   335

Savitha Racha, Megan Buresh, and Michael Fingerhood

> The incidence of opioid use disorder (OUD) and overdose deaths is rising
> yearly within the United States. Many cases are associated with illicitly
> manufactured fentanyl use. In addition to offering patients medications
> for OUD (methadone, buprenorphine, and naltrexone), the approach to
> this epidemic should involve increasing provider awareness and education
> about substance use disorders, expanding urine toxicology screens to test
> for fentanyl, and using low-threshold treatment approaches.

Policy Ahead of the Science: Medical Cannabis Laws Versus Scientific Evidence   347

Gregory Malik Burnett, David A. Gorelick, and Kevin P. Hill

> Forty-one US jurisdictions (37 states) have legalized comprehensive med-
> ical cannabis programs since 1996. The number of qualifying conditions
> per jurisdiction varies from 5 to 29. Five (12%) of 42 qualifying conditions
> have conclusive or substantial evidence of efficacy and are listed in more
> than half of all jurisdictions. Half (50%) of qualifying conditions have no or
> insufficient scientific evidence of benefit from medical cannabis; 9% of
> qualifying conditions have limited evidence of harm from medical
> cannabis. The mean number of qualifying conditions per jurisdiction and
> the proportion of conditions with and without evidence of benefit have
> not changed since 1996.

Practical Considerations for Treating Comorbid Posttraumatic Stress Disorder in the
Addictions Clinic: Approaches to Clinical Care, Leadership, and Alleviating Shame   375

Benjamin Israel, Alicia E. Wiprovnick, Annabelle M. Belcher, Mary B. Kleinman,
Avinash Ramprashad, Max Spaderna, and Eric Weintraub

A practical, common-sense framework for recognizing and addressing co-morbid posttraumatic stress disorder (PTSD) in the substance use disorder (SUD) clinic is outlined. The article focuses on strategies that can help establish trauma-informed care or augment an existing approach. Interventions are organized around the task of ameliorating shame (or shame sensitivity), which represents a transdiagnostic mediator of psychopathology and, potentially, capacity for change. Counter-shaming strategies can guide a trauma-responsive leadership approach. Considering the striking rate of underdiagnosis of PTSD among patients with SUD, implementing routine systematic PTSD screening likely represents the single most consequential trauma-informed intervention that SUD clinics can adopt.

Kratom: Substance of Abuse or Therapeutic Plant?   415

David A. Gorelick

Kratom is the common term for Mitragyna speciosa and its products. Its major active compounds are mitragynine and 7-hydroxymitragynine. An estimated 2.1 million US residents used kratom in 2020, as a "legal high" and self-medication for pain, opioid withdrawal, and other conditions. Up to 20% of US kratom users report symptoms consistent with kratom use disorder. Kratom use is associated with medical toxicity and death. Causality is difficult to prove as almost all cases involve other psychoactive substances. Daily, high-dose use may result in kratom use disorder and opioid-like withdrawal on cessation of use. These are best treated with buprenorphine.

Important Drug-Drug Interactions for the Addiction Psychiatrist   431

Neil Sandson

The misuse of illicit substances, prescribed medications, and alcohol poses obvious health risks to afflicted individuals. When addressing these health risks, the overarching concerns generally relate to the direct effects that various substances can have on the functioning of multiple organ systems: cardiac, pulmonary, central nervous system, and others. What is not always evident, but potentially equally or even more dire, are the risks arising from drug-drug interactions involving illicit drugs and alcohol, whether with each other, or with prescribed medications. This review provides some basics that enable the reader to fruitfully approach the broad topic of drug-drug interactions.

Nicotine Addiction: A Burning Issue in Addiction Psychiatry   451

George Kolodner, Carlo C. DiClemente, and Michael M. Miller

Addressing nicotine addiction has been given a low priority, compared with other substance use disorders (SUDs), by the addiction treatment field. Persons with nicotine addiction are reluctant to attempt to stop using nicotine products—despite recognizing it to be a problem—because they are feeling discouraged by multiple past unsuccessful attempts at quitting.

By understanding that discouragement is a frequent reason that these people are in Precontemplation and by using traditional clinical interventions applied to other SUDs, clinicians could achieve better overall treatment outcomes.

Substance Use Disorders in Postacute and Long-Term Care Settings   467

Abhilash Desai and George Grossberg

Substance use disorders (SUDs) have not been rigorously studied in post-acute and long-term care (PALTC) populations. SUDs are among the fastest growing disorders in the community dwelling older population. Untreated SUDs often lead to overdose deaths, emergency department visits, and hospitalizations due to SUD-related adverse effects, especially exacerbation of comorbid physical and mental health conditions. Primary care providers (PCPs) working in PALTC settings can and should play a key role in its prevention and treatment. This clinical review identifies several practical strategies that PCPs can incorporate in their daily practice to improve lives of PALTC population having SUD.

Update on Gambling Disorder   483

Elina A. Stefanovics and Marc N. Potenza

Gambling disorder (GD) is estimated to be experienced by about 0.5% of the adult population in the United States. The etiology of GD is complex and includes genetic and environmental factors. Specific populations appear particularly vulnerable to GD. GD often goes unrecognized and untreated. GD often co-occurs with other conditions, particularly psychiatric disorders. Behavioral interventions are supported in the treatment of GD. No medications have a formal indication for the GD, although clinical trials suggest some may be helpful. Noninvasive neuromodulation is being explored as a possible treatment. Improved identification, prevention, and treatment of GD are warranted.

Attention-Deficit Hyperactivity Disorder and Therapeutic Cannabis Use Motives   503

Mariely Hernandez and Frances R. Levin

Rates of cannabis use have been rising in the US due to the increasing legalization/decriminalization of cannabis products for medical and recreational use. Individuals with attention-deficit hyperactivity disorder (ADHD) may be at an increased risk of experiencing cannabis use problems due to deficits in self-regulation. This article explores motivations for cannabis use in ADHD populations. Research on the neural correlates and therapeutic potential of cannabis use are reviewed.

Practical Technology for Expanding and Improving Substance Use Disorder Treatment: Telehealth, Remote Monitoring, and Digital Health Interventions   515

Mary M. Sweeney, August F. Holtyn, Maxine L. Stitzer, and David R. Gastfriend

The US opioid crisis and the COVID-19 pandemic have sparked innovation in substance use disorder (SUD) treatment such that telehealth, remote monitoring, and digital health interventions are increasingly feasible and effective. These technologies can increase SUD treatment access and acceptability, even for nontreatment seeking, remote, and underserved populations, and can be used to reduce health disparities. Overall, digital tools will likely overcome many barriers to delivery of evidence-based behavioral treatments such as cognitive behavioral therapy and contingency management, that, along with appropriate medications, constitute the foundation of treatment of SUDs.

Harm Reduction: Not Dirty Words Any More   529

Avinash Ramprashad, Gregory Malik Burnett, and Christopher Welsh

Although many of the tenets of harm reduction have been around for centuries and more traditional harm reduction services such as syringe services programs have been in existence for decades, there has been a recent increase in interest and acceptance of harm reduction as an essential component of a public health approach to substance use. This article provides an overview of harm reduction and its application to alcohol, tobacco, and drug use. It discusses the importance of integrating harm reduction principles and services with traditional psychiatric, medical, and addiction treatment programs.

Individual Paths to Recovery from Substance Use Disorder (SUD): What Are the Implications of the Emerging Recovery Evidence Base for Addiction Psychiatry and Practice?   547

David Best and Mulka Nisic

Although the research base around 12-step effectiveness has been grown markedly in recent years, there has also been growth in the broader evidence base around recovery models, and this article reviews three key components: the transition to a social model of recovery; the emergence of a metric of recovery progress, recovery capital focused on building strengths; and multiple pathways to recovery, involving mutual aid groups, recovery community organizations, and access to jobs, friends, and housing. We conclude with an overview of the practical implications for addiction treatment and sustaining the gains made in specialist treatment services.

The Protective Wall of Human Community: The New Evidence on the Clinical and Public Health Utility of Twelve-Step Mutual-Help Organizations and Related Treatments   557

John F. Kelly

Mutual-help organizations (MHOs) such as alcoholics anonymous (AA) are the most commonly sought source of help for alcohol and other drug (AOD) problems in the United States. Popularity, however, is not commensurate with efficacy; hence, following a call for more rigorous research on AA and 12-step treatments from the Institute of Medicine in 1990 a flurry of clinical trials, cost-effectiveness analyses, and mechanisms studies, have been published during the past 30 years. This body of work has now revealed the true clinical and public health utility attributable to these freely available resources in aiding addiction remission and recovery. AA, and possibly similar organizations, may be the closest thing public health has to a "free lunch" in terms of their ability to facilitate higher rates and longer durations of sustained remission while substantially reducing health care costs.

Technological Addictions   **577**

James Sherer and Petros Levounis

Modern technology rewards constant engagement and discourages sparing use, opening the door to unhealthy use and even addiction. The technological addictions (TAs) are a newly described set of disorders that come with the technological advances that define the new era. Internet gaming disorder (IGD) is already codified as a proposed diagnosis in the 5th Edition of the Diagnostic and Statistical Manual (DSM-5) of the American Psychiatric Association. Others, such as social media addiction (SMA), are in the earlier stages of our understanding. This article provides an overview of the more common TAs including their evaluation and treatment techniques.

Thirty Years of *The ASAM Criteria*: A Report Card   **593**

David R. Gastfriend and David Mee-Lee

The American Society of Addiction Medicine Criteria (ASAM) Criteria has profoundly influenced addiction treatment and reimbursement, with its growing toolkit of ASAM CONTINUUM software, ASAM-CARF Level of Care Certification Program, educational programs, and publications. A retrospective accounting shows that the field has made considerable strides, but has far to go. Providers and payers still need to (1) improve consistency in their use of standardized, multidimensional patient assessment; (2) improve flexibility in providing and reimbursing person-centered, individualized services; (3) improve measurement in treatment planning for determination of progress; and (4) focus on outcomes and value in the care they deliver.

PSYCHIATRIC CLINICS OF NORTH AMERICA

FORTHCOMING ISSUES

December 2022
Geriatric Psychiatry
Louis J. Marino, Jr and George Zubenko,
Editors

March 2023
Treatment Resistant Depression
Manish K. Jha and Madhukar H. Trivedi,
Editors

June 2023
Obsessive Compulsive and Related Disorders
Wayne K. Goodman and Eric A. Storch,
Editors

RECENT ISSUES

June 2022
Workforce and Diversity in Psychiatry
Altha J. Stewart and Howard Y. Liu,
Editors

March 2022
**COVID 19: How the Pandemic Changed
Psychiatry for Good**
Robert L Trestman and Arpan Waghray,
Editors

December 2021
Ethics in Psychiatry
Rebecca Weintraub Brendel and Michelle
Hume, *Editors*

SERIES OF RELATED INTEREST

Child and Adolescent Psychiatric Clinics of North America
https://www.childpsych.theclinics.com/
Neurologic Clinics
https://www.neurologic.theclinics.com/
Advances in Psychiatry and Behavioral Health
https://www.advancesinpsychiatryandbehavioralhealth.com/

THE CLINICS ARE AVAILABLE ONLINE!
Access your subscription at:
www.theclinics.com

Preface

Challenges and Advances in the Field of Addiction Psychiatry

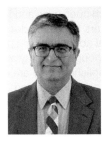 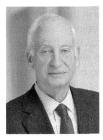 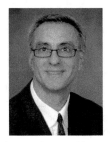

Sunil Khushalani, MD, DLFAPA, FASAM	George Kolodner, MD, DLFAPA, FASAM	Christopher Welsh, MD

Editors

Addiction Psychiatry is one of the very few fields in medicine where the disorders to be studied, understood, and treated keep growing in number rapidly. Many substances, behaviors, and technologies keep getting added to the mix of things to which people can develop a problematic addiction: social media, online gambling, or kratom are a few examples.

In general, the health care system in the United States has been designed to deal with acute conditions much better than it deals with chronic illnesses or population health. As health care costs have risen over the last few decades, there has been a greater awareness of where the system falls short in quality, safety, access to, and delivery of care, especially for chronic conditions, such as psychiatric illnesses and addictions. This system failure becomes very apparent if one were to still look at the gap between how many people suffer from opioid use disorders, those dying from overdoses, and the number of individuals who are getting comprehensive and ongoing treatment. Another example of this gap is the number of individuals who suffer from both trauma and addictions that get recognized or get comprehensive care for these chronic co-occurring conditions.

The global COVID-19 pandemic has exposed the fault lines in our care system for psychiatric conditions and addictions even more: the challenges keep growing and outpacing our capacity to deal with these chronic conditions as a whole. Many US health care system vulnerabilities have become more visible in the spotlight of these devastating and overwhelming problems. These problems have appeared anew or worsened during the pandemic and have become more apparent despite the advances in addiction psychiatry. Some advances, such as neuropsychiatry, drug-drug interactions, or technological avenues to combat addiction, are exciting.

Psychiatr Clin N Am 45 (2022) xiii–xiv
https://doi.org/10.1016/j.psc.2022.05.011
0193-953X/22/© 2022 Published by Elsevier Inc.

psych.theclinics.com

Our society has an ambivalent relationship with addictive substances: this is very apparent as we look at how society has dealt with substances such as cannabis or psychedelics over the last two centuries. These substances can indeed cause problems, but they also have some therapeutic potential. The challenge for the medical field is that the speed at which social forces make these agents available is faster than what science can corroborate.

In the current issue of *Psychiatric Clinics of North America*, we have highlighted some of the ongoing challenges and advances in addiction psychiatry. The purpose of this is to approach the challenges in the entire landscape with open eyes and to underscore the point that progress is being made in various corners to help us deal with addictions better as a system. We have included some material about new and promising developments, especially ones with clinical relevance. Although they may not yet have enough supportive evidence to consider them to be established, they are credible enough and have enough potential that they deserve to be introduced more broadly to practitioners. We have updated some old issues, such as the treatment of opioid use disorder, ADHD, and the use of medical cannabis. We have also highlighted some problems and solutions that have become more prominent and mainstream in the past decade, such as harm reduction, technology addictions, and technology-based treatments.

It makes us feel hopeful even in the context of monumental threats and demanding circumstances. We hope you will enjoy reading this issue as much as we have enjoyed putting it together.

Sunil Khushalani, MD, DLFAPA, FASAM
Morristown, NJ, USA

Behavioral Health, Atlantic Health System
Department of Psychiatry
University of Maryland School of Medicine
465 South Street, Suite 204
Morristown, NJ 07960, USA

George Kolodner, MD, DLFAPA, FASAM
Triple Track
Georgetown University School of Medicine
3204 Klingle Road NW
Washington, DC 20008, USA

Christopher Welsh, MD
Division of Addiction Research and Treatment
Department of Psychiatry
University of Maryland School of Medicine
22 S. Greene Street, S-1-D-04
Baltimore, MD, 21201, USA

E-mail addresses:
khushalani@me.com (S. Khushalani)
gkolodner@tripletrack.com (G. Kolodner)
cwelsh@som.umaryland.edu (C. Welsh)

Neuropsychiatric Model of Addiction Simplified

Wilson M. Compton, MD, MPE*, Eric M. Wargo, PhD, Nora D. Volkow, MD

KEYWORDS

• Neurobiology • Addiction • Addiction cycle • Reinforcement

KEY POINTS

• Developmental neuroscience helps to explain the risk for onset of substance use and substance use disorders (SUDs).
• Severe SUDs involve changes in limbic and prefrontal brain areas after chronic drug exposure.
• The addiction cycles involves reinforced, learned associations between drugs and cues that trigger the anticipation of that reward (known as incentive salience), as well as heightened dysphoria during withdrawal, and weakened prefrontal cortical circuits needed for inhibiting habitual responses.

INTRODUCTION

Observations that specific brain regions are important in specific behavioral patterns have been known at least since the remarkable case of Phineas Gage,[1] and the ways that the use of alcohol and other substances can negatively impact the behavior have been noted for centuries (or even millennia). What was missing until recent decades has been a comprehensive understanding of the neurobiological underpinnings of addiction; yet, this knowledge is essential for clinicians and patients.

Advances in neuroscience research at the anatomic, electrophysiological, and neuroimaging levels have all contributed to establishing central nervous system models that help to explain the signs, symptoms, and course of addictive disorders in the context of relevant environmental contributing factors. Both obvious and counterintuitive aspects of addiction can now be understood through research into the neurobiology of decision-making, choice, habit formation, and brain development. This

Disclaimer: The views expressed in this article are those of the authors and do not necessarily represent the views of the National Institute on Drug Abuse, the National Institutes of Health, or the US Department of Health and Human Services.
National Institute on Drug Abuse, 301 North Stonestreet Avenue, MSC 6025, Bethesda, MD 20892-6025, USA
* Corresponding author.
E-mail address: wcompton@nida.nih.gov

Psychiatr Clin N Am 45 (2022) 321–334
https://doi.org/10.1016/j.psc.2022.05.001
0193-953X/22/Published by Elsevier Inc.
psych.theclinics.com

evolving and growing body of work can be intimidating for clinicians and patients, but the exploration of the basic concepts can help to reduce the mystery of addictive behaviors and provide frameworks for the prevention and treatment of substance use disorders (SUDs).

Although there are multiple frameworks through which to view and consider addiction (a term corresponding to the definition of moderate to severe SUD in DSM 5),[2] including philosophic and psychosocial frameworks, most researchers in addiction medicine consider addiction to be a chronic, relapsing, but treatable biopsychosocial disorder of the brain. What this means is that the clinical components of addictive disorders are reflected in changes in specific brain neurotransmitter systems and functional networks, knowledge of which can help clinicians ground their practice in neuroscience. Shared effects of various substances are apparent for major neurobiological models of addiction, such as those delineated by Koob and Volkow,[3] but it is also important to understand the unique neurobiological effects of different classes of drugs.

In this review, we focus on the key elements of addiction and describe neurobiological underpinnings of these features. A full review of neurobiology is beyond the scope of this overview. Instead, we focus on the major maturational and neuroplastic processes that underlie the onset and natural history of SUD both in general populations, where SUDs may improve without access to formal treatment and in treatment-seeking cases, which tend to have a chronic, relapsing course. We then describe the alterations in brain circuitry that help explain the loss of control over drug use in those who have developed an addiction as they relate to the 3 stages of the addiction cycle: *binge/intoxication*, *withdrawal/negative affect*, and *preoccupation/anticipation* (or craving).[4] We lastly describe areas whereby future research is needed to fill in gaps in knowledge.

ONSET AND NATURAL HISTORY OF SUBSTANCE USE DISORDERS

The science of human development underpins our understanding of the onset of SUD.[5] Environmental factors that influence an individual's risk for substance use and developing a SUD include not only substance exposures themselves but also characteristics of the family, neighborhood, school, and cultural context for which the individual grows up and lives. These environmental influences interact in complex ways with genes as well as brain maturation.[6] Propensity to use substances may arise before the first use of alcohol, nicotine, or other substances. Early-life environments that are stressful have been demonstrated to increase the subsequent likelihood of use of substances and SUD, in both preclinical (animal) and clinical research.[7] For example, the Adverse Childhood Experiences (ACES) retrospective cohort study of primary care patients (N = ~8600) demonstrated that patients who reported more early childhood abuse and neglect experiences were more likely to report using substances during teen or adult years, to have a SUD, and to have initiated drug use at an early age.[8]

While a complete, mechanistic explanation is not fully developed, it is apparent that genetic factors underlie significant risk for SUDs,[9] and that interactions of biology and the environment play a key role in these trajectories from early childhood toward SUD in the teens and in adult life. Epigenetic modifications of gene expression have been shown to link early developmental adversity to sensitivity to stress and associated behavioral disorders.[10] Importantly, altered brain development associated with adverse environments can sometimes be ameliorated.[11] A study in rural Georgia of participants in a prevention trial found a strong correlation between number of teen years in poverty and diminished volume of brain structures that contribute to academic functioning, social development, learning, memory, mood, and stress reactivity (left dentate gyrus, CA3 subfield of the hippocampus, and left amygdala) by the early 20s among those who were in the study control group.[12] In contrast, those volumetric declines were not seen in those in the group whose families had received an experimental family-focused intervention when they were in middle school (ie, early adolescence).[12] These results support the premise that family-based interventions may mitigate the developmental impacts of what otherwise would be a toxic social environment (poverty), even without changing other aspects of that environment.

Interventions as early as the prenatal and infancy periods have also been demonstrated to improve later behavioral, cognitive, and health outcomes. For instance, large randomized studies show that providing guidance to low-income, first-time mothers during pregnancy and in the first 2 years of a child's life through home visitation by nurses can have a range of lasting positive impacts on the child—not only reduced abuse and neglect but also reduced substance use onset and improved cognitive and behavioral outcomes into the teen years.[13] These and other longitudinal, prevention intervention studies document the importance of risk factors for the onset of substance use and the potential benefits of effective interventions that successfully address such risk factors.[14]

A key question is why substance use so typically starts during adolescence, a period of risk for many behavioral concerns.[5,6] Developmental neuroscience has documented that brain development is uneven, with limbic structures involved in emotional responsivity and reward maturing earlier than prefrontal cortical areas involved in decision making, impulse control, and judgment (Fig. 1).[15] Circuitry of the prefrontal cortex does not completely reach maturity until the mid-20s.[16] One result of this developmental mismatch is an increased propensity for risk-taking among youth.[17] While this can be seen as developmentally appropriate, as this time of life is when an individual is challenged to become independent from parents and fashion their self-identity, the propensity for novel experiences and risk-taking can have very negative outcomes. The uneven maturation of the adolescent brain also increases susceptibility to environmental influences dominant during the teen years, such as peer influence.[18] The hazards are compounded by the fact that, as it is not fully mature, the adolescent brain is more vulnerable to lasting effects of substance use, including increased risk of addiction.[19] The risk for developing a SUD is highest for those who initiate substances in the early teens, and addiction is most likely to begin in the late teen years.[20]

Most substance use begins with tobacco, alcohol, and then cannabis—before other substances such as cocaine or opioids are used. Most who misuse opioids have already used these so-called "gateway substances" during adolescence.[21,22] While multiple studies attest to overlapping onset of substance use,[23,24] neurobiological gateway mechanisms for nicotine have the most evidence. By increasing midbrain dopamine neurons' firing rate, nicotine can amplify the reinforcing effects of other substances and nondrug rewards (see later in discussion).[22,25]

Because of the complex interacting biological, psychosocial, and developmental risk factors and various protective factors that may mitigate them (such as attentive parenting and strong social supports), only a subset of people who use drugs—even in their teen years—go on to develop a SUD.[26,27] For instance, using DSM-III-R or DSM-IV definitions, retrospective US national studies have estimated that about 9% of cannabis users will ever develop cannabis dependence, with higher rates for those with early onset, frequent use, or use of more potent forms of cannabis. Similarly, 15% to 23% of alcohol users develop alcohol dependence, 17% to 21% of cocaine users develop cocaine dependence and 32% to 67% of tobacco users develop nicotine dependence.[26,27]

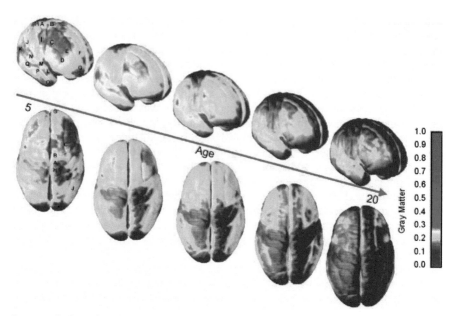

Fig. 1. Right lateral and top views of the dynamic sequence of gray matter maturation over the cortical surface. The side bar shows a color representation in units of gray matter volume. The following regions were selected for analyses in each hemisphere: A, precentral gyrus and primary motor cortex; B, superior frontal gyrus, posterior end near central sulcus; C, inferior frontal gyrus, posterior end; D, inferior frontal sulcus, anterior end in the ventrolateral prefrontal cortex; E, inferior frontal sulcus in the dorsolateral prefrontal cortex; F, anterior limit of superior frontal sulcus; G, frontal pole; H, primary sensory cortex in postcentral gyrus; I, supramarginal gyrus (area 40); J, angular gyrus (area 39); K, occipital pole; L–N, anterior, middle, and posterior portions of STG; O–Q, anterior, middle, and posterior points along the inferior temporal gyrus anterior end. (*Reproduced from* Gogtay N., Giedd J.N., Lusk L., et al., Dynamic mapping of human cortical development during childhood through early adulthood, *PNAS*, **101** (21), 2004, 8174–8179.)

Of those who develop a SUD, many report the current remission of their symptoms. Over 20 million persons in the US report being in recovery from problematic substance use; most of these persons either did not avail themselves of formal treatment or it was inaccessible to them, yet they may have years or decades without symptoms of SUD.[20,28,29] In some cases, SUDs resolve on their own as a result of maturation or because of changing life circumstances or environments—the famous desistence of opioid use among Vietnam war soldiers returning to the US is one example.[30] However, a recent longitudinal study following 11 early cohorts of the annual Monitoring the Future study found that most of the high school seniors who had reported SUD symptoms when surveyed in the late 1970s or early 1980s still reported SUD symptoms more than 3 decades later, at age 50—indicating a long-term course for many SUDs that emerge early in life (ie, in the teen years).[31]

Among persons admitted to treatment of SUD (especially severe SUD), a chronic, relapsing course is well documented.[2,32,33] Use of substances in the year following treatment interventions varies but has been estimated to be 40% to 60%,[34] with longer studies suggesting multiple cycles of heavy use, periodic abstinence, interspersed with incarceration for many.[32,33,35,36] While treatment is a broad predictor of remission,[28,34,35] the underlying chronic, relapsing pattern remains and may be understood based on the neurobiology of the addiction cycle (**Fig. 2**).[37,38]

NEUROPLASTIC CHANGES IN ADDICTION AND THE ADDICTION CYCLE

Among the changes apparent with chronic drug intake is the formation of *tolerance* and physical *dependence*. While not synonymous with addiction, tolerance and dependence develop when the body adapts to the frequent presence of an exogenous substance by counteracting its intracellular signaling responses, such as the levels of adenyl cyclase, and by dialing down its own related endogenous signaling system— endorphins and dynorphins in the case of opioid drugs, or downregulating cannabinoid CB1 receptors in the case of cannabis, and so on. The resulting tolerance is the need for increasing doses of the drug to produce the desired effect; and the resulting physical dependence leads to the emergence of withdrawal symptoms when the drug is interrupted. While tolerance and withdrawal (ie, physical dependence) are typically part of addiction, many substances, including multiple prescription medications, may produce dependence and tolerance without producing addiction. Furthermore, the severity and duration of withdrawal symptoms depend on the specific drug consumed.

Addiction, per se, arises when the individual loses control over use of the substance (ie, spending a great deal of time using a substance, using larger amounts than intended, and so forth). It is driven by the formation of associations between the drug and environmental as well as internal cues that trigger craving, or *incentive salience*; neurobiological changes that lead to intensified dysphoria during withdrawal, as well as increased preoccupation with the drug; and reduction of self-inhibitory

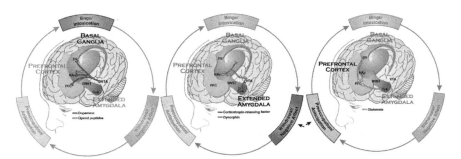

Fig. 2. The three stages of addiction: *Binge/Intoxication*, the stage at which an individual consumes an intoxicating substance and experiences its rewarding or pleasurable effects, primarily involves basal ganglia structures; *Withdrawal/Negative Affect*, the stage at which an individual experiences a negative emotional state in the absence of the substance, involves stress hormone responses and the extended amygdala; and *Preoccupation/Anticipation*, the stage at which one seeks substances again after a period of abstinence, involving interactions of the prefrontal cortex, the extended amygdala, and the basal ganglia. Notes: Blue represents the basal ganglia involved in the Binge/Intoxication stage. Red represents the extended amygdala involved in the Negative Affect/Withdrawal stage. Green represents the prefrontal cortex involved in the Preoccupation/Anticipation stage. Not shown is the neurotransmitter norepinephrine which is also activated in the extended amygdala during withdrawal. PFC - prefrontal cortex, DS - dorsal striatum, NAc - nucleus accumbens, BNST - bed nucleus of the stria terminalis, CeA - central nucleus of the amygdala, VTA - ventral tegmental area. (*Reproduced from* U.S. Department of Health and Human Services (HHS), Office of the Surgeon General, Facing Addiction in America: The Surgeon General's Report on Alcohol, Drugs, and Health. Washington, DC: HHS, 2016.)

control over drug taking despite, in many cases, an awareness that the drug has assumed too much importance and is harming health and other aspects of the individual's life like relationships, school, or work.[2,37–40]

As displayed in **Fig. 2**, 3 areas of the brain are critical for these processes: the *basal ganglia*, the *extended amygdala*, and the *prefrontal cortex*.[37] Changes in circuits in these brain areas play key roles in 3 repeating stages of the addiction cycle, respectively: *binge/intoxication*, the acute rewarding and reinforcing effects on taking the drug; *withdrawal/negative affect*, the unpleasant physical and emotional symptoms associated with a period of abstinence; and *preoccupation/anticipation*, craving the drug in response to internal and external cues. Dynamic relationships across these 3 stages help explain patterns of heavy consumption, followed by abstinence (can be brief or extended), and then recurrent use to alleviate negative internal states or in response to anticipatory motivation. Classes of substances differ in how they produce their effects, especially in the binge/intoxication phase, as well as in how and to what extent they disrupt the relevant circuits, but the overall patterns are consistent across substances.

Binge/intoxication. Either immediately or soon after taking a drug (rapidity depending on the substance's specific properties and mode of administration), the individual experiences rewarding euphoria (ie, positive reinforcement) and, in the case of a person with dependence or addiction, relief from withdrawal symptoms (ie, negative reinforcement). The exact neurobiological correlates of experienced pleasure or the drug "high" are debated and may differ for different substances (see Future Directions, later in discussion), but well understood is the role of dopamine signaling in neurons projecting from the ventral tegmental area (VTA) to the nucleus accumbens (NAC) in building associations between drug-taking and reward, reinforcing those associations each time drug-taking is repeated, and reinforcing associations between the drug and internal and external cues.[41] Multiple preclinical studies in rodents have identified the neuronal and neurochemical actions of drugs on this dopaminergic VTA-NAC circuit (see Koob and Volkow[4] for a full description of these pathways). While the mechanisms of action vary by drug, enhancing dopamine activity in the basal ganglia is responsible for the reinforcing properties of all substances whose misuse can result in addiction.

When an association between dopamine and positive reinforcement was first discovered in rodent studies in the 1970s,[42,43] it was believed that dopamine was the neurotransmitter responsible for rewarding feelings that drive drug seeking. Over subsequent decades, dopamine came to be thought of as the "pleasure chemical," and this idea was expressed widely in the media and popular science explanations of drug addiction. In the past 2 decades, the science of dopamine has departed from this popular conception with the discovery that dopamine has more to do with reinforcement learning and motivated goal-seeking, and probably not drugs' hedonic effects, which engage other neurotransmitter systems including endogenous opioids and cannabinoids.[44] Dopamine signaling in the basal ganglia controls the salience of cues (external or internal) that engender action.[45] It is released in the NAC both in the anticipation of rewards and when rewards exceed expectation, and it is diminished when rewards do not materialize or are less than expected.

The development of incentive salience is a crucial neuroplastic response to natural rewards such as food and one that is hijacked by drugs. Through conditioning and expectation of reward, a memory is formed that will incentivize behaviors to consume the reward (eg, food or drugs). The conditioned memories that drive incentive salience toward conditioned stimuli are fundamental to survival but also facilitate the development of an addiction. When drugs are repeatedly administered, dopamine comes to be released when the individual encounters or experiences the cues associated with the drug before its consumption, energizing the behaviors to obtain it.[46] Incentive salience has the motivational effect of driving drug-seeking during the anticipation/preoccupation phase (described later in discussion).

Depending on the class of drug, dopaminergic signaling in the basal ganglia may be enhanced through several different mechanisms including: direct or indirect increases in activity of VTA-dopamine neurons, increasing terminal dopamine release, blocking dopamine reuptake, or enhancing the postsynaptic actions of dopamine on NAC neurons. An additional neuroplastic mechanism shared among most drugs with their repeated administration is the increase of the ratio of the glutamate receptor, α-amino-3-hydroxy-5-methyl-4-isoxazolepropionic acid (AMPA) receptor, to that of the N-methyl-D-aspartate (NMDA) receptor, which results in enhanced excitatory transmission onto VTA-dopamine neurons.[47,48] See **Box 1** for summaries of the specific mechanisms of action of major drug classes.

Another important component of the binge/intoxication stage is the release of both dopamine and glutamate (an excitatory neurotransmitter) in the dorsal striatum, which is implicated in behavioral reinforcement.[61,62] This is another mechanism through which learning processes contribute to the development of compulsive drug use. Indeed, addiction is sometimes compared with a well-learned skill, one that is difficult to unlearn (see Future Directions later in discussion).

Withdrawal/negative Affect

Koob and Volkow highlight the importance of negative emotional states and memories in the addiction cycle, based on both the expressed responses of human subjects and from fMRI studies correlated with amygdala and hippocampus activation during craving episodes.[4]

As the drug leaves the system and its acute effects wane, an individual who has developed an addiction may experience not only the physical symptoms of withdrawal, which are usually relatively short term but also protracted negative emotional withdrawal symptoms that are part of the long-lasting adaptations in addiction. The negative emotional state during the withdrawal stage of the addiction cycle is caused by increased sensitivity of the extended amygdala to stress, mediated in part through enhanced corticotropin-releasing factor (CRF), norepinephrine, and dynorphin signaling. The feelings of stress caused by this activity in the extended amygdala, compounded in some cases by intense physical symptoms of drug withdrawal, are one reason why it is incorrect to think of people with addiction as simply hedonically driven, motivated by the euphoria or high caused by drug intoxication. To a significant degree, people with addiction are motivated to experience relief, to escape the stress and suffering of withdrawal, which in many cases can be intense or even unbearable.

Preoccupation/anticipation

A core feature of SUD, especially the more severe forms (ie, addiction), is craving, sometimes described as an overwhelming need and urgent compulsion to use a substance after a period of abstinence (short or long).[2,39,40] This preoccupation/anticipation stage in the addiction cycle involves the reciprocal interaction of the dopaminergic pathways of the prefrontal cortex, the brain area most associated with goal-directed behaviors, self-inhibition, and judgment, with both the extended amygdala and the basal ganglia.

Signaling in dopaminergic and glutamate connections between the prefrontal cortex and basal ganglia motivate drug seeking in response to cues. Inhibitory connections between the prefrontal cortex and the dorsal striatum that have been weakened by

Box 1
Reinforcement (dopamine signaling) mechanisms for major drug classes

OPIOIDS
Opioids, including morphine heroin, fentanyl, and prescription analgesics such as oxycodone, increase dopamine signaling in the basal ganglia indirectly through their actions at specific opioid receptors, especially the mu opioid receptor. Preclinical research shows that the activation of mu-opioid receptors on gamma aminobutyric acid (GABA) cells in the VTA disinhibits dopamine neurons increasing their activity and enhancing dopamine release in the NAC.[49]

ALCOHOL
Alcohol's reinforcing effects have been associated with processes involving multiple molecular targets, including the enhancement of opioid signaling through mu-opioid receptors. Alcohol also enhances GABAergic neurotransmission via its direct effects on GABA-A receptors which are believed to contribute to reward and to its anxiolytic effects.[4]

STIMULANTS (COCAINE AND AMPHETAMINE-LIKE SUBSTANCES)
The reinforcing effects of stimulants are mediated by their direct effects on dopamine neurons. Cocaine enhances dopamine levels primarily by inhibiting the dopamine transporter, thus reducing the reuptake of dopamine from the synapse. Amphetamine-like substances, however, both inhibit the transporter and directly increase vesicular dopamine release.[47] In either case, the net effect is to increase dopamine in the NAC. The effects of this class of drugs are also mediated by increases in the activation of the other monoamine systems, serotonin and norepinephrine.[47] The bias toward a particular monoamine system depends on the specific stimulant. For example, cathinones (bath salts) have a greater effect on serotonin than does amphetamine, which is biased toward dopamine and norepinephrine systems.[50]

BENZODIAZEPINES
Benzodiazepines are allosteric modulators of GABA-A receptors, meaning that their binding shifts the way the receptor responds to its standard ligands. Although both GABA and dopamine neurons in the VTA express these receptors, benzodiazepines bind to those containing the alpha-1 subunit, which is only found on GABA neurons in the VTA and is lacking in VTA-dopamine neurons.[51–53] The resulting inhibition of VTA-GABA neurons enhances dopamine release. In human studies, benzodiazepines enhance the subjective effects of opioids, including "high" and "liking," indicating that these drugs' rewarding properties may be synergistic, accounting for their common couse.[54] Combining the 2 classes of drugs has also been implicated in increasing the risk for overdose, due to their shared effect of inhibiting respiration.[54–56]

NICOTINE
The reinforcing effects of nicotine are mediated by multiple receptors in the VTA and NAC,[4] and its actions at nicotinic acetylcholine receptors (nAChR) alpha-4 beta-2 subtype seem to be integral to these effects.[57] In addition to increasing dopamine discharge rate, nicotine changes the pattern of discharge to favor a phasic or bursting mode.[58] Dopamine bursting promotes the formation of associations between stimuli and rewards, and this may be the basis for reinforcement-enhancing effects of nicotine in combination with other substances.[25,59] Analyzing data from 2 cohort studies, Kandel and Kandel found that cocaine dependence was highest in users who had first smoked cigarettes and that concurrent smoking around the time of cocaine initiation was associated with more persistent cocaine use and addiction—consistent with the priming effect they found in an animal model. Conversely, cocaine does not seem to prime the nicotine response.[22] Nicotine's linkages to later addiction to other classes of drugs such as opioids are not fully established.

CANNABINOIDS
Cannabinoids activate type 1 cannabinoid receptors (CB1) in the VTA, but the mechanism by which this activation facilitates dopamine release is not well understood. Cannabis receptor pharmacology research is providing clues. For example, in light of the sometimes contradictory reinforcing and aversive effects of cannabis, Spiller and colleagues document the importance of the balance of both CB1 and CB2 receptor activation in cannabis effects.[60] Their work suggests that reinforcing and aversive effects may be mediated by differential CB1 and CB2 receptor expression.

chronic substance use let the habitual response—taking the drug—win out. These weakened inhibitory signals are especially powerless in the face of the dysphoric feelings generated by the stress neurotransmitters in the extended amygdala. This shift in the balance of what is colloquially called the "Go" and "Stop" systems coordinated by the prefrontal cortex helps explain addiction's chronic, relapsing course.[63]

FUTURE DIRECTIONS

Much is known about the neurobiology of addiction, at least in broad terms—including the development of incentive salience and compromised self-inhibition that underpins compulsive drug use. But there are areas whereby our knowledge remains limited. One, oddly enough, is the neurobiology of pleasure itself. Greater understanding that dopamine has to do mainly with reinforcement but not with hedonic perception has left a gap in our understanding of just what is pleasurable about rewards. Some research points to so-called "hedonic hotspots" in the orbitofrontal cortex, insula, NAC, ventral pallidum, and pontine parabrachial nucleus that have been identified in conjunction with "liking" in animal models.[64] Liking here is distinguished from the anticipatory (and dopamine-related) signal of "wanting." Activity in hedonic hotspots during pleasurable experience involves endogenous opioid, endocannabinoid, and orexin (but not dopamine) signaling,[44] and how different drugs interact with these hotspots remains to be seen. But it is almost certainly the case that the neurobiology of pleasure, including the drug high, will not be a simple story of one neurotransmitter flooding the brain with good feelings.

Another gap in our understanding is the neurobiology of recovery from addiction. We understand how the brain changes when a SUD develops, but we still know very little about how the brain restores balance among the systems disrupted during active drug use. Longitudinal clinical research suggests that stable recovery is more likely with lengthy periods of supported abstinence.[33,65] Yet, susceptibility to relapse even after years of abstinence is not rare, strongly indicating that some neuroplastic changes, for instance, learned associations between drugs and rewards that were formed during the development of the disorder, weaken only very gradually. Addiction is often likened to riding a bicycle: You may not have ridden one in years; yet, if you get on one, you'll be able to ride it quite well. Among the many avenues of addiction treatment research being pursued, one is to find ways of identifying and weakening those learned associations between a drug and its craving-inducing cues.[66] It may also be the case that different drug use disorders may have different long-term impacts on those who have recovered from them, and it is likely the case that individual differences will play a role. There could be many neurobiological trajectories of recovery.

SUMMARY

The medical framing of addiction as a chronic, relapsing brain disorder has been slow to win adherents outside of medicine, and studies show that even clinicians cling to stigmatizing views that see people with addiction as bad or weak.[67] The medical framing has been crucial to research explicating addiction neurobiology and has been essential to developing effective treatments, such as those that currently exist for opioid use disorder. However, as learning mechanisms are so central to the processes that make drug use compulsive in people with addiction, some critics argue that the medical framing is overly reductive and pessimistic, and even disempowering to persons who may hear "brain disorder" or "brain disease" and assume that it somehow means nontreatable or incurable, which is not the case.[68,69] These terminological (and in some cases, philosophic) questions will continue to be fruitful areas of debate and inquiry. If anything, framing addiction as a learned behavior (as well as a disease) helps make the case for greater societal and health care investment in prevention: It may be the case that the surest way to keep people from riding bikes is to keep them from learning to ride them in the first place.

Addiction occurs in a minority of people who use drugs repeatedly, as a result of combinations of biological and psychosocial risk factors. The pathways to addiction involve changes in neurocircuits in limbic and prefrontal regions, and some of these neuroplastic changes may be slow to resolve or "change back" even with months or years of abstinence, warranting calling addiction a chronic brain disorder with high risk of relapse. This understanding of addiction has been crucial to marshaling biomedical research to find and develop treatments. Educating the public, policy-makers, and clinicians about the efficacy of these treatments is a crucial part of eroding the stigma that has prevented their wider adoption.

CLINICS CARE POINTS

- Developmental neuroscience helps to demonstrate both the negative power of risk environments and the positive power of prevention interventions.

- Treatments that reduce the rewarding and reinforcing properties of substances address a key component of the neurobiological binge/intoxication phase of the addiction cycle.

- Both acute withdrawal syndromes and longer-term withdrawal-related negative affect are key risk factors for relapse.

- Providing support to patients in recovery in times of stress addresses a key risk factor for relapse, as elucidated in multiple neuroscience studies.

DISCLOSURE

W.M. Compton reports long-term stock holdings in General Electric Company, 3M Companies, and Pfizer, Inc. unrelated to the article. Other authors have no disclosures to report.

REFERENCES

1. O'Driscoll K, Leach JP. No longer Gage": an iron bar through the head. Early observations of personality change after injury to the prefrontal cortex. BMJ 1998; 317(7174):1673–4.
2. American Psychiatric Association. Diagnostic and statistical manual of mental disorders, Fifth Edition, Text Revision (DSM-5-TR). Washington, DC: American Psychiatric Press; 2022.
3. Koob GF, Volkow ND. Neurobiology of addiction: a neurocircuitry analysis. Lancet Psychiatry 2016;3(8):760–73.
4. Koob GF, Volkow ND. Neurocircuitry of Addiction. Neuropsychopharmacology 2010;35:217–38.
5. National Research Council and Institute of Medicine. From neurons to neighborhoods: the science of early childhood development. Committee on Integrating the Science of Early Childhood Development. Washington, DC: National Academy Press; 2000.
6. Volkow ND, Boyle M. Neuroscience of addiction: relevance to prevention and treatment. Am J Psychiatry 2018;175:729–40.

7. Hughes K, Bellis MA, Hardcastle KA, et al. The effect of multiple adverse childhood experiences on health: a systematic review and meta-analysis. Lancet Public Health 2017;2(8):e356–66.
8. Dube SR, Felitti VJ, Dong M, et al. Childhood abuse, neglect, and household dysfunction and the risk of illicit drug use: the Adverse Childhood Experiences study. Pediatrics 2003;111(3):564–72.
9. Walker DM, Nestler EJ. Neuroepigenetics and addiction. Handbook Clin Neurol 2018;148:747–65.
10. Enoch M-A. The role of early life stress as a predictor for alcohol and drug dependence. Psychopharmacology 2011;214(1):17–31.
11. Nelson CA, Zeanah CH, Fox NA, et al. Cognitive recovery in socially deprived young children: the Bucharest Early Intervention Project. Science 2007;318:1937–40.
12. Brody GH, Gray J, Yu T, et al. Family-centered prevention ameliorates the longitudinal association of poverty with hippocampal and amygdalar volumes in adulthood. JAMA Pediatr 2017;171(1):46–52.
13. Olds DL, Kitzman HJ, Cole RE, et al. Enduring effects of prenatal and infancy home visiting by nurses on maternal life course and government spending: follow-up of a randomized trial among children at age 12 years. Arch Pediatr Adolesc Med 2010;164(5):419–24.
14. Catalano RF, Fagan AA, Gavin LE, et al. Worldwide application of prevention science in adolescent health. Lancet 2012;379(9826):1653–64.
15. Spear LP. The adolescent brain and age-related behavioral manifestations. Neurosci Biobehav Rev 2000;24:417–63.
16. Gogtay N, Giedd JN, Lusk L, et al. Dynamic mapping of human cortical development during childhood through early adulthood. PNAS 2004;101(21):8174–9.
17. Steinberg L. Risk taking in adolescence: new perspectives from brain and behavioral science. Curr Dir Psychol Sci 2007;16(2):55–9.
18. Albert D, Chein J, Steinberg L. Peer influences on adolescent decision making. Curr Dir Psychol Sci 2013;22(2):114–20.
19. Squeglia LM, Jacobus J, Tapert SF. The influence of substance use on adolescent brain development. Clin EEG Neurosci 2009;40(1):31–8.
20. Compton WM, Thomas YF, Stinson FS, et al. Prevalence, correlates, disability, and comorbidity of DSM-IV drug abuse and dependence in the United States: results from the national epidemiologic survey on alcohol and related conditions. Arch Gen Psychiatry 2007;64(5):566–76.
21. Robins L, Compton W, Horton J. Is heroin the worst drug? Implications for drug policy. Addict Res Theor 2000;8(6):527–47.
22. Kandel DB, Kandel ER. The Gateway Hypothesis of substance abuse: developmental, biological and societal perspectives. Acta Paediatr 2015;104:130–7.
23. Han B, Compton WM, Blanco C, et al. National Trends in Substance Use and Use Disorders Among Youth. J Am Acad Child Adolesc Psychiatry 2017;56(9):747–54.
24. DuPont RL, Han B, Shea CL, et al. Drug use among youth: national survey data support a common liability of all drug use. Prev Med 2018;113:68–73.
25. Perkins KA, Karelitz JL, Boldry MC. Nicotine acutely enhances reinforcement from non-drug rewards in humans. Front Psychiatry 2017;8:65.
26. Lopez-Quintero C, Hasin DS, de Los Cobos JP, et al. Probability and predictors of remission from life-time nicotine, alcohol, cannabis or cocaine dependence: results from the National Epidemiologic Survey on Alcohol and Related Conditions. Addiction 2011;106(3):657–69.

27. Anthony J, Warner L, Kessler R. Comparative epidemiology of dependence on tobacco, alcohol, controlled substances, and inhalants: Basic findings from the National Comorbidity Survey. Exp Clin Psychopharmacol 1994;2:244–68.

28. Jones CM, Noonan RK, Compton WM. Prevalence and correlates of ever having a substance use problem and substance use recovery status among adults in the United States, 2018. Drug Alcohol Depend 2020;214:108169.

29. Hasin DS, Stinson FS, Ogburn E, et al. Prevalence, correlates, disability, and co-morbidity of DSM-IV alcohol abuse and dependence in the United States: results from the National Epidemiologic Survey on Alcohol and Related Conditions. Arch Gen Psychiatry 2007;64(7):830–42.

30. Robins LN, Helzer JE, Hesselbrock M, et al. Vietnam veterans three years after Vietnam: how our study changed our view of heroin. Am J Addict 2010;19(3): 203–11.

31. McCabe SE, Schulenberg JE, Schepis TS, et al. Longitudinal analysis of sub-stance use disorder symptom severity at age 18 and substance use disorder in adulthood. JAMA Netw Open 2022;5(4):e225324.

32. Dennis ML, Foss MA, Scott CK. An eight-year perspective on the relationship be-tween the duration of abstinence and other aspects of recovery. Eval Rev 2007; 31(6):585–612.

33. Dennis ML, Scott CK, Funk R, et al. The duration and correlates of addiction and treatment careers. J Subst Abuse Treat 2005;28(2):S51–62.

34. McLellan AT, Lewis DC, O'Brien CP, et al. Drug dependence, a chronic medical illness: implications for treatment, insurance, and outcomes evaluation. JAMA 2000;284(13):1689–95.

35. Scott CK, Foss MA, Dennis ML. Pathways in the relapse—treatment—recovery cycle over 3 years. J Subst Abuse Treat 2005;28(2):S63–72.

36. Hser YI, Longshore D, Anglin MD. The life course perspective on drug use: A conceptual framework for understanding drug use trajectories. Eval Rev 2007; 31(6):515–47.

37. U.S. Department of Health and Human Services (HHS), Office of the Surgeon General. Facing addiction in America: the Surgeon General's report on alcohol, drugs, and health. Washington, DC: HHS; 2016.

38. Feltenstein MW, See RE, Fuchs RA. Neural Substrates and Circuits of Drug Addiction. Cold Spring Harb Perspect Med 2021;11(4):a039628.

39. Li Q, Wang Y, Zhang Y, et al. Craving correlates with mesolimbic responses to heroin-related cues in short-term abstinence from heroin: an event-related fMRI study. Brain Res 2012;1469:63–72.

40. Kakko J, Alho H, Baldacchino A, et al. Craving in Opioid Use Disorder: From Neurobiology to Clinical Practice. Front Psychiatry 2019;10:592.

41. Koob GF. Hedonic valence, dopamine and motivation. Mol Psychiatry 1996;1: 186–9.

42. Olds J, Milner P. Positive reinforcement produced by electrical stimulation of septal area and other regions of rat brain. J Comp Physiol Psychol 1954;47: 419–27.

43. Corbett D, Wise RA. Intracranial self-stimulation in relation to the ascending dopaminergic systems of the midbrain: a moveable electrode mapping study. Brain Res 1980;185(1):1–15.

44. Olney JJ, Warlow SM, Naffziger EE, et al. Current perspectives on incentive salience and applications to clinical disorders. Curr Opin Behav Sci 2018;22: 59–69.

45. Viviani R, Dommes L, Bosch J, et al. Signals of anticipation of reward and of mean reward rates in the human brain. Sci Rep 2020;10:4287.
46. Schultz W. Multiple reward signals in the brain. Nat Rev Neurosci 2000;1: 199–207.
47. Korpi ER, den Hollander B, Farooq U, et al. Mechanisms of action and persistent neuroplasticity by drugs of abuse. Pharmacol Rev 2015;67:872–1004.
48. Saal D, Dong Y, Bonci A, et al. Drugs of abuse and stress trigger a common synaptic adaptation in dopamine neurons. Neuron 2003;37:577–82.
49. Johnson SW, North RA. Opioids excite dopamine neurons by hyperpolarization of local interneurons. J Neurosci 1992;12:483–8.
50. Verrico CD, Miller GM, Madras BK. MDMA (ecstasy) and human dopamine, norepinephrine, and serotonin transporters: implications for MDMA-induced neurotoxicity and treatment. Psychopharmacology (Berl) 2007;189:489–503.
51. Kalivas PW, Duffy P, Eberhardt H. Modulation of A10 dopamine neurons by gamma-aminobutyric acid agonists. J Pharmacol Exp Ther 1990;253:858–66.
52. Okada H, Matsushita N, Kobayashi K, et al. Identification of GABAA receptor subunit variants in midbrain dopaminergic neurons. J Neurochem 2004;89:7–14.
53. Tan KR, Brown M, Labouebe G, et al. Neural bases for addictive properties of benzodiazepines. Nature 2010;463:769–74.
54. Jones JD, Mogali S, Comer SD. Polydrug abuse: A review of opioid and benzodiazepine combination use. Drug Alcohol Depend 2012;125(1–2):8–18.
55. Jones CM, McAninch JK. Emergency department visits and overdose deaths from combined use of opioids and benzodiazepines. Am J Prev Med 2015; 49(4):493–501.
56. Afzal A, Kiyatkin EA. Interactions of benzodiazepines with heroin: respiratory depression, temperature effects, and behavior. Neuropharmacology 2019;158: 107677.
57. Picciotto MR, Zoli M, Rimondini R, et al. Acetylcholine receptors containing the beta2 subunit are involved in the reinforcing properties of nicotine. Nature 1998;391:173–7.
58. Grenhoff J, Aston-Jones G, Svensson TH. Nicotinic effects on the firing pattern of midbrain dopamine neurons. Acta Physiol Scand 1986;128:351–8.
59. Palmatier MI, Evans-Martin FF, Hoffman A, et al. Dissociating the primary reinforcing and reinforcement-enhancing effects of nicotine using a rat self-administration paradigm with concurrently available drug and environmental reinforcers. Psychopharmacology (Berl) 2006;184:391–400.
60. Spiller KJ, Bi GH, He Y, et al. Cannabinoid CB1 and CB2 receptor mechanisms underlie cannabis reward and aversion in rats. Br J Pharmacol 2019;176(9): 1268–81.
61. Kalivas PW. The glutamate homeostasis hypothesis of addiction. Nat Rev Neurosci 2009;10(8):561–72.
62. Belin D, Jonkman S, Dickinson A, et al. Parallel and interactive learning processes within the basal ganglia: Relevance for the understanding of addiction. Behav Brain Res 2009;199(1):89–102.
63. Volkow ND, Baler RD. NOW vs LATER brain circuits: implications for obesity and addiction. Trends Neurosci 2015;38(6):345–52.
64. Nguyen D, Naffziger EE, Berridge KC. Positive Affect: Nature and brain bases of liking and wanting. Curr Opin Behav Sci 2021;39:72–8.
65. DuPont RL, Compton WM, McLellan AT. Five-year recovery: A new standard for assessing effectiveness of substance use disorder treatment. J Subst Abuse Treat 2015;58:1–5.

66. Young EJ, Briggs SB, Miller CA. The Actin Cytoskeleton as a Therapeutic Target for the Prevention of Relapse to Methamphetamine Use. CNS Neurol Disord Drug Targets 2015;14(6):731–7.
67. Stone EM, Kennedy-Hendricks A, Barry CL, et al. The role of stigma in U.S. primary care physicians' treatment of opioid use disorder. Drug Alcohol Depend 2021;221:108627.
68. Lewis M. Brain change in addiction as learning, not disease. N Engl J Med 2018; 379(16):1551–60.
69. Satel S, Lilienfeld SO. Addiction and the brain-disease fallacy. Front Psychiatry 2013;4:141.

KEY ADDITIONAL READINGS:

Compton WM, Valentino RJ, DuPont RL. Polysubstance use in the U.S. opioid crisis. Mol Psychiatry 2021;26(1):41–50.
Feltenstein MW, See RE, Fuchs RA. Neural Substrates and Circuits of Drug Addiction. Cold Spring Harb Perspect Med 2021;11(4):a039628.
Volkow ND, Boyle M. Neuroscience of addiction: relevance to prevention and treatment. Am J Psychiatry 2018;175:729–40.
Volkow ND, Koob GF, McLellan AT. Neurobiologic Advances from the Brain Disease Model of Addiction. N Engl J Med 2016;374(4):363–71.

Pharmacotherapy of Opioid Use Disorder—Update and Current Challenges

Savitha Racha, MD[1],*, Megan Buresh, MD[1],
Michael Fingerhood, MD[1]

KEYWORDS

- Methadone • Buprenorphine • Naltrexone • Opioid use disorder
- Medications for opioid use disorder • Opioid agonist therapy

KEY POINTS

- Despite the advancements in pharmacotherapy for the treatment of opioid use disorder (OUD), utilization of medications for OUD remains poor and the prevalence of OUD and related overdose deaths continue to increase within the country.
- Increased provider awareness and understanding of OUD and medications for OUD is key to increasing access to treatment.
- Methadone, buprenorphine, and naltrexone are all Federal Drug Administration-approved medications for OUD and should be offered to all patients with OUD.

INTRODUCTION
Nature of the Problem

Despite the development of medications for opioid use disorder (MOUD), overdose deaths continue to increase within the United States. Methadone, buprenorphine, and extended-release naltrexone have been approved by the United States Food and Drug Administration (FDA) for the treatment of opioid use disorder (OUD). Methadone and buprenorphine are proven to reduce withdrawal symptoms, cravings, and pain, ultimately protecting against opioid overdose. However, MOUD are underutilized, and most patients with OUD receive no pharmacotherapy. Underutilization can be attributed to limited access to MOUD (system fragmentation, regulatory and legal requirements, insurance barriers, and so forth) as well as misunderstanding of OUD and stigma.[1]

The first step in accepting MOUD is recognizing OUD as a chronic disease. Historically, people with substance use disorders were thought to have weak morals and deserving of punishment for their behaviors.[2] Despite the advances in addiction

Department of Medicine, Division of Addiction Medicine, Johns Hopkins School of Medicine, 5200 Eastern Avenue, Mason F. Lord Building, East Tower, 2nd Floor, Baltimore, MD 21224, USA
[1] Present address: Comprehensive Care Clinic, 5200 Eastern Avenue, Mason F. Lord Building, East Tower, 2nd Floor, Baltimore, MD 21224, USA
* Corresponding author.
E-mail address: savi220@bu.edu

Psychiatr Clin N Am 45 (2022) 335–346
https://doi.org/10.1016/j.psc.2022.04.001 psych.theclinics.com
0193-953X/22/© 2022 Elsevier Inc. All rights reserved.

medicine, data suggest there is still a significant proportion of people who hold this outdated belief. In a 2016 national public opinion survey, most respondents viewed individuals with OUD as deserving blame for their substance use and lacking self-discipline.[3] This view is not limited to lay people; in that same year, a study assessing stigma toward people with OUD in primary care physicians demonstrated even higher rates of stigma than in the general public.[4]

Prevalence

Within recent years, the incidence of OUD has skyrocketed within the United States. The 2018 National Survey on Drug Use and Health estimated that the number of people with OUD more than doubled between 2002 (214,000) and 2018 (526,000).[5] This increase can be attributed to increased access to prescription opioids and the production of illicit fentanyl.

Opioid analgesics are approved for the treatment of cancer-related pain but they are also prescribed routinely for the treatment of chronic noncancer pain[6] despite limited evidence to support their effectiveness and safety.[7] People with chronic opioid prescriptions are at especially high risk for developing OUD if they have multiple opioid prescribers, high dose prescriptions, and overlapping prescriptions.[8] The formulation of the prescription opioid is also important to consider. Long-acting oral formulations were originally thought to be safer than short-acting formulations due to their controlled-release mechanism but they are still not tamper-resistant[9] and the long half-life increases the risk of oversedation.

Even more concerning is the increase in overdose deaths from opioid use. Between May, 2020 and April, 2021, more than 10000 deaths were attributed to drug overdose and 64% involved illicitly manufactured fentanyls, which was a 26% increase from 2020 to 2021.[10] Fentanyl is a synthetic opioid that was originally developed in 1960 for the treatment of severe cancer pain and perioperative pain.[11] Due to its low production cost, eventually, fentanyl and its analogs were manufactured illicitly and sold as heroin.[12] Fentanyl is highly potent (30–50 times more potent than heroin), has a fast onset of action, and long duration.[13] It is no wonder that overdose deaths have grown significantly since its advent. The number of fentanyl-related overdose deaths increased by 32% between 2010 and 2016[14] and tended to cluster among younger individuals (ages 20–40) living in the northeastern United States.[15] Fentanyl use has also been implicated in the disproportionately higher rates of opioid overdose in minority communities.[16]

Goals

The goal of this article is to describe the pharmacotherapy approach to treating OUD with careful attention to the current challenges of MOUD.

DISCUSSION
Current Studies

Methadone

Methadone was the first FDA-approved medication for the treatment of OUD. It is a synthetic, long-acting, full agonist at the mu-opioid receptor.[17] Methadone treats opioid withdrawal, cravings, and pain. Due to its full agonist properties, abstinence from opioids is not required before starting methadone, which makes it accessible to patients who are unable to tolerate withdrawal or pain during initiation. However, titration of methadone to a therapeutic dose is best achieved during days to weeks due to its long half-life (24 hours) and risk of dose stacking. The therapeutic dose varies greatly among individuals and is targeted to the relief of cravings, withdrawal, and pain.[18]

In the United States, methadone distribution is highly regulated by the government and can only be administered and dispensed for the treatment of OUD in 2 settings: outpatient treatment programs (OTPs) and hospitals.[19] When initiating methadone at an OTP, patients are generally mandated to start with daily observed dosing. Only after demonstrating medication adherence, illicit opioid-free urine tests, and regular counseling attendance can patients qualify for take-home doses. Methadone doses start between 15 and 40 mg and increase by 5 to 20 mg every 3 to 7 days for a therapeutic dose between 80 and 150 mg/d.[20,21] For the hospital setting, however, there is little to no guidance on methadone initiation and titration.

Similar to all other opioid agonists, a missed methadone dose may result in opioid withdrawal. The risk of overdose is greatest within the first 2 weeks of starting methadone therapy[22] and is higher in patients also using sedating substances such as benzodiazepines and alcohol. Besides oversedation and respiratory depression, the other major risks of methadone use are corrected QT interval (QTc) prolongation and hypoglycemia, the last of which is very rare and may be an opioid class effect.[23]

Buprenorphine
Buprenorphine is a synthetic, long-acting, high-affinity partial agonist at the mu-opioid receptor.[24] Due to its agonist activity, similar methadone, buprenorphine treats opioid withdrawal, cravings, and pain and discontinuation results in opioid withdrawal. However, unlike methadone, it has less of an effect on respiratory depression and lower risk of overdose due to its partial activation of the mu-opioid receptor.[25] Other side effects of buprenorphine include nausea and delayed gastric emptying.

Buprenorphine traditionally requires a period of abstinence from opioids before initiation to avoid precipitated withdrawal. Precipitated withdrawal can occur in patients whose receptors are occupied with full opioid agonists at the time of buprenorphine initiation because buprenorphine's higher affinity for the opioid receptor displaces full opioid agonists and lowers the activation of the opioid receptor. However, research has shown that "macrodosing" or initiating high-dose buprenorphine (>12 mg) in the emergency department was not associated with significant precipitated withdrawal symptoms.[26] An alternative method of buprenorphine initiation called "microdosing" does not require abstinence from full opioid agonists and consists of concurrently starting low doses of buprenorphine (intravenous, transdermal, or sublingual) and slowly titrating to a therapeutic sublingual dose over a few days.[27–29]

The most common formulation of buprenorphine is the sublingual film. It is often manufactured as a combination film with naloxone, which only activates if the medication is injected and diminishes the rewarding effect of injected buprenorphine. The typical starting dose of buprenorphine is 4 to 8 mg but additional doses can be given to target relief of withdrawal, cravings, and pain.[20] Titration to a therapeutic dose (12–24 mg total per day, which may be taken in a divided dose) can be achieved within a few days,[30] although some patients may need larger doses, especially those who use higher potency opioids and/or have concomitant pain. A case report from Australia in 2019 (during the fentanyl era) detailed the case of a patient requiring a total daily buprenorphine dose of 40 mg to adequately treat her withdrawal and cravings.[31]

In 2017, the Federal Drug Administration approved an extended-release injectable formulation of buprenorphine for the treatment of OUD. Extended-release buprenorphine has a 43 to 60-day half-life, which increases adherence and decreases diversion risk.[32] A double-blind randomized clinical trial demonstrated that injectable buprenorphine was noninferior to sublingual buprenorphine concerning response rate and opioid-free urine toxicology and superior concerning abstinence from illicit opioids.[33]

Buprenorphine can be administered and dispensed through an OTP but is most commonly prescribed in an office-based setting. As with methadone, patients initiating buprenorphine are generally given shorter prescriptions and more frequent office visits until the OUD stabilizes.[34] In order to prescribe buprenorphine, providers (such as physicians, nurse practitioners, and physician assistants) must obtain a special X-waiver certification from the Drug Enforcement Administration. As of 2021, an X-waiver to prescribe buprenorphine to up to 30 patients can be obtained without specific course training. Prescribing for more than 30 patients (thresholds of 100 or 275) requires additional training. Despite the high nationwide prevalence of OUD, as of early 2020, less than 5% of physicians within the United States were X-waivered.[35] However, with the expansion of X-waiver eligibility to advanced practice providers (eg, nurse practitioners, physician assistance, nurse midwives, and so forth) and removal of the 8-hour training requirement, the total number of buprenorphine prescribers is expected to increase.

Extended-release naltrexone

Naltrexone is a full antagonist at the mu-opioid receptor.[24] Naltrexone blocks the euphoric and analgesic effects of opioids, which eventually extinguishes cravings for opioids. Side of effects of naltrexone include nausea, headache, dysphoria, and transaminitis (especially at high doses). When compared with opioid agonist therapy (OAT), naltrexone has been associated with similar mortality rates.[36] A key barrier to naltrexone use is the recommended 7-day period of abstinence from opioids before initiation.[37] Premature initiation of naltrexone increases the risk of precipitated withdrawal, which is more severe than the precipitated withdrawal from buprenorphine due to naltrexone's full antagonist properties. Extended-release naltrexone is available as a monthly 380 mg intramuscular injection. Naltrexone is also available as a once-daily oral tablet and low (1–25 mg) test doses can be given before initiating extended-release naltrexone to ensure tolerability.

Treatment of fentanyl use disorder

Compared with other opioid-related overdoses, fentanyl-related overdoses are more likely to be associated with rigidity, dyskinesia, and bradycardia.[38] Therefore, when treating patients with fentanyl use presenting with opioid overdose, the provider should maintain a low threshold for oxygen supplementation. The patient may also require larger or repeated doses of naloxone (up to 12 mg) to reverse the effect of fentanyl due to fentanyl's higher affinity for the mu-opioid receptor.[39]

The data on methadone[40] and buprenorphine[41] for the treatment of fentanyl use disorder are limited and suggest that 6-month retention is low for both medications. The data on extended-release naltrexone is even more limited because fewer patients initiate naltrexone compared with buprenorphine but the existing research suggests that it is just as safe and effective as opioid agonist therapy.[42] This makes harm-reduction strategies such as naloxone prescriptions and safe injection sites all the more important when considering interventions for individuals who are using potent synthetic opioids such as fentanyl.[43]

Studies in rats have shown that nalmefene, which is longer acting and more potent than naloxone, is better at treating carfentanil-induced respiratory depression.[44] Another study demonstrated that neurosurgical patients on chronic carbamazepine had increased clearance and decreased plasma concentrations of fentanyl.[45] There is also emerging research on a fentanyl vaccine in rats that reduced fentanyl biodistribution and fentanyl reinforcement.[46] A more recent study showed that purified monoclonal antibodies from vaccinated mice prevented acute lethality from fentanyl.[47] However, there are no data yet on the safety and efficacy of the fentanyl vaccine or monoclonal antibodies in humans.

Approach: Low Threshold Care

Although MOUD are traditionally prescribed at in-person encounters with health-care personnel in ambulatory, rehabilitation, residential, and inpatient settings, other low-barrier treatment delivery systems are now gaining popularity. Telemedicine, which was popularized by the coronavirus-19 pandemic, has significantly increased access to MOUD without compromising face-to-face interactions. For patients who were already connected to local MOUD prescribers, telehealth avoided an interruption in care while promoting social distancing. Telehealth also expanded access to addiction medicine care for patients in rural areas of the United States where there is a low number of MOUD prescribers and a high number of opioid-related deaths.[48] Preliminary data also demonstrate patient satisfaction with telemedicine as a medium to deliver OUD care, likely due to its convenience, privacy, and availability.[49] However, despite overall increases in access, telemedicine is not available in both rural and urban areas to technologically challenged individuals and individuals who cannot afford smart phones, broadband, or access to private spaces.

Interim methadone is a treatment approach in response to counselor shortages and refers to supervised methadone with emergency counseling as opposed to standard methadone, which involves routine counseling. A randomized controlled trial found no significant differences in treatment retention, positive urine tests, or arrests between interim methadone treatment and standard methadone treatment.[50] These findings suggest that methadone alone is an effective intervention for the treatment of OUD and that limited availability of psychosocial supports, especially during the coronavirus-19 pandemic, should not prohibit OTP methadone dispensing.

Effective July 28, 2021, the Drug Enforcement Administration revised its regulations to allow mobile dispensing of schedule II–V narcotic drugs such as buprenorphine and methadone.[51] Mobile treatment has the advantage of being able to reach the most vulnerable populations of people with OUD, namely people with unstable housing and/or justice-involved individuals. With their goal to "meet people where they are," mobile OUD providers travel to their patients' encampments[52] or outside a jail[53] to provide medication (most often buprenorphine), counseling, and referrals to other services. Justice-involved individuals are especially vulnerable to overdose due to their lowered tolerance to opioids. A retrospective cohort analysis demonstrated that increasing access to all FDA-approved MOUD in criminal justice settings was associated with decreased overdose mortality.[54]

Testing for Fentanyl

In the most recent wave, fentanyl analogs seemed in the illicit opioid market in 2013 and were marketed as heroin to consumers.[55] Up until recently, many people with OUD were using fentanyl unknowingly.[56] Because fentanyl is a synthetic opioid, small changes can be made to its chemical structure to manufacture countless new analogs. In a postmortem analysis of 174 synthetic overdose deaths between 2016 and 2019 in Connecticut, toxicology testing identified 10 different novel synthetics.[57] The typical health-care setting immunoassay only tests for nonsynthetic opioids such as morphine and codeine.[58] That plus the constant evolution of the opioid drug market complicates our ability to detect fentanyl and appreciate its true prevalence. Gas chromatography mass spectrometry or liquid chromatography tandem mass spectrometry can definitively detect fentanyl, but the delayed results preclude their clinical utility.[59] Only a few automated fentanyl immunoassays have been validated for clinical use and point of care testing strips have varying degrees of accuracy.

Controversies: Opioid Agonist Therapy as "Substitution Therapy"

Methadone and buprenorphine are likened to illicit opioids because they all activate the mu-opioid receptor, unlike naltrexone that blocks the mu-opioid receptor. A common misguided attitude is that starting opioid agonist therapy means substituting one drug (methadone or buprenorphine) for another (illicit opioid).[60] Hence, there is often more support from providers, programs, and patients for opioid antagonists over opioid agonists. However, there are obvious logistical, pharmacologic, and clinical differences between OAT and illicit opioids. First, OAT is FDA-approved, prescribed, evidence-based, and generally covered by medical insurance. In comparison, heroin and other illicit opioids such as fentanyl are unregulated and costly to the consumer. From a pharmacologic standpoint, methadone and buprenorphine have long half-lives, which provide long-acting relief from withdrawal, cravings, and pain. For example, intravenous heroin has an average half-life of 30 minutes, methadone 24 hours, and sublingual buprenorphine 24 to 48 hours.[60] Buprenorphine is a partial mu-opioid agonist, giving it a ceiling effect, which protects against sedation and respiratory depression. Both methadone and buprenorphine have been shown to decrease all-cause mortality.[61] Additionally, because most formulations of methadone and buprenorphine are administered orally as opposed to intravenously or intranasally such as most illicit opioids, they do not carry the risk of infectious disease transmission or nasal perforation. The opioid agonist properties of methadone and buprenorphine promote positive reinforcement of medication adherence and improved retention in treatment.[62] In general, opioid agonist therapy is more effective, safer, and more affordable than illicit opioids.

SUMMARY
Conclusions and Recommendations

The opioid epidemic in the United States is appropriately gaining public attention. However, negative attitudes toward people with OUD hinder progress and reform. Destigmatizing OUD and MOUD is the first step toward fighting the war on opioids. The second step is to offer MOUD with special attention to patients' preferences, comorbidities, and psychosocial barriers. Providers should maintain a high index of suspicion for fentanyl use and tailor choice and dose of MOUD accordingly. Finally, individual efforts must be supported and expanded by regulatory efforts, such as the Substance Abuse and Mental Health Services Administration's consideration to indefinitely extend methadone take-home flexibility.[63]

Future Directions

Although there have been significant advances in the pharmacotherapy for OUD in recent years, there are still ample avenues for future research. There are multiple guidelines for methadone initiation in the outpatient setting but not for the inpatient setting. With regards to buprenorphine, there are newer formulations (extended release) and methods of initiation (microdosing) but limited data comparing these to standard sublingual buprenorphine initiation. Due to the barriers for naltrexone initiation, there are few studies on the outcomes of patients initiated on naltrexone especially in comparison to opioid agonist therapy. Finally, in the era of illicit fentanyl, there is a need for better detection methods and data on effective MOUD doses.

Methadone case presentation
Case Title: Restarting Methadone Treatment after Overdose.

Case Presentation: MC is a 65-year-old woman with a history of OUD on 100 mg of methadone at an OTP. She presented to the emergency department after being found unconscious and was intubated for acute hypoxic respiratory failure. Her admission urine toxicology tested positive for benzodiazepine, cannabinoid, cocaine, fentanyl, methadone, and codeine/morphine.

Her OTP confirmed that her last dose of methadone was 2 weeks before admission. Because a history could not be obtained while the patient was intubated, methadone was restarted at 30 mg daily. Seven days later, after extubation, the patient was interviewed and denied any withdrawal, cravings, or pain.

Clinical Question: How should MC's methadone be managed going forward?

Discussion: Despite being on a higher methadone dose at her OTP, because MC's current dose is appropriately managing her cravings, withdrawal, and pain after having had enough time to achieve steady state, there is no indication to increase her dose beyond 30 mg. A lower methadone dose may also be safer in this patient whose urine contained other sedating substances such as fentanyl, codeine/morphine, and benzodiazepines. This lower methadone dose should be communicated to her OTP.

Buprenorphine case presentation

Case Title: Perioperative Management of Buprenorphine.

Case Presentation: DT is a 47-year-old man with a history of OUD who has been in stable abstinent recovery on sublingual buprenorphine 8 mg tid for years. He presented to the emergency department with a blast injury to his left upper extremity from handling fireworks. Buprenorphine has been held since admission. He underwent multiple reconstructive surgeries and still has more planned. His perioperative pain is being managed by full opioid agonists and nonopioid analgesics but no MOUD. He wishes to eventually resume buprenorphine for his OUD.

Clinical Question: What is the best way to resume DT's buprenorphine?

Discussion: DT should be restarted on buprenorphine via microdosing once all his surgical procedures are completed and his pain is adequately controlled. He is unlikely to tolerate a period of opioid abstinence due to the extent of his injuries. In comparison to standard buprenorphine initiation, microinduction will allow DT to resume this home medication without causing pain or precipitated withdrawal. Although it would be easier pharmacologically to switch this patient to methadone, this is not in line with the patient's preferences and would be disruptive to his recovery. For future surgeries, DT's home buprenorphine should not be held on admission and should be continued throughout the perioperative period.

Naltrexone case presentation

Case Title: Patient Requesting Naltrexone.

Case Presentation: JL is a 56-year-old man with a history of OUD who inquires about being treated for OUD with naltrexone. He has been on buprenorphine in the past but found that he was still occasionally using opioids and could feel some euphoria. He has a new job and has not used any opioids in 2 weeks but feels he might be vulnerable to use illicit opioids when facing stressful situations. With encouragement from his family, he wants to try injectable naltrexone because he will not have to take this medication daily and knows that he will be safe when he might feel vulnerable.

Clinical Question: Should you prescribe injectable naltrexone for JL?

Discussion: JL understands the use of naltrexone and he has chosen it for treatment of OUD with understanding of how it works and why he believes it is the best option for him. He has support from family. A urine screen should confirm absence of opioids, including fentanyl, and naltrexone can then be initiated with discussion of starting with an oral dose of naltrexone before first injection.

CLINICS CARE POINTS

- The incidence of opioid use disorder (OUD), fentanyl use, and overdose deaths is increasing yearly within the United States
- Many lay individuals and health-care professionals stigmatize people with OUD as well as OUD treatment
- Methadone, buprenorphine, and naltrexone are Federal Drug Administration-approved medications for OUD and have been shown to reduce overdose mortality
- Choice of pharmacotherapy for OUD should be driven by patient preference and not by what is convenient pharmacologically or logistically
- Utilization of medications for OUD is low and can be attributed to system fragmentation, regulatory and legal requirements, insurance barriers, and stigma
- Because initiation of naltrexone is more difficult (especially on an outpatient basis), fewer patients have used it, and therefore, there is less outcome data on naltrexone in comparison to opioid agonist therapies
- Methadone and buprenorphine are fundamentally different from heroin due to their superior safety profile and should not be considered substitutes for heroin
- Fentanyl and various analogs should be tested for in urine toxicology
- Telehealth and mobile treatment are patient-centered approaches that increase access to addiction medicine care in vulnerable populations.

FINANCIAL DISCLOSURES

None.

REFERENCES

1. National Academies of Sciences. In: Mancher M, Leshner AI, editors. Engineering, and medicine; Health and medicine Division; board on Health Sciences Policy; Committee on medication-Assisted treatment for opioid Use disorder. Medications for opioid Use disorder Save lives. . Washington (DC): National Academies Press (US); 2019.
2. Rastegar DA, Fingerhood MI. The American Society of addiction medicine Handbook of addiction medicine. 2nd edition. New York: Oxford university press; 2020.
3. Kennedy-Hendricks A, Barry CL, Gollust SE, et al. Social Stigma Toward Persons With Prescription Opioid Use Disorder: Associations With Public Support for Punitive and Public Health-Oriented Policies. Psychiatr Serv 2017;68(5):462–9.
4. Kennedy-Hendricks A, Busch SH, McGinty EE, et al. Primary care physicians' perspectives on the prescription opioid epidemic. Drug Alcohol Depend 2016; 165:61–70.
5. Substance Abuse and Mental Health Services Administration. Key substance Use and Mental Health Indicators in the United States: results from the 2018 national survey on drug Use and Health. Rockville, (MD): Center for Behavioral Health Statistics and Quality, Substance Abuse and Mental Health Services Administration; 2019. HHS Publication No. PEP19-5068, NSDUH Series H-54.

6. Dowell D, Haegerich TM, Chou R. CDC Guideline for Prescribing Opioids for Chronic Pain–United States, 2016. JAMA 2016;315(15):1624–45.

7. Kalso E, Edwards JE, Moore AR, et al. Opioids in chronic non-cancer pain: systematic review of efficacy and safety. Pain 2004;112(3):372–80.

8. Hoffman KA, Ponce Terashima J, McCarty D. Opioid use disorder and treatment: challenges and opportunities. BMC Health Serv Res 2019;19(1):884.

9. Fletcher J, Tsuyuki R. Don't tamper with oxycodone. CMAJ 2013;185(2):107.

10. O'Donnell J, Tanz LJ, Gladden RM, et al. Trends in and Characteristics of Drug Overdose Deaths Involving Illicitly Manufactured Fentanyls - United States, 2019-2020. MMWR Morb Mortal Wkly Rep 2021;70(50):1740–6.

11. Han Y, Yan W, Zheng Y, et al. The rising crisis of illicit fentanyl use, overdose, and potential therapeutic strategies. Transl Psychiatry 2019;9(1):282.

12. Hibbs J, Perper J, Winek CL. An outbreak of designer drug–related deaths in Pennsylvania. JAMA 1991;265(8):1011–3.

13. Poklis A. Fentanyl: a review for clinical and analytical toxicologists. J Toxicol Clin Toxicol 1995;33(5):439–47.

14. Jones CM, Einstein EB, Compton WM. Changes in Synthetic Opioid Involvement in Drug Overdose Deaths in the United States, 2010-2016. JAMA 2018;319(17): 1819–21.

15. Jalal H, Buchanich JM, Roberts MS, et al. Changing dynamics of the drug overdose epidemic in the United States from 1979 through 2016. Science 2018; 361(6408):eaau1184.

16. James K, Jordan A. The Opioid Crisis in Black Communities. J L Med Ethics 2018;46(2):404–21.

17. Kreek MJ. Methadone-related opioid agonist pharmacotherapy for heroin addiction. History, recent molecular and neurochemical research and future in mainstream medicine. Ann N Y Acad Sci 2000;909:186–216.

18. Effective medical treatment of opiate addiction. National Consensus Development Panel on Effective Medical Treatment of Opiate Addiction. JAMA 1998; 280(22):1936–43.

19. CRS (Congressional Research Service). Opioid treatment programs and related federal regulations. 2018. Available at: https://sgp.fas.org/crs/misc/IF10219.pdf. Accessed February 5, 2022.

20. Schuckit MA. Treatment of Opioid-Use Disorders. N Engl J Med 2016;375(4): 357–68.

21. Durrani M, Bansal K. Methadone. StatPearls. Treasure Island (FL): StatPearls Publishing; 2022.

22. Degenhardt L, Randall D, Hall W, et al. Mortality among clients of a state-wide opioid pharmacotherapy program over 20 years: risk factors and lives saved. Drug Alcohol Depend 2009;105(1–2):9–15.

23. Toce MS, Chai PR, Burns MM, et al. Pharmacologic Treatment of Opioid Use Disorder: a Review of Pharmacotherapy, Adjuncts, and Toxicity. J Med Toxicol 2018; 14(4):306–22.

24. Kleber HD. Pharmacologic treatments for opioid dependence: detoxification and maintenance options. Dialogues Clin Neurosci 2007;9(4):455–70.

25. Dahan A, Yassen A, Romberg R, et al. Buprenorphine induces ceiling in respiratory depression but not in analgesia. Br J Anaesth 2006;96(5):627–32.

26. Herring AA, Vosooghi AA, Luftig J, et al. High-Dose Buprenorphine Induction in the Emergency Department for Treatment of Opioid Use Disorder. JAMA Netw Open 2021;4(7):e2117128. https://doi.org/10.1001/jamanetworkopen.2021. 17128.

27. Thakrar AP, Jablonski L, Ratner J, et al. Micro-dosing Intravenous Buprenorphine to Rapidly Transition From Full Opioid Agonists. J Addict Med 2022;16(1):122–4.

28. Brar R, Fairbairn N, Sutherland C, et al. Use of a novel prescribing approach for the treatment of opioid use disorder: Buprenorphine/naloxone micro-dosing - a case series. Drug Alcohol Rev 2020;39(5):588–94.

29. Baumgartner K, Salmo E, Liss D, et al. Transdermal buprenorphine for in-hospital transition from full agonist opioids to sublingual buprenorphine: a retrospective observational cohort study [published online ahead of print, 2022 Jan 20]. Clin Toxicol (Phila) 2022;1–6.

30. Connery HS. Medication-assisted treatment of opioid use disorder: review of the evidence and future directions. Harv Rev Psychiatry 2015;23(2):63–75.

31. Danilewitz M, McLean M. High-dose buprenorphine for treatment of high potency opioid use disorder. Drug Alcohol Rev 2020;39(2):135–7.

32. Haight BR, Learned SM, Laffont CM, et al. Efficacy and safety of a monthly buprenorphine depot injection for opioid use disorder: a multicentre, randomised, double-blind, placebo-controlled, phase 3 trial. Lancet 2019;393(10173):778–90.

33. Lofwall MR, Walsh SL, Nunes EV, et al. Weekly and Monthly Subcutaneous Buprenorphine Depot Formulations vs Daily Sublingual Buprenorphine With Naloxone for Treatment of Opioid Use Disorder: A Randomized Clinical Trial. JAMA Intern Med 2018;178(6):764–73.

34. Fiellin DA, Pantalon MV, Chawarski MC, et al. Counseling plus buprenorphine-naloxone maintenance therapy for opioid dependence. N Engl J Med 2006; 355(4):365–74.

35. Martin A, Raber JP, Shayer D, et al. Get waivered remote: Nationwide, remote DEA-x waiver course in response to COVID-19. Digit Health 2021;7. https://doi.org/10.1177/20552076211048985. 20552076211048985.

36. Kelty E, Joyce D, Hulse G. A retrospective cohort study of mortality rates in patients with an opioid use disorder treated with implant naltrexone, oral methadone or sublingual buprenorphine. Am J Drug Alcohol Abuse 2019;45(3):285–91.

37. Sullivan M, Bisaga A, Pavlicova M, et al. Long-Acting Injectable Naltrexone Induction: A Randomized Trial of Outpatient Opioid Detoxification With Naltrexone Versus Buprenorphine. Am J Psychiatry 2017;174(5):459–67.

38. Kinshella MW, Gauthier T, Lysyshyn M. Rigidity, dyskinesia and other atypical overdose presentations observed at a supervised injection site, Vancouver, Canada. Harm Reduct J 2018;15(1):64.

39. Schumann H, Erickson T, Thompson TM, et al. Fentanyl epidemic in Chicago, Illinois and surrounding Cook County. Clin Toxicol (Phila) 2008;46(6):501–6.

40. Stone AC, Carroll JJ, Rich JD, et al. Methadone maintenance treatment among patients exposed to illicit fentanyl in Rhode Island: Safety, dose, retention, and relapse at 6 months. Drug Alcohol Depend 2018;192:94–7.

41. Wakeman SE, Chang Y, Regan S, et al. Impact of Fentanyl Use on Buprenorphine Treatment Retention and Opioid Abstinence. J Addict Med 2019;13(4):253–7.

42. Lee JD, Nunes EV Jr, Novo P, et al. Comparative effectiveness of extended-release naltrexone versus buprenorphine-naloxone for opioid relapse prevention (X:BOT): a multicentre, open-label, randomised controlled trial. Lancet 2018; 391(10118):309–18.

43. Kim HK, Connors NJ, Mazer-Amirshahi ME. The role of take-home naloxone in the epidemic of opioid overdose involving illicitly manufactured fentanyl and its analogs. Expert Opin Drug Saf 2019;18(6):465–75.

44. Yong Z, Gao X, Ma W, et al. Nalmefene reverses carfentanil-induced loss of righting reflex and respiratory depression in rats. Eur J Pharmacol 2014;738:153–7.

45. Nozari A, Akeju O, Mirzakhani H, et al. Prolonged therapy with the anticonvulsant carbamazepine leads to increased plasma clearance of fentanyl. J Pharm Pharmacol 2019;71(6):982–7.
46. Raleigh MD, Baruffaldi F, Peterson SJ, et al. A Fentanyl Vaccine Alters Fentanyl Distribution and Protects against Fentanyl-Induced Effects in Mice and Rats. J Pharmacol Exp Ther 2019;368(2):282–91.
47. Smith LC, Bremer PT, Hwang CS, et al. Monoclonal Antibodies for Combating Synthetic Opioid Intoxication. J Am Chem Soc 2019;141(26):10489–503.
48. Lister JJ, Weaver A, Ellis JD, et al. A systematic review of rural-specific barriers to medication treatment for opioid use disorder in the United States. Am J Drug Alcohol Abuse 2020;46(3):273–88.
49. Cole TO, Robinson D, Kelley-Freeman A, et al. Patient Satisfaction With Medications for Opioid Use Disorder Treatment via Telemedicine: Brief Literature Review and Development of a New Assessment. Front Public Health 2021;8. 557275.
50. Schwartz RP, Kelly SM, O'Grady KE, et al. Randomized trial of standard methadone treatment compared to initiating methadone without counseling: 12-month findings. Addiction 2012;107(5):943–52.
51. FederalRegistrar.gov. Registration Requirements for Narcotic Treatment Programs With Mobile Components. 2021. Available at: https://www.federalregister.gov/documents/2021/06/28/2021-13519/registration-requirements-for-narcotic-treatment-programs-with-mobile-components. Accessed March 11, 2022.
52. Wenzel K, Fishman M. Mobile van delivery of extended-release buprenorphine and extended-release naltrexone for youth with OUD: An adaptation to the COVID-19 emergency. J Subst Abuse Treat 2021;120:108149.
53. Krawczyk N, Buresh M, Gordon MS, et al. Expanding low-threshold buprenorphine to justice-involved individuals through mobile treatment: Addressing a critical care gap. J Subst Abuse Treat 2019;103:1–8.
54. Green TC, Clarke J, Brinkley-Rubinstein L, et al. Postincarceration Fatal Overdoses After Implementing Medications for Addiction Treatment in a Statewide Correctional System. JAMA Psychiatry 2018;75(4):405–7.
55. Global Smart Programme. Global smart Update: fentanyl and its analogues—50 Years on. 2017. Available at: https://www.unodc.org/documents/scientific/Global_SMART_Update_17_web.pdf. Accessed February 5, 2022.
56. Amlani A, McKee G, Khamis N, et al. Why the FUSS (Fentanyl Urine Screen Study)? A cross-sectional survey to characterize an emerging threat to people who use drugs in British Columbia, Canada. Harm Reduct J 2015;12:54.
57. Clinton HA, Thangada S, Gill JR, et al. Improvements in Toxicology Testing to Identify Fentanyl Analogs and Other Novel Synthetic Opioids in Fatal Drug Overdoses, Connecticut, January 2016-June 2019. Public Health Rep 2021;136(1_suppl):80S–6S.
58. Kale N. Urine Drug Tests: Ordering and Interpreting Results. Am Fam Physician 2019;99(1):33–9.
59. Armenian P, Vo KT, Barr-Walker J, et al. Fentanyl, fentanyl analogs and novel synthetic opioids: A comprehensive review. Neuropharmacology 2018;134(Pt A):121–32.
60. Miller SC, Fiellin DA, Rosenthal RN, et al. The Asam Principles of addiction medicine. 6th edition. Philadelphia: Wolters Kluwer; 2019.
61. Santo T Jr, Clark B, Hickman M, et al. Association of Opioid Agonist Treatment With All-Cause Mortality and Specific Causes of Death Among People With Opioid Dependence: A Systematic Review and Meta-analysis [published

correction appears in JAMA Psychiatry. 2021 Sep 1;78(9):1044]. JAMA Psychiatry 2021;78(9):979–93.

62. Mattick RP, Kimber J, Breen C, et al. Buprenorphine maintenance versus placebo or methadone maintenance for opioid dependence. Cochrane Database Syst Rev 2004;3:CD002207.

63. SAMHSA.gov. SAMHSA Extends the Methadone Take-Home Flexibility for One Year While Working Toward a Permanent Solution. 2021. Available at: https://www.samhsa.gov/newsroom/press-announcements/202111181000. Accessed March 11, 2022.

Policy Ahead of the Science
Medical Cannabis Laws Versus Scientific Evidence

Gregory Malik Burnett, MD, MBA, MPH[a,b],
David A. Gorelick, MD, PhD, DLFAPA, FASAM[c], Kevin P. Hill, MD, MHS[d,e,]*

KEYWORDS

- Medical cannabis • Drug policy • Cannabinoids • Cannabidiol • Research
- Evidence-based medicine

KEY POINTS

- Three-quarters (37) of US states, the District of Columbia, and 3 territories have legalized medical cannabis.
- Forty-two different conditions in various jurisdictions qualify patients to receive medical cannabis.
- The number of qualifying conditions per jurisdiction varies from 5 to 29.
- Fifty percent of qualifying conditions have no or insufficient evidence of benefit from medical cannabis.
- Nine percent of qualifying conditions have limited evidence of harm from medical cannabis.

INTRODUCTION

Legalization of medical cannabis in the United States has expanded substantially since 1996, when California became the first state to legalize medical cannabis. As of March 2022, 37 states, the District of Columbia (DC), and 3 US territories, Guam, Puerto Rico, and the Virgin Islands, have enacted comprehensive medical cannabis laws. In all but 2 jurisdictions, these laws list a variety of conditions for which a

a Center of Addiction Medicine, University of Maryland Midtown Campus, 827 Linden Avenue 4th Floor, Suite 405, Baltimore MD 21201, USA; b Division of Addiction Research and Treatment, Department of Psychiatry, University of Maryland School of Medicine, 22 S. Greene Street S-1-D-04, Baltimore, MD 21201, USA; c Department of Psychiatry, University of Maryland School of Medicine, PO Box, 21247, MPRC-Tawes Building, Baltimore, MD 21228, USA; d Division of Addiction Psychiatry, Beth Israel Deaconess Medical Center, Gryzmish 133, 330 Brookline Avenue, Boston, MA 02215, USA; e Department of Psychiatry, Harvard Medical School
* Corresponding author.
E-mail address: khill1@bidmc.harvard.edu

Psychiatr Clin N Am 45 (2022) 347–373
https://doi.org/10.1016/j.psc.2022.05.002   psych.theclinics.com
0193-953X/22/© 2022 Elsevier Inc. All rights reserved.

physician can recommend or certify a patient for medical cannabis. In 2 jurisdictions, discretion is left entirely to physicians as to which medical conditions would benefit from medical cannabis therapy, that is, no specific qualifying conditions are listed. In addition, 10 states have legalized medical cannabis only for products with low delta-9-tetrahydrocannabinol (THC)/high cannabidiol (CBD) content. All these state laws conflict with federal law. The cannabis plant and all cannabinoids derived from the plant (with the exception of hemp; see below) are classified in Schedule I of the Controlled Substances Act of 1970. This classification legally defines them as having no accepted medical use in the United States, lack of accepted safety for use under medical supervision, and high potential for abuse. Cannabinoids derived from hemp are legal under the 2018 Farm Bill, which defines hemp as a cannabis plant with less than 0.3% delta-9-THC.[1] Hemp is the source of cannabinoids such as CBD and delta-8-THC that are currently sold legally in the United States.[1]

The legalization of medical cannabis by a political process, passage by state legislature or voter referendum, contrasts with the evidence-based process used by federal regulatory agencies such as the US Food and Drug Administration (FDA) to approve new medications for specific clinical indications. Traditionally, the FDA requires 2 adequately powered, phase 3, randomized controlled clinical trials to provide evidence of efficacy and safety. Three cannabinoid-based products have been approved in the United States through this process: synthetic THC (dronabinol), a synthetic THC analogue (nabilone), and a plant extract containing only CBD (**Table 1**). A plant extract containing a nearly 1:1 ratio of THC: CBD (nabiximols) is approved in Canada, Australia, and several European countries[2] (see **Table 1**).

The scientific literature provides a range of systematic reviews on the evidence surrounding the efficacy of cannabis for a range of clinical conditions.[3–7] However,

Table 1
Cannabis-based products with US Food and Drug Administration approval

Name (Brand Name)		Route of Administration	CSA Schedule	Approved Indications
Synthetic cannabinoids				
Dronabinol (Marinol, Syndros)	Synthetic THC	Oral	III	Severe nausea/vomiting Cachexia/weight loss
Nabilone (Cesamet)	Synthetic THC analogue	Oral	II	Severe nausea/vomiting
Phytocannabinoids				
Cannabidiol (Epidiolex)	Cannabidiol extract	Sublingual	Not scheduled	Seizures associated with Lennox-Gastaut syndrome, Dravet syndrome, tuberous sclerosis complex in patients >1 y of age
Nabiximols (Sativex)	1:1 THC/CBD extract	Oral	NDA pending	Muscle spasms/multiple sclerosis, neuropathic cancer pain

Abbreviations: CSA, Controlled Substances Act; NDA, new drug application.

we are not aware of any study that explicitly compares the qualifying conditions listed in US medical cannabis laws with the strength of scientific evidence supporting cannabis therapy for that condition. This article provides a descriptive statistical analysis of the qualifying conditions listed in medical cannabis legislation and the strength of the scientific evidence for the aforementioned conditions, analyzes the distribution and overlap of various qualifying conditions across jurisdictions, examines the association between the number of qualifying conditions in a jurisdiction and the strength of scientific evidence for the listed conditions, and evaluates any changes in the aforementioned variables over time since the first medical cannabis law was enacted in 1996.

METHODS

We obtained the year of enactment and the list of conditions qualifying for medical cannabis from the National Conference of State Legislatures,[8] which keeps up-to-date information with direct access to the legislative texts on its Web site. Qualifying conditions were categorized as medical or psychiatric. Similar conditions described with different wording in state laws were combined for clarity in reporting. Phytocannabinoids were defined as products from the whole plant or extracts enriched in one or more specific cannabinoids. Synthetic cannabinoids were nabilone and dronabinol (synthetic THC).

The scientific evidence for the use of medical cannabis for each qualifying condition was obtained from recent systematic reviews.[3–5,7,9–15] The strength of scientific evidence was evaluated using the framework provided by the National Academies of Science, Engineering, and Medicine[5]: conclusive, substantial, moderate, limited, or no evidence in relation to benefits and harms (**Table 2**). Conditions for which a cannabis product was approved for treatment by the FDA or similar national regulatory authority were graded as having conclusive evidence of benefit. We used the most favorable grade of evidence for any diagnosis within the qualifying condition, regardless of the type or formulation of cannabis product that produced the effect and regardless of whether the beneficial effect was only on secondary symptoms (eg, pain, sleep, agitation, anxiety) rather than on the disease process itself. For purposes of evaluating changes over time, jurisdictions were grouped into 3 periods based on first enactment of comprehensive medical cannabis legislation: 1996 to 2007, 2008 to 2015, and 2016 to 2021. These intervals were chosen to have roughly equivalent numbers of jurisdictions in each interval. The 10 jurisdictions with medical cannabis legislation allowing for only low THC/CBD-based products were excluded from the analysis. Formal statistical testing was not done due to the small sample sizes and limited heterogeneity across qualifying conditions, jurisdictions, and time.

RESULTS
Prevalence of US Medical Cannabis Programs

As of March, 2022, 37 states, DC, Puerto Rico, Guam, and the US Virgin Islands have enacted comprehensive medical cannabis legislation (Appendices 1 and 2).[8] These programs were enacted at a rate of 4 to 8 jurisdictions every 5 years from 1996 to 2015. The rate of enactment increased to 14 new jurisdictions during the period from 2016 to 2020. Three new programs were enacted in 2021. In addition, 10 jurisdictions (all states) have medical cannabis legislation allowing only for low THC/CBD-based products. Thus, only 3 states (Idaho, Kansas, Nebraska) and 2 US territories

Table 2 Grading strength of scientific evidence for therapeutic efficacy of medical cannabis	
Evidence Grade	Description
Conclusive evidence	Strong evidence from randomized controlled trials to support the conclusion that cannabis or cannabinoids are an effective or ineffective treatment. There are many supportive findings from good-quality studies with no credible opposing findings. A firm conclusion can be made, and the limitations to the evidence, including chance, bias, and confounding factors, can be ruled out with reasonable confidence
Substantial evidence	Strong evidence to support the conclusion that cannabis or cannabinoids are an effective or ineffective treatment for the health end point of interest. For this level of evidence, there are several supportive findings from good-quality studies with very few or no credible opposing findings. A firm conclusion can be made, but minor limitations, including chance, bias, and confounding factors, cannot be ruled out with reasonable confidence.
Moderate evidence	Some evidence to support the conclusion that cannabis or cannabinoids are an effective or ineffective treatment for the health end point of interest. For this level of evidence, there are several supportive findings from good- to fair-quality studies with very few or no credible opposing findings. A general conclusion can be made, but limitations, including chance, bias, and confounding factors, cannot be ruled out with reasonable confidence.
Limited evidence	Weak evidence to support the conclusion that cannabis or cannabinoids are an effective or ineffective treatment for the health end point of interest. For this level of evidence, there are supportive findings from fair-quality studies or mixed findings with most favoring one conclusion. A conclusion can be made, but there is significant uncertainty due to chance, bias, and confounding factors.
No or insufficient evidence	No or insufficient evidence to support the conclusion that cannabis or cannabinoids are an effective or ineffective treatment for the health end point of interest. For this level of evidence, there are mixed findings, a single poor study, or health end point has not been studied at all. No conclusion can be made because of substantial uncertainty due to chance, bias, and confounding factors.

Source: [5]

(American Samoa, Northern Mariana Islands) currently have no form of medical cannabis program.

Qualifying Conditions for Medical Cannabis

Qualifying medical conditions

Among the 41 jurisdictions with comprehensive medical cannabis programs, 42 different conditions are designated as qualifying: 35 (83%) medical (see Appendix 1) and 7 (17%) psychiatric (see Appendix 2). These qualifying conditions are not necessarily specific diagnoses but can be symptoms (eg, pain, nausea/vomiting) or medical status (eg, terminal illness). Two jurisdictions (Oklahoma, Virginia) do not specify any qualifying conditions, leaving the decision to the physician on how best to use medical cannabis therapy. In addition, 18 (44%) jurisdictions allow physicians or state health authorities to recommend medical cannabis for any condition for which it is believed the benefits of cannabis outweigh the harms. The median number of qualifying conditions per jurisdiction is 13, with a range of 5 conditions (South Dakota) to 29 conditions (Illinois) (**Table 3**). There was no meaningful change in the mean number of qualifying conditions per jurisdiction between the 1996 to 2007 period and the 2016 to 2021 period.

The type and number of qualifying medical conditions vary substantially across jurisdictions (see **Table 3**). Nine medical conditions have been adopted by more than 50% of jurisdictions: multiple sclerosis/muscle spasms (98%), cancer (90%), human immunodeficiency virus/AIDS (90%), epilepsy/seizures (88%), glaucoma (83%), intractable/chronic pain (83%), cachexia/wasting syndrome (73%), Crohn disease/inflammatory bowel disease (68%), severe nausea/vomiting (60%), and amyotrophic lateral sclerosis (ALS) (58%). All but Crohn disease and ALS were included in the original medical cannabis legislation passed in 1996. Crohn disease was adopted in 2004, and ALS was adopted in 2008. Eight conditions have been adopted by 25% to 50% of jurisdictions: Parkinson disease (43%), Alzheimer disease (40%), hepatitis C (38%), autism spectrum disorder (38%), terminal illness (38%), and neurologic pathology/trauma (35%). These conditions were adopted between 1998 and 2007, except autism spectrum disorder, which was first adopted in 2016. Six conditions have been adopted by 10% to 24% of jurisdictions: arthritis (23%), peripheral neuropathy (15%), Huntington disease (15%), fibromyalgia (15%), sickle cell anemia (15%), and migraine headache (15%). which were adopted between 2004 and 2012, expect for arthritis, which was designated a qualifying condition in 1996. The remaining 11 conditions have been adopted by less than 10% of jurisdictions, all occurring between 2010 and 2014 (**Table 4**).

Qualifying psychiatric conditions

The inclusion of qualifying psychiatric conditions is a more recent and less common phenomenon than medical qualifying conditions (see Appendix 2). The earliest qualifying psychiatric condition was posttraumatic stress disorder (PTSD), first adopted in 2011. PTSD is the only psychiatric condition adopted by more than 25% of jurisdictions (**Table 5**).

Strength of Scientific Evidence for Medical Cannabis

The strength of scientific evidence for each qualifying condition is listed in **Box 1**. The number of qualifying conditions with each level of evidence is listed in **Table 6**. Evidence is summarized separately for phytocannabinoids (ie, plant derived) and 2 synthetic cannabinoids (nabilone, dronabinol).

Among the 35 qualifying medical conditions, 5 (14%) qualifying conditions have conclusive or substantial evidence of benefit, 5 (14%) qualifying conditions have moderate evidence of benefit, 4 (11%) qualifying conditions have limited evidence of benefit, 21 (60%) qualifying conditions have no or insufficient evidence of benefit, and 2 (6%) qualifying conditions have limited evidence of harm.

Among the 7 qualifying psychiatric conditions, 1 (14%) has moderate evidence of benefit, 2 (28%) have limited evidence of benefit from medical cannabis, 2 (28%) have no or insufficient evidence of benefit, 1 (14%) condition has limited evidence of harm, and 1 psychiatric condition (PTSD) has limited evidence for harm with phytocannabinoids and limited evidence of benefit with synthetic cannabinoids. The following discussion provides additional details about the evidence relating to each qualifying psychiatric condition.

Table 3
Number and strength of evidence for medical cannabis qualifying conditions by US jurisdiction

Year Law Enacted	Jurisdiction	Number of Conditions	% of Conditions with at Least Moderate Evidence	% of Conditions with No or Insufficient Evidence
1996	California	10	30	40
1998	Oregon	8	38	25
1998	Washington	13	38	38
1999	Alaska	8	38	38
1999	Maine	10	40	40
2000	Hawaii	13	38	46
2001	Colorado	10	30	30
2001	Nevada	9	44	33
2004	Montana	13	38	31
2004	Vermont	8	38	38
2006	Rhode Island	11	45	36
2007	New Mexico	16	31	44
2008	Michigan	19	37	37
2010	Arizona	13	46	38
2010	District of Columbia	9	22	56
2010	New Jersey	15	40	33
2011	Delaware	15	40	33
2012	Connecticut	19	32	42
2013	Massachusetts	8	25	38
2013	New Hampshire	19	32	42
2014	Illinois	29	31	45
2015	Maryland	6	67	33
2014	Minnesota	13	46	23
2014	New York	17	29	41
2016	Arkansas	15	47	40
2016	Louisiana	12	33	33
2016	North Dakota	15	47	33
2016	Ohio	15	47	27
2016	Pennsylvania	18	33	33
2017	Florida	11	36	27
2017	Puerto Rico	21	38	29
2018	Missouri	18	33	39
2018	Oklahoma[a]	0	—	—
2018	Utah	11	45	27
2018	Guam	8	38	25
2019	West Virginia	7	71	14
2019	US Virgin Islands	20	20	25
2020	Virginia[a]	0	—	—
2021	Alabama	17	35	35

(continued on next page)

Table 3 (continued)				
Year Law Enacted	Jurisdiction	Number of Conditions	% of Conditions with at Least Moderate Evidence	% of Conditions with No or Insufficient Evidence
2021	Mississippi	16	25	38
2021	South Dakota	5	60	40

[a] Physician is able to recommend medical cannabis for any medical condition.

Anxiety is graded as having moderate evidence of efficacy, based on 31 published studies (including 17 randomized controlled trials).[7,9,11] Efficacy was shown for anxiety accompanying other conditions (cannabis plant, THC, THC: CBD combinations) and for social anxiety (oral cannabidiol in two 1-day studies). No study evaluated other specific anxiety disorders such as panic disorder.

Autism spectrum disorder is graded as having limited evidence of efficacy based on 4 open-label observational studies using CBD-enriched cannabis plant extracts.[15] All studies showed improvement in secondary symptoms such as anxiety, sleep, and agitation. One study also showed improvement in core autism symptom domains such as communication, social interaction, and cognition.

Depression is graded as having limited evidence of harm based on 40 published studies (including 22 randomized controlled trials).[7,9,11] All studies evaluated patients with depressed mood associated with other conditions; none evaluated primary depressive disorder. No study showed a beneficial effect of a cannabis product. Some studies with THC-predominant products found worse mood at higher doses.

Obsessive compulsive disorder is graded as having no or insufficient evidence of efficacy based on 1 small randomized, placebo-controlled clinical trial that found no benefit from smoked cannabis.[9]

Opioid use disorder is graded as having limited evidence of efficacy based on 3 small randomized clinical trials (2 placebo controlled) using oral dronabinol (synthetic THC) or CBD.[9] All 3 studies showed significant reduction in opioid craving and withdrawal symptoms. No study evaluated opioid use.

Panic disorder (listed independently from anxiety by a few states) is graded as having no or insufficient evidence of efficacy. We are not aware of any published studies evaluating medical cannabis as treatment of panic attacks or panic disorder.[7,9,11]

PTSD (listed independently from anxiety in several states) is graded as having moderate evidence of efficacy, based on 12 published studies (including 1 randomized clinical trial).[7,9,11,14] The randomized placebo-controlled clinical trial found that nabilone (synthetic THC analogue) significantly improved overall well-being and reduced disturbed dreaming but did not alter other core PTSD symptoms such as enhanced startle response, irritability, and impaired concentration. Some small, open-label studies found improvement in several core PTSD symptoms (cannabis plant, CBD). In 2 studies, a small proportion of patients experienced worsening symptoms.

Association of frequency of listing with strength of evidence

The 6 most commonly listed (at least 80% of jurisdictions) qualifying conditions have more favorable strength of evidence of benefit than do the 18 least commonly

Table 4
Prevalence and strength of evidence for qualifying medical conditions

Year Law Enacted	Medical Condition	# Of Jurisdictions with Approval	% of Jurisdictions with Approval	Evidence Grade Phytocannabinoids	Evidence Grade Synthetic Cannabinoids
1996	Multiple sclerosis/muscle spasms	39	95	2	1
1996	HIV/AIDS	36	88	0.5	0
1996	Cancer	36	88	0	0
1996	Epilepsy/seizures	35	85	0	0
1996	Intractable/chronic pain	33	80	2	0
1996	Glaucoma	33	80	-0.5	0
1996	Cachexia/wasting syndrome	29	71	0	0
2004	Crohn disease/IBD	27	66	1	0
1996	Severe nausea/vomiting	24	59	2	0
2008	ALS	23	56	0	0
2007	Parkinson disease	17	41	0.5	0
1999	Alzheimer disease	16	39	1	0.5
1999	Hepatitis C	15	37	0	0
2004	Terminal illness	15	37	0	0
2013	Neurologic malformation/trauma	14	34	0.5	0
2013	Tourette syndrome	9	22	0.5	1
1996	Arthritis (severe)	9	22	0	0
2010	Muscular dystrophy	7	17	0	0
2012	Fibromyalgia	6	15	1	1
2004	Peripheral neuropathy	6	15	0	0
2007	Huntington disease	6	15	0	0
2012	Sickle cell anemia	6	15	0	0.5
2011	Migraine	5	12	1	0

Year	Condition			Score
2013	Systemic lupus erythematosus	3	7	0
2011	Cirrhosis	2	5	0
2013	Polycystic kidney disease	2	5	0
2013	Ehlers-Danlos syndrome	2	5	0
2014	Obstructive sleep apnea	1	2	1
2010	Dysmenorrhea	1	2	0
2012	Cystic fibrosis	1	2	0
2013	Fibrous dysplasia	1	2	0
2013	Interstitial cystitis	1	2	0
2013	Sjögren syndrome	1	2	0
2014	Macular degeneration	1	2	0
2013	Chronic pancreatitis	1	2	−0.5

Legend

Score	Interpretation
−2	Conclusive or substantial evidence of harm
−1	Moderate evidence of harm
−0.5	Limited evidence of harm
0	No or insufficient evidence to support or refute benefit or harm
0.5	Limited evidence of benefit
1	Moderate evidence of benefit
2	Conclusive or substantial evidence of benefit

Abbreviations: HIV, human immunodeficiency virus; IBD, inflammatory bowel disease.

Table 5
Prevalence and strength of evidence of qualifying psychiatric conditions

Year Law Enacted	Psychiatric Condition	# Of Jurisdictions Listing	% of Jurisdictions Listing	Evidence Grade Cannabinoids	Evidence Grade Synthetic Cannabinoids
2011	PTSD	31	76	−0.5	0.5
2016	Autism spectrum disorder	15	37	0.5	0
2018	Opioid use disorder	7	17	0	0.5
2015	Anxiety	5	12	1	1
2015	Depression	2	5	0	−0.5
2019	Obsessive compulsive disorder	1	2	0	0
2021	Panic disorder	1	2	0	0

Legend

Score	Interpretation
−2	Conclusive or substantial evidence of harm
−1	Moderate evidence of harm
−0.5	Limited evidence of harm
0	No or insufficient evidence to support or refute benefit or harm
0.5	Limited evidence of benefit
1	Moderate evidence of benefit
2	Conclusive or substantial evidence of benefit

> **Box 1**
> **Medical cannabis qualifying conditions by strength of evidence**
>
> Conclusive or substantial evidence of benefit
> Cachexia/wasting syndrome, epilepsy/seizures, multiple sclerosis/muscle spasms, severe nausea/vomiting, intractable/chronic pain
>
> Moderate evidence of benefit
> Alzheimer disease, anxiety, Crohn disease/inflammatory bowel disease, fibromyalgia, migraine, obstructive sleep apnea, posttraumatic stress disorder (synthetic), Tourette syndrome
>
> Limited evidence of benefit
> Autism spectrum disorder, human immunodeficiency virus/acquired immunodeficiency syndrome, neurologic malformation/trauma, opioid use disorder, Parkinson disease
>
> No or insufficient evidence to support or refute benefit or harm
> Amyotrophic lateral sclerosis, arthritis, cancer, cachexia/wasting syndrome, cirrhosis, cystic fibrosis, dysmenorrhea, Ehlers-Danlos syndrome, fibrous dysplasia, hepatitis C, Huntington disease, interstitial cystitis, macular degeneration, muscular dystrophy, obsessive compulsive disorder, panic disorder, peripheral neuropathy, polycystic kidney disease, sickle cell anemia, Sjögren syndrome, systemic lupus erythematosus, terminal illness
>
> Limited evidence of harm
> Depression, glaucoma, chronic pancreatitis, posttraumatic stress disorder (phyto)
>
> Moderate evidence of harm
> None
>
> Substantial evidence of harm
> None

listed (less than 20% of jurisdictions) qualifying conditions. Two of the most commonly listed conditions have conclusive or substantial evidence of efficacy, whereas only 3 of the least commonly listed conditions have moderate evidence of efficacy. The 5 qualifying conditions with conclusive or substantial evidence of efficacy are more commonly listed (greater than 50% of jurisdictions) than are the 3 qualifying conditions with limited evidence of harm (2 in <10% of jurisdictions) (see **Table 6**).

The mean (standard deviation [SD]) proportion of qualifying conditions per jurisdiction with at least moderate evidence of efficacy is 39% (11%), with a range of 22% (DC) to 71% (West Virginia) (see **Table 5**). Conversely, the mean (SD) proportion of qualifying conditions per jurisdiction with no or insufficient evidence of efficacy is 35% (8%), with a range of 14% (West Virginia) to 56% (DC) (see **Table 5**) Neither do these proportions seem to have changed meaningfully since 1996 (see **Table 4**) nor does there seem to be any association between the number of qualifying conditions adopted by a jurisdiction and the proportion with at least moderate evidence of efficacy (see **Table 3**).

DISCUSSION

The 42 different qualifying conditions for which patients may be certified for medical cannabis use in the 37 states, the DC, and 3 territories that have enacted medical cannabis laws have been reviewed. The number of conditions in each jurisdiction varies widely from as few as 5 qualifying conditions to as many as 29 qualifying

Table 6 Strength of evidence associated with medical cannabis treatment		
Phytocannabinoids	Number of Qualifying Conditions	% of Qualifying Conditions
Conclusive or substantial evidence of benefit	3	7
Moderate evidence of benefit	6	14
Limited evidence of benefit	4	10
No or insufficient evidence to support or refute benefit or harm	25	60
Limited evidence of harm	4	10
Moderate evidence of harm	0	0
Substantial evidence of harm	0	0
Synthetic Cannabinoids (Dronabinol/Nabilone)	Number of Qualifying Conditions	% of Qualifying Conditions
Conclusive or substantial evidence of benefit	2	5
Moderate evidence of benefit	5	12
Limited evidence of benefit	4	10
No or insufficient evidence to support or refute benefit or harm	32	76
Limited evidence of harm	1	2
moderate evidence of harm	0	0
Substantial evidence of harm	0	0

conditions; 2 jurisdictions do not require any specific qualifying condition for medical cannabis therapy. The level of scientific evidence supporting each of these qualifying conditions varies widely as well. Many of the qualifying conditions have little evidence supporting their use. About 50% of qualifying conditions have no or insufficient evidence of benefit from medical cannabis, and another 9% have limited evidence of harm.

US medical cannabis laws are in conflict with federal law and often with science as well. The stipulation of medical conditions with little evidence supporting the efficacy of medical cannabis is a by-product of a political process whereby citizens lobby elected officials for the inclusion of conditions often based on anecdotal evidence of benefit. Not only does such use incur the possibility of adverse effects from cannabis with little prospect of benefit but also there are instances in which a discrepancy between policy and science may lead to adverse outcomes. For example, eschewing the effective FDA-approved medications for opioid use disorder in favor of medical cannabis is not evidence based and may have adverse consequences for the patient.[16]

Our analysis revealed other patterns as well. Among the most commonly listed and earliest-adopted conditions are those for which there is the strongest evidence for cannabinoid (including the FDA-approved cannabinoids) pharmacotherapy, including cachexia/weight loss, muscle spasticity associated with multiple sclerosis, nausea and vomiting, chronic pain, and seizures. However, some conditions with evidence demonstrating that medical cannabis pharmacotherapy can be harmful were still listed by many jurisdictions, including glaucoma, which is listed as a qualifying condition in 80% of jurisdictions with medical cannabis laws. In contrast, some psychiatric conditions for which there is limited evidence of benefit from medical cannabis are not listed as qualifying conditions in any jurisdiction, for example, schizophrenia and tobacco use disorder.[7,9,11] Although there have been US jurisdictions with medical cannabis laws since 1996, little has changed regarding qualifying conditions. The median number of qualifying conditions per jurisdiction and the proportion of conditions supported by evidence has not changed meaningfully since 1996.

Limitations

This analysis has some limitations. The authors did not conduct their own systematic review of strength of evidence, but relied on published reviews, which may have overlooked some studies. The relationship between the year each law was enacted and the year evidence was published was not assessed. The level of evidence may have changed in the years following passage of a given medical cannabis law, and this may have led to overestimation of the concordance between qualifying conditions and the strength of the evidence supporting the use of medical cannabis for that condition. The authors were generous in applying the evidence relevant to any condition. Benefit in improving secondary symptoms was given the same weight as improving the disease process itself. For some diseases there is evidence only for secondary symptom improvement, for example, cancer and neurodegenerative disorders. If one particular cannabinoid formulation or dose had evidence for a specific diagnosis, the authors gave that grade of evidence to the qualifying condition that included that diagnosis. For example, CBD has conclusive evidence, including FDA approval, as treatment of several syndromes of childhood seizures. Therefore, the authors gave a grade of "conclusive or substantial" evidence of benefit for epilepsy/seizures as a qualifying condition. Given that jurisdictions allow any potency and formulation of cannabis product to be recommended, this may tend to overestimate the concordance between condition and strength of evidence.

CONCLUSION

Millions of Americans use cannabis and cannabinoids to treat a host of medical and psychiatric conditions.[16] Many of these conditions are specified in medical cannabis laws as conditions for which patients can be recommended or certified for medical cannabis use. In many jurisdictions, the law allows physicians to certify medical cannabis use for broad and undefined conditions (eg, terminal or debilitating illness) or for any condition they choose. Because there is limited or no scientific evidence for the efficacy of medical cannabis for most conditions (and evidence of harm for a few), the state-level legal status of medical cannabis runs far ahead of the science in these instances.

This conflict between local law and the strength of evidence for efficacy puts patients and physicians in a difficult position. Cannabis and cannabinoids like CBD remain popular, so patients are either interested in using them to treat their maladies or are already doing so. Patients may opt for medical cannabis pharmacotherapy for a given medical condition when it is listed in a state law but not evidence based. In such instances, patients may suffer adverse outcomes and/or fail to receive any therapeutic benefit from medications FDA approved for their disease condition. Furthermore, physicians often must explain that use of medical cannabis, despite being allowable under local law, may not be in their patient's best interest.

There is a dire need for rigorous research to adequately evaluate the benefits and harms of medical cannabis for a broad range of conditions. This evaluation requires both increased resources for clinical research (including adequately designed and powered phase 2 and phase 3 controlled clinical trials) and altering federal laws and regulations that hinder the ability to conduct clinical studies with cannabis and cannabinoids. Many stakeholders who profit from cannabinoid sales, including jurisdictions with legalized medical cannabis and companies that sell medical cannabis products, have largely failed to contribute to the evidence base. The rate and scope of cannabinoid research must keep pace with cannabis policy if we are going to maximize the potential benefits and minimize the potential harms of medical cannabis.

SUMMARY

In the context of changing cannabis policies in the United States, 37 states, the DC, and 3 territories have enacted medical cannabis laws as of March 2022. The number of qualifying conditions stipulated by each state and the strength of scientific evidence supporting the use of medical cannabis for each of these conditions vary widely. The evidence supporting the use of medical cannabis for many of these conditions is weak: 50% of qualifying conditions have no or insufficient evidence of benefit from medical cannabis; 9% of qualifying conditions have limited evidence that medical cannabis may cause harm if used for that condition. Despite intense interest in medical cannabis, the implementation of medical cannabis laws and proportion of qualifying conditions with evidence supporting them has not changed meaningfully since the first medical cannabis law was passed in 1996. As a result, patients and physicians are in difficult positions as they try to use medical cannabis safely and effectively for appropriate medical conditions.

CLINICS CARE POINTS

- Physicians should be knowledgeable about the current evidence of the benefits and harms of medical cannabis so that they can have informed discussions with their patients.

- Physicians should be cautious about recommending medical cannabis in the absence of at least moderate evidence of benefit.

- When recommending medical cannabis, physicians should follow the same clinical approach as when prescribing conventional medication—careful diagnosis, evaluation for comorbidity, and balancing benefits and harms, including potential drug-drug interactions

DISCLOSURE

Dr G.M. Burnett has no disclosures. Dr D.A. Gorelick receives royalties from Wolters Kluwer for writing medical articles about cannabis and honoraria from Springer Nature and Colorado State University—Pueblo for serving as Editor-in-Chief of the Journal of Cannabis Research. Dr K.P. Hill is a consultant to Greenwich Biosciences and is an author with Wolters Kluwer.

REFERENCES

1. Abernethy A. Hemp production & 2018 Farm Bill. US Food Drug Adm; 2019. Available at: https://www.fda.gov/news-events/congressional-testimony/hemp-production-and-2018-farm-bill-07252019.

2. Boivin M. Nabiximols (Sativex®). In: Narouze SN, editor. Cannabinoids and pain. Cham (Switzerland): Springer; 2021. p. 119–26.

3. Inglet S, Winter B, Yost SE, et al. Clinical Data for the Use of Cannabis-Based Treatments: A Comprehensive Review of the Literature. Ann Pharmacother 2020;54(11):1109–43.

4. Montero-Oleas N, Arevalo-Rodriguez I, Nuñez-González S, et al. Therapeutic use of cannabis and cannabinoids: an evidence mapping and appraisal of systematic reviews. BMC Complement Med Ther 2020;20(1):12.

5. National Academies of Sciences, Engineering, and Medicine. The Health effects of cannabis and cannabinoids: the current state of evidence and recommendations for research. Washington, DC: The National Academies Press; 2017. https://doi.org/10.17226/24625.

6. Lim K, See YM, Lee J. A Systematic Review of the Effectiveness of Medical Cannabis for Psychiatric, Movement and Neurodegenerative Disorders. Clin Psychopharmacol Neurosci 2017;15(4):301–12.

7. Sarris J, Sinclair J, Karamacoska D, et al. Medicinal cannabis for psychiatric disorders: a clinically-focused systematic review. BMC Psychiatry 2020;20(1):24.

8. National Conference of State Legislatures. State Medical Cannabis Laws. Available at: https://www.ncsl.org/research/health/state-medical-marijuana-laws. aspx. Accessed February 2, 2022.

9. McKee KA, Hmidan A, Crocker CE, et al. Potential therapeutic benefits of cannabinoid products in adult psychiatric disorders: A systematic review and meta-analysis of randomised controlled trials. J Psychiatr Res 2021;140: 267–81.

10. Liang AL, Gingher EL, Coleman JS. Medical Cannabis for Gynecologic Pain Conditions: A Systematic Review. Obstet Gynecol 2022;139(2):287–96.

11. Black N, Stockings E, Campbell G, et al. Cannabinoids for the treatment of mental disorders and symptoms of mental disorders: a systematic review and meta-analysis. Lancet Psychiatry 2019;6(12):995–1010.

12. Abrams DI, Couey P, Dixit N, et al. Effect of Inhaled Cannabis for Pain in Adults With Sickle Cell Disease: A Randomized Clinical Trial. JAMA Netw Open 2020; 3(7):e2010874.

13. Poudel S, Quinonez J, Choudhari J, et al. Medical Cannabis, Headaches, and Migraines: A Review of the Current Literature. Cureus 2021. https://doi.org/10.7759/cureus.17407.

14. Rehman Y, Saini A, Huang S, et al. Cannabis in the management of PTSD: a systematic review. AIMS Neurosci 2021;8(3):414–34.

15. da Silva Junior EA, Medeiros WMB, Torro N, et al. Cannabis and cannabinoids use in autism spectrum disorder: a systematic review. Trends Psychiatry Psychother 2021. https://doi.org/10.47626/2237-6089-2020-0149.

16. Hill KP, Gold MS, Nemeroff CB, et al. Risks and Benefits of Cannabis and Cannabinoids in Psychiatry. Am J Psychiatry 2022;179(2):98–109.

APPENDIX I: MEDICAL CANNABIS QUALIFYING MEDICAL CONDITIONS BY JURISDICTION

Medical Cannabis Qualifying Medical Conditions by Jurisdiction

Year Law Passed	Year Law Effective	Jurisdiction	ALS	Alzheimer Disease	Arthritis	Cancer	Cachexia/Wasting Syndrome	Crohn Disease/IBD	Cirrhosis	Cystic Fibrosis
1996	1996	California			*	*	*			
1998	1999	Alaska				*	*			
1998	2010	District of Columbia	*	*		*	*		*	
1998	1998	Oregon				*	*			
1998	1998	Washington				*	*	*		
1999	1999	Maine	*	*		*		*		
2000	2001	Colorado				*	*			
2000	2000	Hawaii	*		*	*	*	*		
2000	2001	Nevada				*	*			
2004	2004	Montana				*	*	*		
2004	2004	Vermont				*	*			
2006	2006	Rhode Island		*		*	*	*		
2007	2007	New Mexico	*			*	*	*		
2008	2008	Michigan	*	*	*	*	*	*		
2010	2010	Arizona	*	*		*	*	*		
2010	2010	New Jersey	*			*		*		
2011	2011	Delaware	*	*		*	*		*	
2012	2012	Connecticut	*		*	*	*	*		
2012	2013	Massachusetts	*			*	*	*		*
2013	2014	Illinois	*	*	*	*	*	*		
2013	2013	New Hampshire	*	*	*	*	*	*		

Medical Cannabis Qualifying Medical Conditions by Jurisdiction (Cont.)

Year Law Passed	Year Law Effective	Jurisdiction	Qualifying Medical Condition — ALS	Alzheimer Disease	Arthritis (Severe)	Cancer	Cachexia/Wasting Syndrome	Crohn Disease/IBD	Cirrhosis	Cystic Fibrosis
2015	2017	Maryland				*				
2014	2014	Minnesota			*					
2014	2021	New York		*	*					
2014	2015	Guam			*					
2015	2017	Puerto Rico		*	*	*				
2016	2016	Arkansas		*	*	*				
2016	2017	Florida			*					
2016	2016	Louisiana			*	*				
2016	2016	North Dakota	*	*		*	*	*		
2016	2016	Ohio	*	*		*		*		
2016	2016	Pennsylvania	*			*		*		
2017	2019	West Virginia					*			
2018	2018	Missouri	*	*		*	*	*		
2018	2018	Oklahoma								
2018	2018	Utah	*	*		*	*	*		
2019	2019	US Virgin Islands	*	*	*	*	*	*		
2020	2022	Mississippi				*	*	*		
2020	2022	South Dakota					*			
2021	2022	Alabama	*			*	*	*		
2021	2022	Virginia								

Medical Cannabis Qualifying Medical Conditions by Jurisdiction (Cont.)

Year Passed	Year Effective	Jurisdiction	Qualifying Medical Condition						
			Dysmenorrhea	Ehlers-Danlos Syndrome	Epilepsy/Seizures	Fibromyalgia	Fibrous Dysplasia	Glaucoma	Hepatitis C
1996	1996	California			*			*	
1998	1999	Alaska			*			*	
1998	2010	District of Columbia			*			*	
1998	1998	Oregon							
1998	1998	Washington			*			*	*
1999	1999	Maine			*			*	*
2000	2001	Colorado			*			*	
2000	2000	Hawaii			*			*	
2000	2001	Nevada			*			*	
2004	2004	Montana			*			*	
2004	2004	Vermont			*			*	-
2006	2006	Rhode Island			*			*	*
2007	2007	New Mexico			*			*	*
2008	2008	Michigan			*			*	*
2010	2010	Arizona			*			*	*
2010	2010	New Jersey	*		*			*	
2011	2011	Delaware			*			*	
2012	2012	Connecticut			*	*		*	
2012	2013	Massachusetts							
2013	2014	Illinois		*	*	*		*	*
2013	2013	New Hampshire		*	*		*	*	*
2015	2017	Maryland			*				
2014	2014	Minnesota			*			*	

Medical Cannabis Qualifying Medical Conditions by Jurisdiction (Cont.)

| | | | Qualifying Medical Condition | | | | | | |
Year Law Passed	Year Law Effective	Jurisdiction	Dysmenorrhea	Ehlers-Danlos Syndrome	Epilepsy/Seizures	Fibromyalgia	Fibrous Dysplasia	Glaucoma	Hepatitis C
2014	2021	New York			*				
2014	2015	Guam			*			*	
2015	2017	Puerto Rico			*	*		*	*
2016	2016	Arkansas			*	*		*	*
2016	2017	Florida			*			*	
2016	2016	Louisiana			*			*	
2016	2016	North Dakota	*		*	*		*	*
2016	2016	Ohio				*		*	*
2016	2016	Pennsylvania			*			*	
2017	2019	West Virginia							
2018	2018	Missouri			*			*	*
2018	2018	Oklahoma							
2018	2018	Utah							
2019	2019	US Virgin Islands			*			*	*
2020	2022	Mississippi			*			*	
2020	2022	South Dakota			*				
2021	2022	Alabama			*				
2021	2022	Virginia							

Medical Cannabis Qualifying Medical Conditions by Jurisdiction (Cont.)

| | | | Qualifying Medical Condition | | | | | | |
Year Law Passed	Year Law Effective	Jurisdiction	HIV/AIDS	Huntington Disease	Interstitial Cystitis	Systemic Lupus Erythematosus	Macular Degeneration	Migraine	Multiple Sclerosis/ Muscle Spasms
1996	1996	California	*						*

(continued on next page)

APPENDIX I: MEDICAL CANNABIS QUALIFYING MEDICAL CONDITIONS BY JURISDICTION (continued)

Medical Cannabis Qualifying Medical Conditions by Jurisdiction (Cont.)

Year Law Passed	Year Law Effective	Jurisdiction	Qualifying Medical Condition						
			HIV/AIDS	Huntington Disease	Interstitial Cystitis	Systemic Lupus Erythematosus	Macular Degeneration	Migraine	Multiple Sclerosis/ Muscle Spasms
1998	1999	Alaska	*						*
1998	2010	District of Columbia	*						*
1998	1998	Oregon	*						*
1998	1998	Washington	*						*
1999	1999	Maine	*						*
2000	2001	Colorado	*						*
2000	2000	Hawaii	*			*			*
2000	2001	Nevada	*						*
2004	2004	Montana	*						*
2004	2004	Vermont	*						*
2006	2006	Rhode Island	*						*
2007	2007	New Mexico	*	*					*
2008	2008	Michigan	*						*
2010	2010	Arizona	*						*
2010	2010	New Jersey	*						*
2011	2011	Delaware	*					*	*
2012	2012	Connecticut	*					*	*
2012	2013	Massachusetts	*						*
2013	2014	Illinois	*		*	*		*	*
2013	2013	New Hampshire	*			*			*
2015	2017	Maryland							*

Year Law Passed	Year Law Effective	Jurisdiction	HIV/AIDS	Huntington Disease	Interstitial Cystitis	Systemic Lupus Erythematosus	Macular Degeneration	Migraine	Multiple Sclerosis/Muscle Spasms
2014		Minnesota					*		*
2014		New York		*					*
2014		Guam							*
2015		Puerto Rico						*	*
2016		Arkansas							*
2016		Florida							*
2016		Louisiana							*

Medical Cannabis Qualifying Medical Conditions by Jurisdiction (Cont.)

Year Law Passed	Year Law Effective	Jurisdiction	HIV/AIDS	Huntington Disease	Interstitial Cystitis	Qualifying Medical Condition			
						Systemic Lupus Erythematosus	Macular Degeneration	Migraine	Multiple Sclerosis/Muscle Spasms
2016	2016	North Dakota	*						*
2016	2016	Ohio	*						*
2016	2016	Pennsylvania	*	*					*
2017	2019	West Virginia	*						
2018	2018	Missouri	*	*				*	*
2018	2018	Oklahoma							
2018	2018	Utah	*						*
2019	2019	US Virgin Islands	*	*					*
2020	2022	Mississippi	*	*					*
2020	2022	South Dakota							
2021	2022	Alabama	*						*
2021	2022	Virginia							

Medical Cannabis Qualifying Medical Conditions by Jurisdiction (Cont.)

Year Law Passed	Year Law Effective	Jurisdiction	Muscular Dystrophy	Severe Nausea/Vomiting	Neurologic Malformation/Trauma	Qualifying Medical Condition			
						Obstructive Sleep Apnea	Intractable/Chronic Pain	Chronic Pancreatitis	Parkinson Disease
1996	1996	California		*			*		

(continued on next page)

APPENDIX I: MEDICAL CANNABIS QUALIFYING MEDICAL CONDITIONS BY JURISDICTION (continued)

Medical Cannabis Qualifying Medical Conditions by Jurisdiction (Cont.)

Year Law Passed	Year Law Effective	Jurisdiction	Muscular Dystrophy	Severe Nausea/ Vomiting	Neurologic Malformation/ Trauma	Obstructive Sleep Apnea	Intractable/ Chronic Pain	Chronic Pancreatitis	Parkinson Disease
1998	1999	Alaska	*				*		
1998	2010	District of Columbia							
1998	1998	Oregon	*		*		*		
1998	1998	Washington	*ˆ	*	*		*		
1999	1999	Maine	*						
2000	2001	Colorado		*			*		
2000	2000	Hawaii		*			*		
2000	2001	Nevada		*			*		
2004	2004	Montana	*	*	*		*		–
2004	2004	Vermont		*			*		
2006	2006	Rhode Island		*			*		
2007	2007	New Mexico		*			*		*
2008	2008	Michigan		*	*		*		*
2010	2010	Arizona		*			*		
2010	2010	New Jersey	*				*		
2011	2011	Delaware		*			*		
2012	2012	Connecticut	*		*		*		*
2012	2013	Massachusetts							*
2013	2014	Illinois	*	*ˆ	*				*
2013	2013	New Hampshire	*	*	*		*	*	*

Medical Cannabis Qualifying Medical Conditions by Jurisdiction (Cont.)

Year Law Passed	Year Law Effective	Jurisdiction	Muscular Dystrophy	Severe Nausea/Vomiting	Neurologic Malformation/Trauma	Obstructive Sleep Apnea	Intractable/Chronic Pain	Chronic Pancreatitis	Parkinson Disease
2015	2017	Maryland		*^			*		
2014	2014	Minnesota				*	*		
2014	2021	New York	*		*		*		*
2014	2015	Guam			*				
2015	2017	Puerto Rico			*		*		*
2016	2016	Arkansas		*			*		*
2016	2017	Florida					*		*
2016	2016	Louisiana	*				*		*

Medical Cannabis Qualifying Medical Conditions by Jurisdiction (Cont.)

Year Law Passed	Year Law Effective	Jurisdiction	Muscular Dystrophy	Severe Nausea/Vomiting	Neurologic Malformation/Trauma	Obstructive Sleep Apnea	Intractable/Chronic Pain	Chronic Pancreatitis	Parkinson Disease
2016	2016	North Dakota	*	*	*		*		
2016	2016	Ohio		*			*		*
2016	2016	Pennsylvania					*		*
2017	2019	West Virginia		*			*		
2018	2018	Missouri							*
2018	2018	Oklahoma							
2018	2018	Utah		*					
2019	2019	US Virgin Islands		*	*		*		*
2020	2022	Mississippi	*		*		*		*
2020	2022	South Dakota		*			*		
2021	2022	Alabama		*			*		*
2021	2022	Virginia							

(continued on next page)

APPENDIX I: MEDICAL CANNABIS QUALIFYING MEDICAL CONDITIONS BY JURISDICTION (continued)

Year Law Passed	Year Law Effective	Jurisdiction	Qualifying Medical Condition						
			Peripheral Neuropathy	Polycystic Kidney Disease	Sickle Cell Anemia	Sjögren Syndrome	Terminal Illness	Tourette Syndrome	Any Condition Approved by MD/SHA
1996	1996	California							*
1998	1999	Alaska							*
1998	2010	District of Columbia							*
1998	1998	Oregon							*
1998	1998	Washington		*'					
1999	1999	Maine							
2000	2001	Colorado							*
2000	2000	Hawaii							
2000	2001	Nevada							*
2004	2004	Montana	*				*		
2004	2004	Vermont							
2006	2006	Rhode Island							*
2007	2007	New Mexico	*				*		
2008	2008	Michigan						*	
2010	2010	Arizona							
2010	2010	New Jersey					*	*	
2011	2011	Delaware					*		
2012	2012	Connecticut			*		*		*
2012	2013	Massachusetts							
2013	2014	Illinois		*		*	*	*	
2013	2013	New Hampshire							*

Year Law Passed	Year Law Effective	Jurisdiction	Peripheral Neuropathy	Polycystic Kidney Disease	Sickle Cell Anemia	Sjögren Syndrome	Terminal Illness	Tourette's Syndrome	Any Condition Approved by MD/SHA
2014	2015	Maryland							*
2014	2014	Minnesota					*	*	
2014	2021	New York	*				*		*
2014	2015	Guam	*						*
2015	2017	Puerto Rico	*				*		*
2016	2016	Arkansas	*					*	*
2016	2017	Florida					*		
2016	2016	Louisiana							

Medical Cannabis Qualifying Medical Conditions by Jurisdiction

Year Law Passed	Year Law Effective	Jurisdiction	Peripheral Neuropathy	Polycystic Kidney Disease	Sickle Cell Anemia	Sjögren Syndrome	Terminal Illness	Tourette's Syndrome	Any Condition Approved by MD/SHA
									Qualifying Medical Condition
2016	2016	North Dakota							*
2016	2016	Ohio			*			*	
2016	2016	Pennsylvania	*		*		*	*	
2017	2019	West Virginia					*		
2018	2018	Missouri			*		*	*	*
2018	2018	Oklahoma							*
2018	2018	Utah					*		
2019	2019	US Virgin Islands					*		
2020	2022	Mississippi			*				
2020	2022	South Dakota							*
2021	2022	Alabama			*		*	*	
2021	2022	Virginia							*

Abbreviations: AIDS, acquired immunodeficiency syndrome; ALS, amyotrophic lateral sclerosis; HIV, human immunodeficiency virus; IBD, inflammatory bowel disease; MD, physician; SHA, state health authority.
Source:[8]

Appendix II Medical Cannabis Qualifying Psychiatric Conditions by Jurisdiction

Medical Cannabis Qualifying Psychiatric Conditions by Jurisdiction

Year Law Passed	Year Law Effective	Jurisdiction	Qualifying Psychiatric Condition							
			Anxiety	Autism Spectrum Disorder	Depression	Obsessive Compulsive Disorder	Opioid Use Disorder	Panic Disorder	PTSD	Any Condition Approved by MD/SHA
1996	1996	California								*
1998	1999	Alaska								*
1998	2010	District of Columbia								*
1998	1998	Oregon								*
1998	1998	Washington							*	
1999	1999	Maine								
2000	2001	Colorado	*				*		*	*
2000	2000	Hawaii							*	
2000	2001	Nevada							*	*
2004	2004	Montana							*	
2004	2004	Vermont								
2006	2006	Rhode Island							*	*
2007	2007	New Mexico							*	
2008	2008	Michigan	*			*			*	
2010	2010	Arizona							*	
2010	2010	New Jersey	*				*		*	
2011	2011	Delaware		*					*	
2012	2012	Connecticut							*	
2012	2013	Massachusetts					*		*	
2013	2014	Illinois	*						-	*
2013	2013	New Hampshire							*	*

Year Law Passed	Year Law Effective	Jurisdiction	Anxiety	Autism Spectrum Disorder	Depression	Obsessive Compulsive Disorder	Opioid Use Disorder	Panic Disorder	PTSD	Any Condition Approved by MD/SHA
2015	2017	Maryland							*	*
2014	2014	Minnesota	*						*	*
2014	2021	New York	*				*		*	*
2014	2015	Guam	*						*	*
2015	2017	Puerto Rico	*		*				*	*
2016	2016	Arkansas							-	*
2016	2017	Florida							*	*
2016	2016	Louisiana	*						*	*

Medical Cannabis Qualifying Psychiatric Conditions by Jurisdiction (Cont.)

Year Law Passed	Year Law Effective	Jurisdiction	Anxiety	Autism Spectrum Disorder	Depression	Obsessive Compulsive Disorder	Opioid Use Disorder	Panic Disorder	PTSD	Any Condition Approved by MD/SHA
2016	2016	North Dakota		*					*	*
2016	2016	Ohio							*	
2016	2016	Pennsylvania	*	*			*		*	
2017	2019	West Virginia	*	*					*	
2018	2018	Missouri		*					*	*
2018	2018	Oklahoma		*						*
2018	2018	Utah		*					*	
2019	2019	US Virgin Islands		*		*	*		*	
2020	2022	Mississippi		*			*		*	*
2020	2022	South Dakota								
2021	2022	Alabama		*	*			*	*	*
2021	2022	Virginia								*

Abbreviations: MD, physician; PTSD, posttraumatic stress disorder; SHA, state health authority.
Source: Ref.[8]

Practical Considerations for Treating Comorbid Posttraumatic Stress Disorder in the Addictions Clinic
Approaches to Clinical Care, Leadership, and Alleviating Shame

Benjamin Israel, MD[a],*, Alicia E. Wiprovnick, PhD[b],
Annabelle M. Belcher, PhD[b], Mary B. Kleinman, MS, MPH[c],
Avinash Ramprashad, MD[b], Max Spaderna, MD[d],
Eric Weintraub, MD[d]

KEYWORDS

• Trauma • Substance use • PTSD • Shame • Screening • Treatment • Leadership
• Burnout

KEY POINTS

• Posttraumatic stress disorder (PTSD) co-occurs frequently with substance use disorder (SUD) and makes treatment more difficult and complex. Yet, PTSD in this high-risk population frequently is not diagnosed or directly treated.

• PTSD underdiagnosis can be reduced through systematic screening. Practical, validated PTSD screening tools are reviewed.

• Shame—and reactions to shame—contributes substantially to SUD-PTSD psychopathology. The authors review common shame reactions and illustrate shame-alleviating strategies for clinical use.

• The authors illustrate selected strategies for alleviating shame and posttraumatic symptoms.

• Strategies to reduce the impacts of secondary PTSD and burnout among SUD clinic employees are introduced.

[a] Division of Consultation-Liaison Psychiatry, Department of Psychiatry, University of Maryland School of Medicine, 4801 Yellowwood Ave, Ste 2E1, Baltimore, MD 21209, USA; [b] Division of Addiction Research and Treatment, Department of Psychiatry, University of Maryland School of Medicine, 655 West Baltimore Street, Baltimore, MD 21201, USA; [c] Department of Psychology, University of Maryland at College Park, Biology/Psychology Building, 4094 Campus Drive, College Park, MD 20742, USA; [d] Division of Addiction Research and Treatment, University of Maryland School of Medicine, 655 West Baltimore Street, Baltimore, MD 21201, USA
* Corresponding author.
E-mail address: bisrael@som.umaryland.edu

Psychiatr Clin N Am 45 (2022) 375–414
https://doi.org/10.1016/j.psc.2022.05.003
0193-953X/22/© 2022 Elsevier Inc. All rights reserved.

INTRODUCTION

Psychological trauma is widely viewed as a root cause of addiction[1,2] and underlies many of the clinical challenges, comorbid physical and mental conditions, and staffing dilemmas in substance use disorder (SUD) clinics. This article aims to illustrate common ways in which such challenges manifest in the SUD clinic setting and to offer a practical, common-sense framework for addressing trauma and addictions together. After discussing the clinical overlap between SUD and posttraumatic stress disorder (PTSD), the authors outline the framework and offer trauma-responsive tools that can be implemented individually or in combination. This approach considers the interplay between 3 entwined dynamics: (1) the causal, epidemiologic, and neurobiological relationships connecting trauma exposure, PTSD, and SUD; (2) the ways in which patients suffering from PTSD and/or SUD may experience and cope with internalized stigma and shame; and (3) the impacts that treating trauma may have on clinic employees, including experienced clinicians.

The connection between PTSD and SUD is clear, albeit complex. Patients with PTSD are more likely to have or develop an SUD,[3,4] patients with SUD are likely to have more severe symptoms of PTSD,[5] traumatized patients with SUD are more vulnerable to developing multiple addictions,[6] and the clinical course of patients with comorbid SUD and PTSD (SUD-PTSD) typically is more complex than in substance-dependent patients without PTSD.[7] Furthermore, trauma cues predict increased substance use and relapse.[8]

Trauma exposure in the SUD population is widespread. Gielen and colleagues,[9] for example, found that more than 97% of patients with SUD across 11 clinical sites reported experiencing one or more traumatic events. It has been argued that the high-risk lifestyle involved with heavy drug use may expose patients with SUDs to more traumatic events and increase their risk for developing PTSD; however, evidence supporting this relational pathway is mixed.[10] Evidence suggesting that trauma exposure and/or PTSD directly or indirectly contribute to the development of SUD is more consistent and clear.[2,10–12]

Despite the high prevalence of PTSD among patients with SUD, comorbid PTSD evades recognition by SUD providers in general.[9] This trend is not unique to practitioners in the SUD field, but rather is endemic to mental health treatment settings.[13,14] Overall, studies assessing detection of PTSD in various clinical environments demonstrate striking discrepancies between PTSD rates as measured by validated instruments versus the rate of diagnosed PTSD. For example, the study by Gielen and colleagues[9] of more than 400 patients with SUD identified approximately 36% as having current PTSD; yet only 2.1% of these patients carried a charted PTSD diagnosis. Similar rates of PTSD underdiagnosis have been demonstrated in community settings, inpatient wards, and training environments.[13–16] In a parallel process, psychiatric and medical clinicians often underdiagnose SUD.[17,18]

Organizing a Practical Approach to Treating Substance Use Disorder-Posttraumatic Stress Disorder: the Significance of Shame and Shame Reactions

We propose that understanding *shame* is central to shaping trauma-responsive care and can help address challenges in SUD treatment such as internalized stigma or cognitive distortions that relapses represent failures. Although not typically emphasized in medical or psychiatric training, shame (and reactions to it) plays a unique role in the development of psychiatric disorders and has been examined as a transdiagnostic target variable for assessment and treatment.[19–23]

Severe, maladaptive shame can be contagious; it contributes to treatment resistance, fuels relational problems, and drives patients to act out.[20] Patients suffering from extreme shame states may induce shame reactions in their providers and staff who in turn may feel their efforts to help their clients have been undermined. Correspondingly, we will address the impacts that treating a high volume of patients with SUD-PTSD may have on clinicians and SUD clinic staff through secondary posttraumatic stress (SPS) and burnout syndromes.

Rather than focus on symptom clusters, which vary across individuals and over time, the authors organize recommendations around strategies to ameliorate shame states experienced by patients, clinicians, and non-clinical staff alike. Two basic strategies for alleviating shame states are described: (1) cultivating *competency* experiences and (2) developing a sense of relatedness or *belonging* with others. For a concise review of the developmental features and phenomenology of shame, features distinguishing shame states from related emotions such as fear and guilt, and the experience of shame following trauma, the readers are referred to Herman.[20]

Although most people attempt to hide feelings of shame, shame *reactions* are more readily observable and map onto 4 broad categories. Originally described by Nathanson,[24] these categories provide the basis for a validated instrument measuring shame reactivity.[25] Nathanson's categories or "Compass" of shame (**Fig. 1**) are (1) *withdraw* and isolate so that others cannot witness the person in their ashamed state; (2) *avoid* the shame through maladaptive or thrill-seeking behaviors such as drug use, impulsive

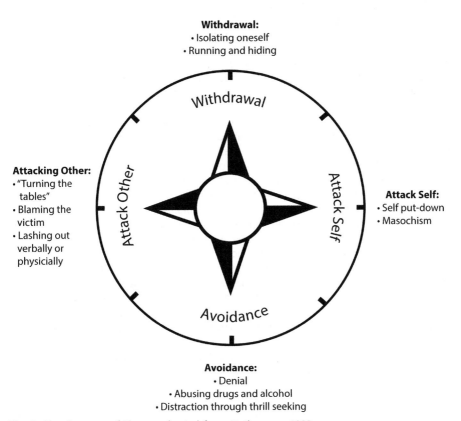

Fig. 1. The Compass of Shame adopted from Nathanson, 1992.

sex, and gambling; (3) *attack self* by berating or physically harming oneself; and (4) *attack others* through verbal aggression, physical violence, or both.

These responses to shame often overlap within the same individual. Furthermore, they correlate with high-risk behaviors often observed in patients with SUD-PTSD. Through the case vignette, the utility of identifying shame reactions in approaching patient care is discussed. These principles are later extended in a discussion of clinical leadership. Because experiencing shame may uniquely predict the desire for self-change among nonclinical subjects,[26] approaches targeted to reduce shame to a tolerable intensity among patients with SUD-PTSD may be well supported from a motivational perspective. The term used to describe shame reduction—*countershaming*—is meant to convey that shame is alleviated most effectively when it is not only regulated but also replaced with an incompatible experience such as competency or belonging[1].

CLINICAL CASE: PATIENTS, CLINICIANS, AND SHAME REACTIONS

Ms Y is a 40-year-old woman with past psychiatric diagnoses of anxiety disorder, attention-deficit/hyperactivity disorder (ADHD), opioid use disorder, major depressive disorder, and schizoaffective disorder. She transferred to the SUD clinic after her previous provider refused to prescribe methadone alongside high doses of benzodiazepine and stimulant medications. She asserted that her medication regimen had been stable for years and therefore was low risk. She refused to try an alternative evidence-based regimen and stated she would seek her medications elsewhere if the clinic did not prescribe them. She often presented while intoxicated on cannabis.

Her psychosocial problems were extensive. She had been emotionally and physically abused in most of her close relationships. She was estranged from her siblings and children. She had been homeless in the past but now was working part-time and able to rent a small apartment. She hoped to improve her life and asserted that remaining "stable" on her medications was central to this aim.

In the clinic, Ms Y often treated staff with dismissiveness, irritability, impatience, and occasionally open hostility. Discussions about her medications frequently led appointments with her doctor to run over time. Staff members avoided her and thought that her behavior diverted attention away from other patients. Her doctor, therapist, and social worker feared that her leaving the clinic would lead to decompensation and loss of employment and housing, so they reluctantly continued her medications and other treatments without fully assessing their effects.

Six months after establishing care, she arrived at the clinic appearing somnolent. She denied relapsing on nonprescribed opioids and told her social worker that she had woken up from a bad dream overnight and could not return to sleep. She agreed to complete a brief screening for PTSD, on which she answered "yes" to all 6 screening questions. During the screen, she mentioned (without prompting) that her father had abused her, physically and sexually, and that her mother periodically abandoned Ms Y, for weeks at a time, when she relapsed on heroin. Ms Y appeared increasingly restless as this discussion unfolded and started rubbing her abdomen. With prompting, she agreed to change the subject and soon appeared more comfortable.

The social worker reported the screen at a team meeting. Team members noticed that Ms Y often appeared hypervigilant, assessing clinic doors and windows closely.

---

[1] For simplicity, the authors do not focus on related affective experiences—confidence, pride, empathy, amicability, caring, tenderness, and many others.

When they asked about her nightmares, she stated flatly that they were like rewatching her father attempt suicide. Her mother later blamed Ms Y for her father's death, assaulted her, then relapsed, and never returned home. Ms Y described flashbacks as resembling a "film reel" playing in the front of her head, many hours per day, which she could not turn off. She described somatoform flashbacks in her abdomen and genital areas. She often heard her father's voice yelling at her. She avoided visiting areas in the city where she had been assaulted or abused.

During a subsequent visit, her doctor positioned his stool between the patient and the door to the examination room. Ms Y suddenly appeared terrified, screamed, and shook her umbrella at him, leading him to terminate the interview. She soon appeared calmer and apologized, and then left the clinic without her prescriptions. She missed several subsequent appointments. She later returned, unexpectedly, stating she had "gotten by on my own" and now wished to resume treatment. Staff noticed lacerations on her left arm, which were healing. She attributed these to a fall.

Ms Y soon acknowledged that during her absence she relapsed on nonprescribed opioids and lost her job. She could no longer afford rent and had moved into a women's shelter. Although she was embarrassed over her relapse, on returning she expressed motivation to learn from what had happened. She continued to exhibit posttraumatic reactivity but overall treated staff with greater consideration. She adhered to her pre-scribed medications, smoked cannabis less often, and eventually agreed to consider alternative medications. Following continued assessment, her providers removed her previous diagnoses of anxiety disorder, ADHD, and schizoaffective disorder—these were thought to be redundant or incorrect—and made a diagnosis of PTSD.

Case Discussion

Ms Y's case illustrates clinical and managerial challenges that treating patients with SUD-PTSD may present. On an overt level, intense anger,[27] impulsivity,[28] and/or alex-ithymia[29] may complicate therapeutic relationships and interfere with care. Such symptoms and behaviors correlate with classic shame responses[2] and may be misat-tributed to other conditions, resulting in misdiagnosis and suboptimal care.

Like any other clinical device, the Compass of Shame should be used as a tool to help make sense of a complex situation, not as an augur of truth. All instances of her-oin use, for example, do not represent shame-avoidance reactions. The Compass's points must be considered within a larger constellation of symptoms, behaviors, his-torical information, and medical data.

In response to shame reactions, counter-shaming interventions may be used simi-larly to the use of intravenous fluids on a burn recovery unit. The onset of hypotension in a burn survivor suggests fluid loss. Most providers would increase the rate of intra-venous hydration before investigating why the patient became hemodynamically un-stable. Similarly, the onset of shame-related behaviors in a trauma survivor suggests that symptoms have been activated in a clinically significant way, and that counter-shaming can help. Clarification of the behavior's origin may be pursued later.

Many of Ms Y's behaviors likely represented shame reactions. Her repeated sub-stance use exemplifies *shame avoidance*. Her outward aggression toward staff and threats to quit treatment illustrate *attack-other* behaviors. More pernicious *attack-other* responses were manifested through passive aggression: she continually requested unsafe medications, coaxed providers to spend extended time with her (thus diverting resources away from peers), angered and repelled members of staff (diverting further resources), and instilled fear that she would decompensate if the

---

[2] Respectively: attack-other, avoid, withdraw.

clinic terminated care. After yelling at her provider[3] she apologized and abruptly *withdrew* from the clinic. When she returned, her presentation suggested she had *avoided* her inner experience through substance abuse and *attacked herself* through self-injury. Her behaviors, especially *avoid* and *attack-other* reactions, provoked analogous responses among employees, who then struggled to maintain the standard of care.

Several details in Ms Y's case suggest she was suffering from "complex" PTSD (c-PTSD). c-PTSD was added to the International Classification of Diseases, 11th edition, to incorporate manifestations of PTSD that repeated and/or extreme traumatic events frequently caused.[30,31] Ms Y's history of violent relationships, estrangement, legal problems, and difficulty maintaining income and housing are more common in individuals with extensive childhood trauma (often communicated as adverse childhood events[32] [ACEs]). Her experiences of posttraumatic intrusions are complex, especially her somatoform flashbacks, experiences of a film playing in her mind, and hallucinations of her father's voice. The picture invites screening for dissociation, which, if present, can further inform diagnosis and referral to supplemental care.

THE LINK BETWEEN ADDICTION AND TRAUMA
A Brief Note on Epidemiology

It is difficult to overstate the preponderance of studies that have demonstrated a link between childhood trauma and the development of PTSD and/or SUD. The link is probably causal, overall, rather than correlative.[11] ACEs unequivocally escalate risk for both conditions.[1,33–36] When patients with ACEs develop PTSD, they may experience worse psychiatric and substance use outcomes[37] and benefit less from SUD treatment.[38–41]

About 30% to 60% of SUD meet criteria for PTSD at least once in their life.[4] In 2 large national samples, approximately one-third to half of patients with PTSD also met criteria for SUD.[6,40] Mills and colleagues[6] observed that patients with sedative and opioid use disorders were approximately 23 times more likely to have PTSD compared with individuals without SUD. Many patients with SUD-PTSD struggle to access SUD treatment.[41] For a focused review of convergent epidemiologic features of SUD and PTSD, including characteristics of treatment-seeking patients with SUD, the readers are referred to McCauley and colleagues.[4]

The Shared Neurobiology of Posttraumatic Stress Disorder and Substance Use Disorder

Given the high rate of comorbidity between PTSD and SUD, as well as the common experience of associated shame, it is perhaps unsurprising that the neurobiological correlates of SUD and PTSD overlap considerably. For PTSD, decades of research implicate aberrant hypothalamic-pituitary-adrenal axis activity, hyperreactivity of fear- and anxiety-related systems, and structural diminutions and functional aberrations in several brain regions including the amygdala, hippocampus, and prefrontal cortical areas governing emotion and attention.[42] For addiction, a well-accepted heuristic model implicates 3 functional domains—incentive salience, state/trait negative emotionality, and executive function—each of which is subserved by 3 neurobiological cores: respectively, the basal ganglia (BG), the amygdala plus its extended projections, and the prefrontal cortex.[43]

---

[3] This is a good example of a behavior that maps readily onto an *attack-other* shame script, yet based on the clinical context—in which a hypervigilant trauma survivor was made to feel trapped inside a small room—it mostly likely represents a fear response, not a shame reaction.

Despite the high clinical and prima facie neurobiological overlap between PTSD and addiction, there is a near vacuum of review literature (or, for that matter, controlled clinical trials) investigating the shared neurobiology of the 2 conditions[4]. Although a comprehensive review of the neurobiology of PTSD and addiction lies outside of the scope of this discussion, we have attempted to distill some of the most robust findings of the brain aberrations associated with PTSD and addiction, focusing on regions that are common to the 2 conditions in **Table 1**.

Although the authors propose that shame plays a central role both phenomenologically and in approaching the treatment of SUD and PTSD, it is worth noting that research on shame has largely been constrained to the domain of social cognition,[46] with little attention applied to investigations of the underlying neurobiology. The few investigations that do exist, however, implicate several of the brain regions found to be important in PTSD and SUD, and include the amygdala, the insula, and anterior cingulate cortex.[47,48]

How Stigma Creates and Perpetuates Shame in Substance Use Disorder-Posttraumatic Stress Disorder

The public understanding of SUD has shifted from a moral model toward a disease model that emphasizes risk factors, psychobiological processes, and the need for treatment.[12,49–52] Yet, due in part to the moral model's lasting effects, patients with SUD continue to face the greatest degree of stigma among sufferers of any health condition worldwide.[53] Stigma, defined as "an attribute that is deeply discrediting that reduces someone from a whole and usual person to a tainted, discounted one,"[54] operates at multiple levels—self, public, and structural—all of which contribute to social devaluation, inequality, and discrimination.[55]

Patients with SUD-PTSD may experience stigma as internalized, enacted, or both. *Internalized stigma* refers to a process through which an individual believes negative messages about their condition and applies those messages to themselves. Patients may also observe others (family members, employers, health care providers, and so on) as *enacting stigma* through discrimination or bias." Internalized stigma corresponds with negative outcomes including poorer quality of life, reduced sense of meaning, and emotional suffering.[56] Internalized stigma exemplifies a self-attacking response to shame (see **Fig. 1**). Enacted stigma enhances the stigma's internalization and often reinforces its public perception, contributing to a vicious cycle.[57]

Together, internalized and enacted stigma likely contribute to poor health outcomes in patients with SUDs through overlapping mechanisms, including by weakening social bonds, interfering with attempts to secure housing and employment, and creating barriers to medical, psychiatric, and/or SUD treatments.[58] Comparatively few studies have examined stigma among patients with PTSD; however, the available studies suggest that patients with PTSD often do suffer from stigma. For example, 1 investigation found that traumatized veterans score similarly to patients with schizophrenia (one of the most stigmatized psychiatric diagnoses[59]) on a validated assessment for measuring stigma experiences (correlations were highest on subscales measuring self-stigma, lower on subscales assessing enacted stigma).

The high prevalence of SUD-PTSD naturally invites questions about intersectional stigma and its manifestations in the clinic. Although internalized stigma functions in part as a *self-attack* shame response, and the relationship between shame and aggression is well established,[60] the extent to which enacted stigma may

---

[4] Anecdotally, a search in PubMed by one of the authors [A.M.B.] for clinical studies using the search terms "addiction," "PTSD," and "neurobiology" yielded only 55 records.

Table 1
Shared neurobiology of posttraumatic stress disorder and substance use disorder: select clinical findings of enduring brain structural and functional changes

Brain Region		PTSD Clinical Findings (References)	SUD Clinical Findings (References)
Noncortical limbic regions	Amygdala (and extended amygdala)	• Increased rCBF in response to trauma-associated cues in combat-related PTSD • Meta-analytic finding of increased amygdala activity in mixed clinical samples with PTSD111[a,b]	• Increased amygdala activation (CBF) in response to drug-related cues • Decreased bilateral amygdala morphometry in AUD that normalized with abstinence
	Hippocampus	• Decreased volume of right[44] and bilateral[45] hippocampus in patients with combat-related PTSD • Decreased volume of left[44,118] and bilateral[119-121][3] hippocampus in early abuse-related PTSD • Decreased hippocampal neuronal density in a mixed cohort with combat and early abuse-related PTSD[122]	• Alcohol dependence associated with smaller subiculum and Ca1 subfields[123] • Smaller gray matter volume of the right hippocampus in crack cocaine-dependent subjects[124] • Methamphetamine abstinence associated with increases in hippocampal volume[125]
Prefrontal cortex PFCx	vmPFCx	• Decreased volume of rostral vmPFCx in combat-related PTSD[126] • Hypoactivation of the vmPFCx in early abuse-related[127] and combat-related[128] PTSD • Meta-analytic findings of hypoactivity of vmPFCx in mixed clinical samples	• Decreased gray matter volume in prefrontal lobe in polysubstance SUD[129] • Decreased prefrontal rCBF in chronic cocaine use[130] • Decreased prefrontal metabolic activity in chronic cocaine use[131]
	ACC	• Decreased volume of ACC in early abuse-[132] and combat-related[133] PTSD • Hypoactivation of the ACC in combat-related PTSD[134] • Hypoactivity of dorsal and rostral ACC in mixed clinical samples	• Increased ACC activation (CBF) in response to drug-related cues • Decreased volume of the ACC in cocaine-dependent subjects[135]
Basal ganglia		• Differential activation of basal ganglia (especially in the putamen and GP) in individuals with PTSD vs trauma-exposed controls[136] • Overactivity of the striatum during emotion processing among individuals with PTSD[137]	• Decreased BG activation (CBF) in response to drug-related cues • Decreased striatal dopamine response and D2 receptor availability in early and protracted cocaine withdrawal[131,138] • Decreased striatal D2 receptor availability in opioid-dependent subjects[139]
Insula		• Hyperactivation of the insula in intimate partner violence-related PTSD[140,141]	• Disruption of nicotine addiction in persons who have had stroke with lesions of the insula[142]

- Meta-analytic finding of increased insula activity in mixed clinical samples with PTSD[45]

- Increased insula activation (PET) in response to internally driven drug craving in cocaine[143] and heroin[144] dependence
- Decreased volume of the insula in cocaine-dependent subjects[135]

This is neither intended to be a comprehensive listing of all brain regions involved in either PTSD or SUD nor meant to serve as an all-encompassing literature review of all studies. Rather, this table is meant to point readers to the neurobiological changes associated with PTSD and SUD, focusing only on those that are common to both conditions, with references for the earliest and most important pieces of evidence.

Abbreviations: ACC, anterior cingulate cortex; AUD, alcohol use disorder; BG, basal ganglia; CBF, cerebral blood flow; fMRI=functional magnetic resonance imaging; GP, globus pallidum; PET, positron emission tomography; PFCx, prefrontal cortex; rCBF, regional cerebral blood flow; vmPFCx, ventromedial prefrontal cortex.

[a] Data derived from a meta-analysis of 14 independent studies analyzing PET or fMRI results conducted with populations with clinically diagnosed PTSD.
[b] Meta-analysis of pooled structural data from 13 separate studies.

incorporate *attack-other* shame responses (ie, do stigmatizers cope with shame in part through maltreating the stigmatized?) is less clear based on existing empirical evidence.

It is not uncommon for SUD providers to harbor stigma against patients with SUD.[61] In our view, clinician-harbored stigma is best addressed in a sensitive and countershaming manner by clinical supervisors. Although stigma cannot be eradicated by one provider or clinic alone, the way in which clinic staff and employees communicate with patients and with each other can alleviate stigma and reduce its negative effects on treatment. Changing stigmatizing or shaming language and attitudes can help move away from outdated, punitive views of addiction.[62]

CLINICAL APPROACH: SCREENING, DIAGNOSIS, SUMMARY OF EXISTING TRAUMA + ADDICTIONS MODELS
Screening Tools for Posttraumatic Stress Disorder

Despite broad agreement among academicians that comorbid PTSD should be treated concurrently with SUD, most clinics do not detect, and therefore do not directly treat, most co-occurring cases of PTSD. Patients with SUD and untreated, comorbid PTSD typically engage less in treatment and suffer worse outcomes than when PTSD is treated. If trauma began in childhood and led to development of complex PTSD, or if dissociative symptoms play a significant role, then the deleterious impact of untreated PTSD on treatment is further amplified.[63–65]

Considering that PTSD detection within SUD clinics is low, that the rate of comorbid PTSD is high, and that the potential benefits of treating comorbid PTSD are substantial, the single, possibly most consequential trauma-informed intervention that an SUD clinic can make is the systematic implementation of routine screening for PTSD. This intervention can be achieved economically using one of the following brief validated screening tools.

First, the Primary Care PTSD screen for DSM-5 (PC-PTSD-5) consists of 1 trauma screening item and 5 symptom items that ask broadly about intrusions, avoidance symptoms, negative alterations to cognitions/mood, and arousal/reactivity.[66] Breslau's short screening scale for PTSD comprises 7 items and may achieve higher specificity than the PC-PTSD-5, although its sensitivity is lower.[67,68] The Short Posttraumatic Stress Disorder Rating Interview (SPRINT) demonstrates high sensitivity and specificity. SPRINT comprises 8 screening questions and 2 follow-up questions.[69] These tools may be used for both initial and follow-up (eg, annual) screening. All screens include recommended cutoff scores, which may help inform referrals to specialized evaluation for PTSD. Characteristics of validated brief screens for PTSD are summarized in **Table 2**.

In select cases, clinics may opt to augment evaluation using a longer assessment such as the 20-item PTSD symptom checklist (PTSD Checklist for DSM-5 [PCL-5]).[70,71] For certain cases, clinics may opt to use the gold-standard Clinician-Administered PTSD Scale for the DSM-5 (CAPS).[72] CAPS requires training to use and takes 45 to 60 minutes to administer. Dissociative symptoms, which occur commonly, may mimic certain symptoms of substance intoxication or withdrawal, and are associated with higher impairment, can be surveyed using the Dissociative Experiences Scale-II[73,74] or the Multiscale Dissociation Inventory.[75]

In general, we recommend against asking questions about specific traumatic events. None of the screenings that the authors suggest include detailed questions about trauma history, which are not necessary for symptom screening purposes or

Table 2
Validated screening measures for posttraumatic stress disorder

Instrument	Number of Items	Response Type	Scoring Method	Recommended Cutoff for "Positive" Screen	Sensitivity	Specificity	Source Reference
Brief screen							
PC-PTSD	1–6[a]	Yes/no	Sum of "yes" responses	3	0.95	0.85	Prins et al., 2016[66]
Short Form of the PTSD Checklist – Civilian Version	6	Likert scale (0–4)	Sum of responses	14	0.92	0.72	Lang and Stein, 2005[145]
Breslau Screen	7	Yes/no	Sum of "yes" responses	4	0.80–0.85	0.97–0.84	Breslau et al. 1999,[146] Kimerling et al., 2006[68]
SPRINT	8[b]	Likert scale (0–4)	Sum of responses	14–17	0.95–0.89	0.96–0.97	Connor and Davidson, 2001[69]
Selected moderate-length tools (provide both screening and symptom severity scores)							
PCL-5	20	Likert scale (0–4)	Sum of responses[c]	31–33 (Recommended cutoff for possible PTSD diagnosis)	0.81	0.71	Blevins et al., 2015[70]
PDS	24[c]	Likert scale (0–4)	Sum of responses for items 1–20	28	0.79	0.78	Foa et al., 2016[147]

Abbreviations: PC-PTSD, Primary Care PTSD Screen PCL-5, PTSD Checklist for DSM-5; PDS, Posttraumatic Diagnostic Scale.
[a] Includes first question about history of traumatic experience (yes/no) that determines further inquiry about symptoms.
[b] Includes 2 follow-up questions.
[c] This assessment contains an additional 2 questions focused on clarifying trauma history and identifying a single traumatic event ("index trauma"). The last 4 questions ask about level of distress, interference, onset, and duration of symptoms.

for guiding basic clinical interventions. Furthermore, patients may find probing questions about trauma to be shaming and/or symptomatically activating. If it becomes necessary to collect a more complete trauma history, we suggest using a validated screening instrument such as the 24-Item Trauma History Questionnaire,[76] which is relatively brief and captures basic information about the frequency and duration of traumatic events. Many clinicians and researchers screen using the ACE questionnaire, which comprises 10 yes or no questions.[32] These tools differ somewhat in what they assess and may be used in a complementary manner. There is a dearth of validated questionnaires that screen for traumatic experiences related to racism, classism, discrimination related to gender identity or sexual orientation, or refugee status.

Existing Treatment Models for Substance Use Disorder-Posttraumatic Stress Disorder

Evidence-based models for SUD-PTSD treatment have been reviewed recently.[77] Accordingly, we offer a targeted review of established treatments. Arguably, the most researched and widely disseminated approach designed to treat SUD-PTSD is Seeking Safety (SS),[78] which can be implemented in both group and individual formats. SS focuses on safety and stabilization skills for PTSD and covers many topics that assist in recovery from both disorders such as healthy relationships, coping with triggers, and grounding skills.[78] SS includes 25 topics and typically runs 12 to 25 sessions.

Trauma-processing treatments such as cognitive processing therapy, eye movement desensitization and reprocessing (EMDR), and prolonged exposure (PE) have been applied to people with co-occurring SUD-PTSD.[79–81] However, these treatments are focused on processing memories and cognitions related to traumatic events; they do not prioritize safety or sobriety skills. Rather, they require patients to abstain from using substances before and after sessions and while completing assigned practice between sessions, because maintaining avoidance through substance use reduces treatment effectiveness. This requirement can be challenging for many patients with SUD-PTSD, for whom substance use represents a strongly conditioned symptom avoidance behavior. Trauma processing sessions are typically conducted in an individual therapy format.

PE has been adapted for SUD-PTSD as Concurrent Treatment of PTSD and SUD using Prolonged Exposure (COPE), which incorporates elements of relapse prevention to PE. When following the manualized protocol, sessions 1 to 2 focus on relapse prevention and psychoeducation and sessions 3 to 12 involve imaginal and in vivo exposure. Overall focus on sobriety skills is limited.

Interventions designed for isolated SUD, such as mindfulness-based relapse prevention (MBRP), may also help patients with SUD-PTSD. MBRP is an 8-week group intervention that may be incorporated readily into SUD-PTSD treatment. MBRP is particularly effective for individuals with high negative affect.[82] Evidence from the first clinical trial assessing the effectiveness of MBRP in PTSD is forthcoming.[83] Other mindfulness-based interventions, such as mindfulness-based stress reduction, have led to reductions in symptoms of PTSD.[84] Modalities such as acceptance and commitment therapy (ACT) and dialectical behavioral therapy also use mindfulness, and initial evidence suggests they may be effective for SUD-PTSD.[85,86] Saliently, an ACT-based group intervention targeting shame improved SUD outcomes and treatment retention.[87]

Diverging from these approaches, treatment modalities targeting isolated SUD (ie, SUD without comorbid PTSD) often emphasize avoidance-based coping skills such as distraction or evasion of external reminders of substance use. Although useful in some instances, an overreliance on avoidance-based coping may entrench symptoms of PTSD. In addition, many addiction treatment programs incorporate 12-step work and/or group attendance. The focus on powerlessness in 12-step programs may repel some trauma survivors who have been harmed by people in positions of authority, who in recovery may wish to exert greater control over their circumstances.[88] Furthermore, the emphasis on "character defects" in some 12-step programs may be experienced as shaming rather than normalizing to traumatized individuals.

Current treatment approaches for SUD-PTSD have several limitations. First, existing treatment models (with the notable exception of SS) have emerged from either the SUD or the PTSD treatment camp and do not consistently focus on treating both disorders. Most treatment models for PTSD require extensive training (especially EMDR, PE, and COPE), limiting accessibility to providers due to cost or availability. SS offers a flexible training model, yet studies supporting the efficacy of SS required rigorous provider training and supervision standards. Furthermore, PE has high dropout rates and is not tolerable for some patients.[89] Practical, common-sense interventions that can help establish or enhance trauma-responsive care to patients with SUD-PTSD are outlined in the following section.

CLINICAL APPROACH: COMMON-SENSE INTERVENTIONS THAT ANY CLINICIAN OR CLINICAL STAFF MEMBER CAN USE

For SUD clinics in the early stages of incorporating trauma-responsive care, or for providers who wish to augment the tools they already use, we propose that PTSD recovery interventions can be conceptualized from the vantage point of identifying and ameliorating shame. In PTSD recovery, the stages of treatment are organized in a triphasic model,[90] which is analogous to the Stages of Change framework for targeting SUD recovery interventions[91] and provides the basis for gold-standard treatment guidelines for c-PTSD and dissociation.[92,93] The triphasic model divides treatment into 3 stages—(1) stabilization of safety, symptoms, and functioning; (2) remembrance and grieving of traumatic losses, which includes trauma narrative exposure or "memory processing" work; and (3) reconnecting with others. For practical reasons, we will limit the discussion to the stabilization phase of treatment.

Stabilizing Interventions: Posttraumatic Stress Disorder Symptom Management Skills and Safeguarding Clinical Boundaries

Stabilization-phase interventions for PTSD are concerned with managing intrusive sensations and memories, enhancing regulation of mood and/or anxiety associated with posttraumatic triggers, improving social and occupational functioning, and, most of all, maintaining safety. In approaching stabilization-phase interventions, individual interventions may help alleviate a transient posttraumatic symptom. By contrast, internalization and mastery of the intervention across relationships, work, and treatment enables the patient to develop interlinking experiences of competency, confidence, and pride, which are phenomenologically distinct from the relief of symptoms. The outcome of this process is akin to the lowering of the "tide" of PTSD; symptomatic "waves" may still occur but overall are less disruptive. We propose that this second dynamic—in which the evocation of competency reduces shame sensitivity and helps patients transform their relationship with their disorder—may help explain the increasing application of skills- and competency-based treatment models for treating PTSD.[94]

Training manuals for treating PTSD offer many skills for reducing posttraumatic symptoms. Although these skill sets overlap, for simplicity's sake we will divide symptom management skills for PTSD into 3 categories: grounding, containment, and affective de-escalation. **Table 3** provides specific examples of each of these skill sets. As patients learn these techniques, they may (1) develop a sense of control over their symptoms and, upon mastery, (2) cultivate enduring competency in managing their broader posttraumatic syndrome. Many patients, on stabilizing, opt to repair relationships (or end them), address financial or housing problems, resume schooling, or pursue more satisfying work as they gain confidence that they can regulate their symptoms under moderate or even significant stress.

Coping skills such as mindful grounding exercises can easily be learned by most staff and providers in clinical settings, and these can be taught to patients without delving into the details of a patient's trauma. For clinical staff who choose to teach skills to patients, it is helpful to remember that practicing basic skills is not a replacement for psychotherapy. We recommend that staff who offer coaching on coping skills encourage patients to practice the skills routinely. If a patient complains that a skill "doesn't work for me," despite having practiced the skill, staff should encourage the patient to address the problem with their therapist, rather than personally attempting to work through the issue with the patient. Troubleshooting a skill may require specialized management of posttraumatic triggers or involve a complex relational dynamic that would most effectively be handled in psychotherapy.

Similarly, before approaching any intervention with a traumatized patient, we encourage providers to adhere to conventional clinical boundaries. Doing so may be more challenging when working with this population because, for patients who were traumatized from an early age (such as Ms Y), *their PTSD represents a developmental condition that arose from attachment relationships and circumstances in which safe and healthy boundaries were never established or maintained.* Thus, many patients may exhibit a disorganized attachment style[96,97] in which acting out—positively or negatively—toward clinicians is common and often is experienced by patients as protective against the expectation that even professionally qualified "helpers" will inevitably betray them. In **Box 1**, the basic strategies for maintaining healthy clinical boundaries are presented.

Psychoeducation: Teach Traumatized Patients that They Are Not Defective, and Their Posttraumatic Stress Disorder Symptoms Can Improve

Providing psychoeducation to patients about the symptoms of PTSD and the effects of trauma on the brain can help normalize reactions to trauma and reduce stigma.[99] Patients with PTSD may not understand the cause of their symptoms or how their PTSD and SUD symptoms may interrelate. Without sufficient education, patients may resort to maladaptive, self-attacking shame scripts in an effort to cope with their trauma, telling themselves that they are broken, "not normal," or "going crazy."[100]

Accordingly, psychoeducation represents an essential component of trauma-informed and trauma-processing therapies such as SS, cognitive processing therapy, and PE.[78,100,101] Psychoeducation should include information on symptoms of PTSD, how PTSD impacts the brain leading to hyperarousal, and how avoidance serves to maintain symptoms of PTSD. **Table 4** illustrates sample psychoeducational topics, which may be helpful to discuss with patients with SUD-PTSD.

In patients with SUD-PTSD, substance use can be formulated as a manifestation of phobic avoidance and, in many cases, as a shame-avoidance script. Considering the high rate of trauma exposure among patients with SUD, the regularity of clinical contact often required for treatment, and the emphasis on recovery and change that SUD

Table 3
Selected posttraumatic stress disorder symptom management skills

Skill Type	Target Symptoms	Example
Grounding	Derealization, depersonalization, disconnection from physical senses, hypervigilance, intrusive thoughts/memories	"Dropping anchor"[95]: Mindfulness based, 3 steps (A-C-E) 1. A: *Acknowledge* your thoughts and feelings. Label how you are feeling, emotionally, and acknowledge what thoughts are passing through your mind. 2. C: *Connect* with your body. In addition to providing a countermeasure to dissociative symptoms, connecting purposefully with your senses can help block or reduce rumination, intrusive thoughts, and/or intrusive memories. Connecting to your body can involve any physical movement such as pushing your feet into the floor, moving your fingers and toes, breathing mindfully, or doing some stretching. Similarly, you might notice any smells or tastes present in this moment. 3. E: *Engage* in what you are doing. This step can help you become more present focused and regain your sense of control; this could involve observing who and what else are in the room, noticing any sounds in the environment, and giving full attention to what you are doing.
Containment	Intrusive memories (flashbacks) and thoughts	1. Physical containment: Write down the thought or memory that is intruding on a loose piece of paper (without getting into potentially activating details). Then, fold up the paper and store it in a box for use when needed or ready during therapy. This can be your "containment box," which you may wish to personalize as you develop your own way to use it. 2. Containment vault: Imagine a strong, secure, pristinely organized safety vault. Only you can lock or unlock its door. Whenever you have an uncomfortable thought or memory, notice that you can place it very comfortably and easily in a place inside the vault that feels right to you. You can even shrink down the thought or memory to make it fit just right. Before using your vault for containing flashbacks, it will be important to practice locking it, unlocking it, and placing neutral or pleasant objects inside, perhaps such as a baseball or a stuffed animal you liked as a child. Then reopen the vault and make sure you can find and retrieve what you have put inside.
De-escalating	Affective reactivity and emotional flooding (often coincides with posttraumatic intrusions)	1. Progressive muscle relaxation: Once you're able to notice where your emotions are in your body (eg, after grounding or dropping anchor), notice that you can slowly change the way the emotions feel by tensing your body, one part at a time. Tense one part of your body at a time starting at your feet and working your way up your whole body. Now, each time you exhale, relax one part of your body. Continue relaxing each part of your body until the tension has

(continued on next page)

Table 3
(continued)

Skill Type	Target Symptoms	Example
		dissipated. Some parts of your body might take 2 or 3 breaths to relax all the way. If that happens, it's okay. Simply notice the tension and keep releasing what is comfortable for a few more exhales.
		2. Kitchen dial: Imagine an old-fashioned kitchen dial. Its numbers, 1 through 10, represent how you might feel, with 1 being the most calm and happy and 10 being the most overwhelmed. Notice where the dial is pointing in this moment. To test the dial, let it go up one notch. Then, in the next couple of breaths, let it fall back to where you started. Dialing down to a lower number might be easier if you time it with an exhale.
		To master this skill: practice "dial up, dial down." Start in a calm or neutral mood, then first dial *up* to a level of moderate intensity. Then dial back down to a comfortable setting. When comfortable and grounded, repeat both steps and notice how comfortable it becomes to control the skill in both directions. Notice that dialing up may worry you less as your comfort and skill improves.

Box 1
Tips for maintaining healthy and effective clinical boundaries

1. Minimize physical contact with patients. For example, only shake hands if the patient offers. Avoid hugging or other contact that would be more intimate than a handshake.

2. Maintain professional relationships: clinicians and nonclinical staff should not start friendships or become a "close acquaintance" with clinic patients.

3. Prevent severe boundary violations: clinicians and nonclinical staff should *never* enter an extraclinical financial relationship, romantic relationship, or sexual relationship with a clinic patient, including after the patient recovers and/or terminates care at the clinic.

4. Do not routinely make exceptions to your standard clinical practices. Exceptions may include holding onto an item for the patient, extending session frequency or time, operating outside of the standard telephone policy, having nonprofessional contact of any kind, sharing revealing personal information, sharing personal contact information, connecting on a personal social media account, engaging in conflicts of interest such as treating an established patient's close family member.

5. Remember the adage: most boundary violations begin "between the chair and the door."[98]

---

providers already provide, the SUD clinic offers a well-suited environment for educating patients with SUD-PTSD about trauma and setting reasonable expectations about recovering from both conditions.

Clinical Interviewing: Consider a Counter-Shaming Approach

To organize strategies for alleviating shame, one may be reminded of a cognitive distortion that many patients with SUD have experienced: "I'm defective and unworthy of... love."[102] The first assertion ("I'm defective") captures shame's ability to create a "broken" or disorganized self-experience, which often manifests through a sense of incompetence. Alternatively, patients may complain that they feel like a failure—an experience that childhood sexual abuse may engender[103,104] and which may be reinforced by subsequent setbacks related to the patient's psychiatric disorders or low self-esteem. We propose that experiences of competency can be developed strategically in the SUD clinic and help to alleviate this aspect of maladaptive shame.

The second assertion ("I'm unworthy of love") evokes the sense of being unlikable, unlovable, disgusting, and/or alienated that people experiencing catastrophic shame states often describe. Patients may assert that they do not belong in a treatment group, do not feel welcome at the clinic, do not deserve to get better, or do not deserve help. As a counter-shaming approach, we will propose strategies to enhance patients' sense of belonging in the clinic environment.

Tables 5 and **6** illustrate counter-shaming approaches to clinical interviewing, which adhere to these principles. **Table 7** highlights common language that may reinforce shame and offers possible alternatives. Finally, **Table 8** enumerates shame-based cognitive distortions that patients with SUD-PTSD may endorse. The authors offer possible therapeutic responses.

Like the burn-case analogy introduced earlier, in which rehydration does not cure the injuries but may stabilize a patient's blood pressure and promote healing, applying a counter-shaming approach does not on its own cure PTSD or extinguish symptoms. Rather, it promotes short-term symptom reduction, protects capacity to intellectualize, facilitates mindful discourse, and strengthens the treatment alliance—processes that may promote healthy change and/or enhance other interventions.

Table 4
Sample psychoeducation for patients with posttraumatic stress disorder

Topic	Target Issues or Symptoms	Example
Neurobiology	Sense that the patient is defective for having or not "getting over" trauma Fear that intrusive thoughts and/or flashbacks may be dangerous	A nurse begins educating patients about brain changes that may lead to ongoing psychiatric symptoms, that is, hyperarousal and depressed mood, and how pharmacotherapeutic and/or psychotherapeutic interventions will help to alleviate these experiences. Her patients are relieved to learn that mood swings and flashbacks are common to experience early in sobriety and can be regulated without self-medicating. Most of all, they express relief that their symptoms "make sense," in terms of how their brains work, and they develop more questions about the science of their recovery that they bring to their doctor's visits.
Treatment course	Concerns that past treatments have not worked, or that the patient has "failed" too many times to recover Misunderstandings about the circumstances required to recover from PTSD	A physician informs a patient who recently relapsed on substances and self-harmed: In recovery from trauma, we're all going to prioritize your basic safety. Your PTSD is unlikely to get better, especially in the long term, if you continue to harm yourself—physically, through using substances, through unsafe relationships, through eating disordered behaviors, and so on. A patient in early sobriety asks her social worker about starting memory processing work. He replies: you've worked hard to get sober. Memory processing work will stress your system—that's why it's not the focus right now and might even be harmful to pursue until you've maintained your sobriety, learned to regulate your major PTSD symptoms, and discussed the possibility of processing your traumatic memories with your therapist.
Link between SUDs and PTSD	Newly sober patients may experience intensified symptoms related to their PTSD. Conversely, trauma cues predict increased substance use and relapse.	A therapist explains to her patient: as you get used to being sober from substances, at first you might experience more uncomfortable emotions or intrusive memories. We want to help you hone skills, gain confidence, and make stronger connections in your life. It will get easier to cope without using substances. Many of us in the clinic can help you learn and practice coping skills, and your doctor can talk with you about medications that might help reduce cravings or take the edge off from stress.

Table 5
Counter-shaming approaches in everyday practice

Counter-shaming Strategy	Rationale[a]	Example
Ask permission	*Competency: we value your input and judgment.* *Belonging: your opinions, concerns, and comfort matter here*	"With your permission, can we discuss...." "Would it be okay if I asked you about...." "Does this plan sound acceptable to you...." "Is the number of people in the room/the way we're positioned in the room/the way we're talking about this (so far) acceptable to you...?"
Instill a sense of partnership	*Competency: you are capable of being an active and effective partner in this work* *Belonging: you and I hold different roles in treatment, but fundamentally we are equals and allies*	"While we will only work together for a short time, how can we as partners work to support your goals?" "Can you please help me understand..." "As partners, how can we...." "Together, how can we...." "As a team, how can we..." "Based on what you've shared with me, I'd like to propose...." "If the way we're talking, now or later on, doesn't feel quite right to you, would you please let me know so that I can get back on the same page as you as quickly as possible...." * *It helps to display warmth when working to establish partnership!*
Help the patient feel welcome Show warmth	*Belonging: we're glad you're here, no matter what struggles and challenges you bring with you.*	"Welcome (back)! It's good to see you." "How can we help you...?" "I'm glad you came in for help..." "This is a helping place..." (not a hurting place) "Thank you for helping me understand that." * *Traumatized individuals often exhibit a recognition bias to detect anger, even when viewing neutral faces,[103] so showing warmth can help prevent*

(continued on next page)

Table 5
(continued)

Counter-shaming Strategy	Rationale[a]	Example
		posttraumatic misinterpretations of a clinician's facial expression.
Clarify roles, tasks, and role/task boundaries for staff and patients alike	*Competency: clarifying respective roles and tasks equips patients to make the most of the visit.*	"As your doctor, we'll regularly discuss how treatment is going and address any concerns you have. We may shake hands, but please notice that we won't hug or share any more intimate form of physical contact! I'll be able to connect you with our clinic's therapist and social worker, but I won't attempt to do therapy with you, myself. If you have questions about my background or personal life, please know that I won't get into most of that with you, since I don't think it would be helpful to your recovery...."
* *Remember: in interpersonal trauma, conventional role boundaries are violated. Traumatized patients may therefore benefit from proactive and repeated psychoeducation about the roles and tasks of each treatment team member.*	*Furthermore, because trauma survivors may expect "helpers" such as clinic providers to neglect or betray them, clarifying therapeutic roles and tasks may provide traumatized patients with a secure anchor point from which they can evaluate the clinical relationship autonomously and build trust.*	"My role here is to be helpful to you. We'll work hard to support you in all the ways we can, but the really hard work of getting and staying better is going to be yours."
	Belonging: you deserve to know where you are, who you're talking to, and what our respective tasks are.	"The technical/medical problems are ours to worry about, but the will to get better has to be yours. Let's be clear: we can't make you do anything – in treatment or otherwise – without your will and consent."
Acknowledge obvious limitations within the facility, the clinical situation, or even the clinician.	*Belonging: because we are fundamentally equals, it is only fair that I acknowledge my own/the team's limitations when necessary.*	"I only will know what you share with me..." (*Clinician's limitation: I am not omniscient*) "This can be a difficult place to have a conversation. Is there anything we can do to make it more comfortable for you?" (*Facility limitation: the room or building requires repair, there might be distracting noise, etc. All of this makes clinical work more difficult*)

(Situational limitation: seeking help might feel like a risk, especially to traumatized patients)

Emphasize the patient's rights, dignity, capabilities, and ability to make their own choices	*Competency: you are capable and able to decide what is best for yourself.* *Belonging: even if we disagree, you have dignity, you're welcome here, and you deserve respect.*	"With your permission..." "Can you help me understand..." "What do you think is best..." "With all respect..." "My I run this idea by you..." "What would you prefer out of these options...?"
Educate the patient about their circumstances and options	*Competency: you're capable of making good choices, but like anyone else you require sufficient information to do that.*	"Here's how your addiction/PTSD works in your brain..." "When you have a flashback (or panic attack), you may feel under threat. That's understandable, considering the terrible things you endured. For starters, it's vital to understand that even during flashbacks you're not actually in danger anymore. This knowledge might not make your flashbacks go away, but if it can help you get some distance from these scary experiences, then perhaps it can become more comfortable to use the coping skills you've been practicing..." "To feel more comfortable when flashbacks happen, it can help to..."

a How the strategy fosters counter-shaming experiences of competency and/or belonging.

Table 6
Counter-shaming: techniques for opening an interview with traumatized patients

Counter-Shaming Strategy	Rationale[a]	Example
Explain who you are, what your role is (and what your role is not), offer an estimate of how long the interview will last	Competency: knowing who you're seeing and our time limit equips you to make the most of this visit. Belonging: you deserve to know where you are, who you're talking to, and what our tasks are here.	"As the _____ on your team, my role here is _____. I work with _____ and _____, who are also on your treatment team. We hope that, with all of us working together, this can be a helpful place for you." "We have the next 20 min to work together. Are there any matters you want to make sure we cover in that time?" "My role is to be helpful to you. Your role is to do the work of recovery, which can be very hard. But it's work that only you can do. As partners, perhaps we can learn together how to make this as comfortable as possible and maximize our chances of _____ [patient's stated goal]."
Interview the patient in private. Avoid hallway discussions or curbside conversations.	Belonging: your privacy and dignity matter here.	"Can we please discuss this in my office?" "There is a good space nearby that we can use for this conversation...."
Ask the patient if the circumstances of the interview are acceptable. * Includes position of people and furniture * Includes relative position of the patient vs the provider. Ideally, they should be at the same eye level (ie, generally, one should not stand while the other sits) * Provider's chair should not be nicer than the patient's * Many patients with PTSD prefer to sit near the door (so that others cannot block the patient from escaping and/or in a place that maximizes their ability to	Belonging: while our roles are different, we are fundamentally equals. We value your opinion and comfort.	"Before we begin, may I ask if the way we are sitting/ standing here is acceptable to you?" "Are you comfortable sitting there? Would you prefer to sit closer to the door?" If the provider needs to take notes: "Would it be all right with you if I took some notes, from time to time, while we speak?" "Will you please let me know if, at any point, the way in which we're speaking doesn't feel quite right to you? That way, I can make sure we're on the same page as much as possible." "Is there anything about this place you find strange or uncomfortable?"

surveil the whole room. Accommodating such preferences helps *reduce hypervigilance*. * Includes all that is happening during the interview		
If the patient asks to change aspects of the interview, do what you reasonably can to honor the request. If you can't honor the request, explain the reason and attempt to find a mutually acceptable alternative.	*Competency: your opinion matters.* *Belonging: I'm listening to you and taking what you say seriously.*	"Sure, we can talk about _____ later, but because of the nature of this discussion it's important that we get to it today, even if it only means we cover the headlines rather than the whole story. Does that sound acceptable to you?" "I'm afraid I cannot offer what you're asking. Based on _____, I believe that would not be responsible or safe for us to do. And if we start acting in a way that's not 100% responsible, then we won't be much help to you or anyone else. I won't take it personally if you disagree. In fact, I hope in our work that having a disagreement now and then can be helpful, strange as that might sound! But I'm afraid I can't offer what you're asking me to do."
Acknowledge any aspects of the situation or setting that are challenging or uncomfortable. * For example, the patient may not wish to be in treatment, or the facility may obviously require some maintenance. You don't need to apologize for the difficulty; rather, attempt to partner with the patient around making the situation as comfortable as possible.	*Competency (if the patient is ambivalent about treatment): although you may not wish to be here, we do not take your ambivalence personally and will honor your right to make your own decisions about treatment as we learn to work together.* *Belonging: although the circumstances for meeting may not be ideal, we will strive to make our work together as comfortable as possible*	"I realize it might be uncomfortable talking about your difficulties in this place, with someone you haven't known for very long..." "The problem with the construction outside is on us, not on you, and I can see how that might not make our conversation easier..." "Is there anything we can do here to make this work more comfortable? If we look at this together, then as partners, can you please let me know if we need to slow down or change our approach? For example, taking a break or even changing where in the room we're sitting can help sometimes..."

a How the strategy fosters counter-shaming experiences of competency and/or belonging.

Table 7
Counter-shaming: selected language to avoid

Shame-Inducing Language	Reason to Avoid	Alternative
"Why…"	"Why" questions are often experienced as shaming	"What happened that…" "What was going on that…" "How is it that…" "Can you please help me understand how…" "What do you think happened that…"
"Clean" (from substances)	Implies that when a patient uses, they're "dirty" (or, they were dirty or unworthy when they were using)	"Sober" Action words: "using," "not using," "intoxicated"
"I understand just how you feel…" "What's happening now is that you're feeling _____…"	Trauma survivors may be bewildered by their own symptoms; yet, they know that others cannot truly understand the nature of their suffering. Attempts to declare "understanding" of a patient's posttraumatic experiences (or to define their experiences for them) may backfire and disrupt the treatment alliance.	When patient describes feeling overwhelmed or hopeless: "That sounds very difficult, and I am sorry to hear you've had to carry that weight alone all these years. Even if we spent many hours talking, I don't think I could fully understand what you've been through… that being said, considering what you've shared, do you think we can work together to find a more comfortable way to cope? Perhaps we can discover a way where you don't have to carry the weight quite so much on your own." When intrusive symptoms become activated: "I'm not sure what exactly is happening now, though clearly something has hit a nerve. I'd like to honor that and with your permission take a step back together from what's happening. Once we're back in a more comfortable place, perhaps then we can figure out what's been happening. Would that be okay with you?"
		(continued on next page)

Table 7 (continued)		
Shame-Inducing Language	**Reason to Avoid**	**Alternative**
"Don't worry about that..." "You can trust me..." * Counterintuitive: these statements may appear reassuring but many trauma survivors experience them as the opposite.	Survivors of multiple traumas often expect that people who claim to be helping them will inevitably harm or betray them.	"Thanks for letting me know it's hard to trust me right now. Can I ask you to please keep your eyes on me (or us), to make sure that I (or we) act as safely and as responsibly as I'm (or we're) supposed to?" "Can you please let us know if there is something that doesn't look or feel right to you, so we can be on the same page and make sure we're in the best position to be helpful to you?"

APPROACHES TO CLINICAL LEADERSHIP: TAKING CARE OF ONE'S STAFF

The SUD clinic environment exposes clinicians and nonclinical staff alike to 2 work-related stress syndromes—(1) SPS and (2) employee burnout. These phenomena are best detected through active surveillance and may be dealt with separately or in combination depending on how their effects take form.

Owing to the high prevalence of trauma-related disorders among patients with SUD, SUD staff and treatment providers face an increased risk of experiencing vicarious trauma and SPS.[106] Even trauma specialists are vulnerable to developing posttraumatic reactivity, in which a provider experiences countertransference anger, helplessness, detachment, dismissiveness, and/or shame in response to treating traumatized patients. These processes reduce treatment quality and retention.[107,108] Similarly, providers who are experiencing posttraumatic reactivity themselves may struggle to use counter-shaming interventions.

Burnout syndrome develops in response to problematic relationships between employees and their workplace. Burnout syndrome leads employees to experience exhaustion, detachment, and a reduced sense of accomplishment.[105] In the health care setting, burnout is associated with reduced quality of care, decreased safety, and increased turnover.[109,110] Burnout among SUD clinic staff is common,[111] and SUD counselor turnover rates of 18.5% to 49% measure among the highest in professional services.[112]

Burned-out employees typically detach from their work, as described in Ms Y's case. However, it is not uncommon for staff or providers treating traumatized patients to become *overinvolved* with patients in well-intentioned (and ultimately unconstructive) attempts to regulate their reactions to certain patients. Overinvolvement can take various forms, such as extended session times, staff-patient enmeshment (eg, socializing or nonclinical phone calls), or therapeutic heroics.[113,114] Severe cases in which an employee and patient become romantically and/or sexually involved are notoriously damaging to patients, violate every published professional code of ethics, and may prompt civil litigation.[115,116] Although boundaries are crossed or violated in all instances of therapeutic overinvolvement, the insidious course of most boundary violations can make incidents difficult to detect.[117] Strategies for preventing boundary violations are summarized in **Box 1**.

Table 8
Counter-shaming: ways to challenge shame-based-distortions without inadvertently shaming the patient

Shame-Based Distortions (Shame Reaction: Attack-self)	Basis for Distortion	Possible Response (These Examples Focus on Counter-Shaming Interventions, Rather than Countering the Obvious Cognitive Distortions)
"I'm untreatable…" "I'm a failure…" "I used again and just can't get better…" "No one can help me…"	*Shame: sense of incompetency* Common underlying beliefs: *I'm defective and incapable of getting better, no matter what I try, how hard I work, or who tries to help me. Furthermore, if I start to make progress, then that's frightening, because then treatment will just turn into a bigger chance to fail and show everyone what a lost cause I really am.*	"Thanks for sharing that with me. Would it surprise you if I said that, in my professional view, under the right conditions, you're going to be able to recover and heal?" "As you aptly point out, as partners in this work, we'll need to be careful, and stay on the same page, to maximize our chances of progress." "You describe having setbacks in the past, which if we work together, we'll need to honor and learn from in this work – won't we? What you point out seems clear: there won't be room for pretending that recovery is going to be straightforward or easy, or for avoiding the hard work, is there? As a team, we'll need to figure out how to pace the work and make it comfortable enough." "In my view, it's helpful that you've pointed this concern out so early. With your permission, can we learn together from what's happened before and move forward as a team, but just one step at a time? Does that sound acceptable to you?"[a]
"I'm unlikeable/unlovable…" "Who would want to be my friend…" "No one cares about me…" "I'll never fit in anywhere…" "I'm going to be alone forever…"	*Shame: sense of alienation* Common underlying beliefs: *No one loves me, and if they did then I wouldn't deserve it. Others can see how appalling and underserving of compassion I really am. Anyone who thinks otherwise probably is crazy or shouldn't be trusted. As an unlovable person, the best I can do is hide away (shame: withdraw), hang out with other "losers" like*	"Thanks for sharing that thought with me.[b]" "That sounds really tough, to be having thoughts like that all the time. If I understand correctly, are you saying you sense I might be judging you or having a bad feeling toward you right now?" *The patient takes opportunity to reality check and may answer either yes or no. The clinician then explores and clarifies any "no" responses before proceeding to the next statement.*

me (shame: avoid/withdraw), or escape into drugs (shame: avoid).

If people try to show me love or caring, I might hurt myself (shame: self-attack) or push them away (shame: attack other) to prove how bad and deserving of punishment I am.

"Thanks for verifying with me that you're experiencing the two of us as being equals, though our roles and responsibilities here clearly are different. If, sooner or later, you sense I might be judging or criticizing you, would you please let me know so that we can figure out how to get back on the same page?"

The patient replies "yes."

"That would be helpful to me, since I only know what you share with me. Now, it seems that..."

[a] Interviewing note: This series of layered, overlapping assertions and queries would be interactive in practice and exemplifies the yes-set interviewing technique. Yes sets affirm alignment on goals and tasks and enhance rapport by rapidly establishing agreement on central treatment tasks and the need for change. If the patient answers "no" to any question in the set, then the clinician attempts to clarify the misunderstanding so that alignment may be restored. The clinician may then continue building the set as before. The final question in the set typically aims to move the treatment forward—by one step.

[b] Interviewing note: Alienation statements can be difficult to challenge and may be rooted in a patient's formative attachment experiences. Clarifying that these statements represent *thoughts* rather than emotions illustrates a *cognitive distancing* or *defusion* technique, which aims to help the patient access their capacity to think critically rather than catastrophize or engage in verbal self-attack. In other words, cognitive distancing/defusing encourages the patient to replace regressive, self-defeating reactions with more adaptive responses that incorporate healthy use of intellectualization and isolation of affect. Patients who can intellectualize and isolate affect can reflect more constructively (and competently) about their experiences and approach to treatment. Similarly, they may be more likely to accept a clinician's efforts to challenge shame-based distortions. Here, the interviewer repeats the distancing/defusing statement ("Thanks for sharing that thought... having thoughts...") then pivots into developing a yes-set.

Table 9
Leadership strategies for reducing secondary posttraumatic stress and burnout among substance use disorder clinic employees

Intervention	Rationale	Example
1. Track burnout	a. Enables more precise assessment and management of burnout b. Communicates that management values clinician and employee well-being c. Demonstrates investment in clinician and employee well-being d. Signals openness to discussing clinician and employee well-being	A clinic manager asks all clinicians and employees to complete a validated burnout scale semiannually, anonymously, and on a voluntary basis. Findings are analyzed alongside other data relating to the workplace environment and culture. The manager then reviews her conclusions and action steps in an all-staff meeting.
2. Implement staff groups/forums	a. Protects space for clinicians, clinic staff, and management personnel to relate in healthy and constructive ways b. Creates opportunity for clinicians, staff, and management personnel to identify the clinic's challenges, to acknowledge the difficulties they create, and, when possible, to problem solve together c. Enables clinicians and staff to share and validate challenges that arise from routine SUD clinic work d. Allows managers to model a collaborative work environment and encourage self-care practices	All clinic managers, providers, and staff meet twice monthly in a semistructured meeting focused on the clinic's functioning and on employee well-being. Ground rules are reviewed and include a time limit, expectations for professional behavior, and universal respect. All participants are invited to provide input. Managers and senior clinicians model nonjudgmental, nonpunitive responses when concerns or complaints about the clinic are raised. When attempting to solve a problem, suggestions are welcomed from all attendees, including junior clinicians, assistant clinicians, and nonclinical staff.
3. Maintain routine supervision and instruction	a. Equips staff to maintain a high standard of performance b. Builds staff-wide knowledge of trauma, stigma, and their effects on patients and clinicians alike c. Demonstrates commitment to personal engagement and professional growth d. Provides opportunities for junior clinicians, senior clinicians, and management personnel to enhance rapport	a. In supervision, a recently hired counselor realizes that his focus on spirituality leads some patients to feel alienated. The counselor learns to recognize more often when patients feel alienated and increasingly adopts an evidence-based treatment approach. b. All management personnel and clinicians are asked to participate in an annual workshop focused on identifying and addressing stigma and implicit bias. c. After attending a discussion on vicarious trauma and secondary posttraumatic syndromes, a clinician who has

appeared cynical and dissatisfied with her work attends more carefully to interpersonal boundaries, stops making negative comments to patients and staff, and prioritizes self-care by leaving the clinic on time and beginning a meditation practice.

| 4. Promote workplace dignity and autonomy | a. Enhances perceptions of self-worth, and of others' worth
b. Fosters a sense of belonging and pride
c. May reduce cynicism associated with burnout | a. A clinic incorporates a presentation on workplace dignity and respect into its onboarding procedures.
b. Following up on an employee's request, all staff are invited to a workshop on alleviating shame and stigma. On anonymous feedback, participants report feeling validated personally and professionally by the content of the workshop and by the respectful way in which it was carried out. Staff express enthusiasm and gratitude for the opportunity to practice techniques for treating difficult patients with dignity. Finally, staff members thank management for prioritizing and attending the workshop. The workshop is subsequently offered twice annually and enjoys robust levels of attendance and participation.
c. During a staff meeting, management and senior clinicians realize that they have not empowered several members of junior and support staff to function at the level of their competency and intended authority in the clinic. The matter is addressed individually with the staff members, who express surprise and relief that they no longer need to seek permission or oversight when performing various routine tasks. Over ensuing months, the staff members appear increasingly satisfied and productive in their roles. They offer more positive feedback and support to other team members during meetings. Meanwhile, their supervisors notice they have more time to devote to other tasks, and that some projects require less effort due to support staff's increased productivity. Staff continues to seek guidance from supervisors, but this is generally limited to circumstances involving novel or less frequent tasks. |

(continued on next page)

Table 9
(continued)

Intervention	Rationale	Example
5. Maintain healthy and therapeutic boundaries throughout the clinic	a. Facilitates a safe and effective treatment environment b. Prioritizes staff and clinician self-care (and models self-care to patients), reducing risk for exhaustion c. Reduces risk of overinvolved treatment practices d. Reduces risk of severe boundary violations	a. Clinic managers encourage staff to leave work on time and use all available vacation days b. A clinic's CEO leads a series of discussions with psychiatrists, counselors, and social workers about reasonable caseload size. The clinic later develops and implements caseload guidelines based on these discussions. c. Clinic leadership supports a clinician's decision to terminate care and refer a patient to an outside clinic after the patient became verbally aggressive toward nurses and front desk staff on multiple occasions. d. The importance of maintaining essential personal and clinical boundaries is emphasized during onboarding and reinforced in supervision sessions and staff meetings.

To address burnout, this framework prioritizes maximizing the autonomy, competency, and relatedness among clinicians, assistant clinicians, and nonclinical employees. These priorities are supported by numerous lines of evidence in the study of workplace motivation and well-being.[44] overlap with shame-alleviating principles that we have described, and have been applied previously to the problem of clinician burnout.[45] To reduce vulnerability to SPS, the authors encourage the protection of clinical boundaries, application of shame-alleviating principles by management, and promotion of workplace dignity. We recommend that clinic leadership implement this framework or its components using Leiter and Maslach's[105] principles for preventing and alleviating burnout: (1) interventions are applied with *urgency*, (2) they are *targeted* and *strategic*, (3) interventions are *collaborative*, (4) commitment to addressing burnout is *sustained*, and (5) intervention effects are *evaluated*. Validated measures for assessing employee burnout are widely available. Any clinician or other employee experiencing potentially significant SPS and/or workplace-associated PTSD should seek evaluation and treatment with a qualified professional.

In **Table 9**, a 5-factor framework for supporting SUD clinic employees to moderate risk for burnout and SPS is offered (for employees suffering from severe or clinically significant secondary PTSD, these recommendations are not meant to replace the need for individualized assessment and treatment). From a leadership perspective, reducing burnout and SPS requires willingness by management to engage authentically with staff and participate in interventions.[112]

CONCLUDING REMARKS

We recommend that SUD clinics screen for PTSD systematically. Considering the high lifetime prevalence of PTSD among patients with SUD, screening should be performed upon intake and repeated annually. Screening communicates awareness of and concern for the impacts of trauma. Screening stimulates clinical discussion and problem solving. Psychoeducational, symptom-regulating, and counter-shaming interventions can be used liberally and may improve treatment adherence and retention. Counter-shaming principles may also be used by clinic leadership in efforts to reduce risk for burnout, secondary PTSD, and turnover among clinicians and staff.[44,45]

CLINICS CARE POINTS

- Systematic use of a validated screening measure can help clinicians recognize, discuss, and initiate treatment of PTSD among patients with SUD.

- Basic psychoeducational and symptom reduction interventions can easily be incorporated into SUD-PTSD treatment.

- Hidden shame is readily identifiable and may be clinically significant. Counter-shaming interventions can be used broadly within the SUD clinic environment and may improve treatment adherence and retention.

- Clinic leadership may help reduce risk of burnout, secondary PTSD, and turnover among clinicians and nonclinical staff alike by using shame-alleviating principles targeted to enhance experiences of competency, autonomy, and relatedness.

ACKNOWLEDGMENTS

The authors would like to thank Dr Susan Wait for her comments on an early version of this article. Also, the authors would like to thank members of the nursing and social work teams at the University of Maryland Medical System and at the Trauma Disorders Program at Sheppard Pratt Hospital for their collegiality and guidance in many topics related to this work. The authors thank nursing staff members for sharing their views on and experiences of using shame-alleviating language through workshops and clinical discussions, and for exemplifying the high degree of trauma-responsive care that a devoted multidisciplinary team can offer (and achieve).

DISCLOSURE

The authors have nothing to disclose.

REFERENCES

1. Dube SR, Felitti VJ, Dong M, et al. Childhood abuse, neglect, and household dysfunction and the risk of illicit drug use: the adverse childhood experiences study. Pediatrics 2003;111(3):564–72.

2. Felitti VJ. Ursprünge des Suchtverhaltens: Evidenzen aus einer Studie zu belas-tenden Kindheitserfahrungen [Origins of addictive behavior: evidence from a study of stressful chilhood experiences]. Prax Kinderpsychol Kinderpsychiatr. 2003;52(8):547-59. German. PMID: 14619682.

3. Jacobsen LK, Southwick SM, Kosten TR. Substance Use Disorders in Patients With Posttraumatic Stress Disorder: A Review of the Literature. AJP 2001; 158(8):1184–90.

4. McCauley JL, Killeen T, Gros DF, et al. Posttraumatic Stress Disorder and Co-Occurring Substance Use Disorders: Advances in Assessment and Treatment. Clin Psychol (New York) 2012;19(3). https://doi.org/10.1111/cpsp.12006.

5. Saladin ME, Brady KT, Dansky BS, et al. Understanding comorbidity between PTSD and substance use disorders: two preliminary investigations. Addict Be-hav 1995;20(5):643–55.

6. Mills KL, Teesson M, Ross J, et al. Trauma, PTSD, and Substance Use Disor-ders: Findings From the Australian National Survey of Mental Health and Well-Being. AJP 2006;163(4):652–8.

7. Ouimette PC, Brown PJ, Najavits LM. Course and treatment of patients with both substance use and posttraumatic stress disorders. Addict Behav 1998;23(6): 785–95.

8. Ouimette P, Coolhart D, Funderburk JS, et al. Precipitants of first substance use in recently abstinent substance use disorder patients with PTSD. Addict Behav 2007;32(8):1719–27.

9. Gielen N, Havermans Remco C, Tekelenburg M, et al. Prevalence of post-traumatic stress disorder among patients with substance use disorder: it is higher than clinicians think it is. Eur J Psychotraumatology 2012;3(1):17734.

10. Chilcoat HD, Breslau N. Investigations of causal pathways between PTSD and drug use disorders. Addict Behav 1998;23(6):827–40.

11. Anda RF, Felitti VJ, Bremner JD, et al. The enduring effects of abuse and related adverse experiences in childhood: A convergence of evidence from neurobi-ology and epidemiology. Eur Arch Psychiatry Clin Neurosci 2006;256(3):174–86.

12. Khantzian EJ. The Self-Medication Hypothesis of Substance Use Disorders: A Reconsideration and Recent Applications. Harv Rev Psychiatry 1997;4(5): 231–44.

13. Alexander AA, Welsh E, Glassmire DM. Underdiagnosing Posttraumatic Stress Disorder in a State Hospital. J Forensic Psychol Pract 2016;16(5):448–59.

14. da Silva HC, Furtado da Rosa MM, Berger W, et al. PTSD in mental health outpa-tient settings: highly prevalent and under-recognized. Braz J Psychiatry 2018; 41:213–7.

15. Mueser KT, Goodman LB, Trumbetta SL, et al. Trauma and posttraumatic stress disorder in severe mental illness. J Consult Clin Psychol 1998;66(3):493–9.

16. Zanville HA, Cattaneo LB. Underdiagnosing and nontreatment of posttraumatic stress disorder in community mental health: A case study. Psychol Serv 2009; 6(1):32–42.

17. Bowman S, Eiserman J, Beletsky L, et al. Reducing the Health Consequences of Opioid Addiction in Primary Care. Am J Med 2013;126(7):565–71.

18. Hilton NZ, McKee SA, Ham E, et al. Co-Occurring Mental Illness and Substance Use Disorders in Canadian Forensic Inpatients: Underdiagnosis and Implica-tions for Treatment Planning. Int J Forensic Ment Health 2018;17(2):145–53.

19. Candea D, Szentagotai A. Shame and psychopathology: From research to clin-ical practice. J Cogn Behav psychotherapies 2013;13(1):101–13.

20. Herman JL. Posttraumatic stress disorder as a shame disorder. In: Dearing RL, Tangney JP, editors. Shame in the therapy hour. Washington, DC: American Psychological Association; 2011. p. 261–75.

21. Holl J, Wolff S, Schumacher M, et al. Substance use to regulate intense posttraumatic shame in individuals with childhood abuse and neglect. Dev Psychopathol 2017;29(3):737–49.

22. Luoma JB, Chwyl C, Kaplan J. Substance use and shame: A systematic and meta-analytic review. Clin Psychol Rev 2019;70:1–12.

23. Saraiya T, Lopez-Castro T. Ashamed and Afraid: A Scoping Review of the Role of Shame in Post-Traumatic Stress Disorder (PTSD). J Clin Med 2016;5(11):94.

24. Nathanson DL. Shame and pride: affect, sex, and the birth of the self. New York, NY: W. W. Norton & Company; 1992.

25. Schalkwijk F, Stams GJ, Dekker J, et al. Measuring shame regulation: Validation of the Compass of Shame Scale. Soc Behav Pers 2016;44(11):1775–91.

26. Lickel B, Kushlev K, Savalei V, et al. Shame and the motivation to change the self. Emotion 2014;14(6):1049–61.

27. Olatunji BO, Ciesielski BG, Tolin DF. Fear and loathing: a meta-analytic review of the specificity of anger in PTSD. Behav Ther 2010;41(1):93–105.

28. Young DA, Neylan TC, Zhang H, et al. Impulsivity as a multifactorial construct and its relationship to PTSD severity and threat sensitivity. Psychiatry Res 2020;293:113468.

29. Frewen PA, Dozois DJA, Neufeld RWJ, et al. Meta-analysis of alexithymia in posttraumatic stress disorder. J Trauma Stress 2008;21(2):243–6.

30. Maercker A. Development of the new CPTSD diagnosis for ICD-11. Bord Personal Disord Emot Dysregul 2021;8(1):7.

31. World Health Organization. ICD-11: International Classification of diseases (11th revision). 2019. Available at: https://icd.who.int/. Accessed Februrary 1, 2022.

32. Felitti VJ, Anda RF, Nordenberg D, et al. Relationship of childhood abuse and household dysfunction to many of the leading causes of death in adults: The Adverse Childhood Experiences (ACE) Study. Am J Prev Med 1998;14(4): 245–58.

33. Campbell JA, Walker RJ, Egede LE. Associations Between Adverse Childhood Experiences, High-Risk Behaviors, and Morbidity in Adulthood. Am J Prev Med 2016;50(3):344–52.

34. Chang X, Jiang X, Mkandarwire T, et al. Associations between adverse childhood experiences and health outcomes in adults aged 18-59 years. PLoS One 2019;14(2):e0211850.

35. Afifi TO, Henriksen CA, Asmundson GJG, et al. Childhood maltreatment and substance use disorders among men and women in a nationally representative sample. Can J Psychiatry 2012;57(11):677–86.

36. Pratchett LC, Yehuda R. Foundations of posttraumatic stress disorder: does early life trauma lead to adult posttraumatic stress disorder? Dev Psychopathol 2011;23(2):477–91.

37. Mergler M, Driessen M, Havemann-Reinecke U, et al. Differential relationships of PTSD and childhood trauma with the course of substance use disorders. J Subst Abuse Treat 2018;93:57–63.

38. Fitzpatrick S, Saraiya T, Lopez-Castro T, et al. The impact of trauma characteristics on post-traumatic stress disorder and substance use disorder outcomes across integrated and substance use treatments. J Subst Abuse Treat 2020; 113:107976.

39. Reynolds M, Mezey G, Chapman M, et al. Co-morbid post-traumatic stress disorder in a substance misusing clinical population. Drug Alcohol Depend 2005; 77(3):251–8.
40. Pietrzak RH, Goldstein RB, Southwick SM, et al. Prevalence and Axis I comorbidity of full and partial posttraumatic stress disorder in the United States: results from Wave 2 of the National Epidemiologic Survey on Alcohol and Related Conditions. J Anxiety Disord 2011;25(3):456–65.
41. Goytan A, Lee W, Dong H, et al. The impact of PSTD on service access among people who use drugs in Vancouver, Canada. Subst Abuse Treat Prev Policy 2021;16(1):53.
42. Pitman RK, Rasmusson AM, Koenen KC, et al. Biological studies of post-traumatic stress disorder. Nat Rev Neurosci 2012;13(11):769–87.
43. Koob GF, Volkow ND. Neurobiology of addiction: a neurocircuitry analysis. Lancet Psychiatry 2016;3(8):760–73.
44. Gagné M, Deci EL. Self-determination theory and work motivation. J Organizational Behav 2005;26(4):331–62.
45. Hartzband P, Groopman J. Physician Burnout, Interrupted. N Engl J Med 2020; 382(26):2485–7.
46. Fontenelle LF, de Oliveira-Souza R, Moll J. The rise of moral emotions in neuropsychiatry. Dialogues Clin Neurosci 2015;17(4):411–20.
47. Michl P, Meindl T, Meister F, et al. Neurobiological underpinnings of shame and guilt: a pilot fMRI study. Soc Cogn Affect Neurosci 2014;9(2):150–7.
48. Roth L, Kaffenberger T, Herwig U, et al. Brain Activation Associated with Pride and Shame. Neuropsychobiology 2014;69(2):95–106.
49. Abrams D, Niaura R. Social learning theory of alcohol use and abuse. In: Blanc HT, Leonard KE, editors. Psychological theories of drinking and alcoholism. New York, NY: Guilford Press; 1987. p. 131–78.
50. Alvarez-Monjaras M, Mayes LC, Potenza MN, et al. A developmental model of addictions: Integrating neurobiological and psychodynamic theories through the lens of attachment. Attach Hum Dev 2019;21(6):616–37.
51. Saloner B, McGinty EE, Beletsky L, et al. A Public Health Strategy for the Opioid Crisis. Public Health Rep 2018;133(1_suppl):24S–34S.
52. Volkow ND, Koob GF, McLellan AT. Neurobiologic Advances from the Brain Disease Model of Addiction. N Engl J Med 2016;374(4):363–71.
53. Rundle SM, Cunningham JA, Hendershot CS. Implications of addiction diagnosis and addiction beliefs for public stigma: A cross-national experimental study. Drug Alcohol Rev 2021;40(5):842–6.
54. Goffman E. The presentation of self in everyday life. 1st edition. New York, NY: Anchor Books, Doubleday; 1959.
55. Committee on the Science of Changing Behavioral Health Social Norms, Board on Behavioral, Cognitive, and Sensory Sciences, Division of Behavioral and Social Sciences and Education, National Academies of Sciences, Engineering, and Medicine. Ending discrimination against people with mental and substance Use disorders: the evidence for stigma change. Washington, DC: National Academies Press; 2016. Available at: http://www.ncbi.nlm.nih.gov/books/NBK384915/. Accessed April 23, 2021.
56. Bonfils KA, Lysaker PH, Yanos PT, et al. Self-stigma in PTSD: Prevalence and correlates. Psychiatry Res 2018;265:7–12.
57. Tsai AC, Kiang MV, Barnett ML, et al. Stigma as a fundamental hindrance to the United States opioid overdose crisis response. PLOS Med 2019;16(11): e1002969.

58. Livingston JD, Milne T, Fang ML, et al. The effectiveness of interventions for reducing stigma related to substance use disorders: a systematic review. Addiction 2012;107(1):39–50.
59. Wood L, Birtel M, Alsawy S, et al. Public perceptions of stigma towards people with schizophrenia, depression, and anxiety. Psychiatry Res 2014;220(1–2): 604–8.
60. Elison J, Garofalo C, Velotti P. Shame and aggression: Theoretical considerations. Aggression Violent Behav 2014;19(4):447–53.
61. Kulesza M, Hunter SB, Shearer AL, et al. Relationship between Provider Stigma and Predictors of Staff Turnover among Addiction Treatment Providers. Alcohol Treat Q 2017;35(1):63–70.
62. Zgierska AE, Miller MM, Rabago DP, et al. Language Matters: It Is Time We Change How We Talk About Addiction and its Treatment. J Addict Med 2021; 15(1):10–2.
63. Ford JD, Hawke J, Alessi S, et al. Psychological trauma and PTSD symptoms as predictors of substance dependence treatment outcomes. Behav Res Ther 2007;45(10):2417–31.
64. Hien DA, Nunes E, Levin FR, et al. Posttraumatic stress disorder and short-term outcome in early methadone treatment. J Subst Abuse Treat 2000;19(1):31–7.
65. Najavits LM, Harned MS, Gallop RJ, et al. Six-Month Treatment Outcomes of Cocaine-Dependent Patients With and Without PTSD in a Multisite National Trial. J Stud Alcohol Drugs 2015. https://doi.org/10.15288/jsad.2007.68.353.
66. Prins A, Bovin MJ, Smolenski DJ, et al. The Primary Care PTSD Screen for DSM-5 (PC-PTSD-5): Development and Evaluation Within a Veteran Primary Care Sample. J Gen Intern Med 2016;31(10):1206–11.
67. Davis SM, Whitworth JD, Rickett K. What are the most practical primary care screens for post-traumatic stress disorder? J Fam Pract 2009;58(2):100–2.
68. Kimerling R, Ouimette P, Prins A, et al. BRIEF REPORT: Utility of a Short Screening Scale for DSM-IV PTSD in Primary Care. J Gen Intern Med 2006; 21(1):65–7.
69. Connor KM, Davidson JRT. SPRINT: a brief global assessment of post-traumatic stress disorder. Int Clin Psychopharmacol 2001;16(5):279–84.
70. Blevins CA, Weathers FW, Davis MT, et al. The Posttraumatic Stress Disorder Checklist for DSM-5 (PCL-5): Development and Initial Psychometric Evaluation. J Trauma Stress 2015;28(6):489–98.
71. Bovin MJ, Marx BP, Weathers FW, et al. Psychometric properties of the PTSD Checklist for Diagnostic and Statistical Manual of Mental Disorders-Fifth Edition (PCL-5) in veterans. Psychol Assess 2016;28(11):1379–91.
72. Weathers FW, Bovin MJ, Lee DJ, et al. The Clinician-Administered PTSD Scale for DSM-5 (CAPS-5): Development and initial psychometric evaluation in military veterans. Psychol Assess 2018;30(3):383.
73. Carlson EB, Putnam FW. An update on the Dissociative Experiences Scale. Dissociation: Prog Dissociative Disord 1993;6(1):16–27.
74. Najavits L, Walsh M. Dissociation, PTSD, and Substance Abuse: An Empirical Study. J Trauma Dissociation 2012;13(1):115–26.
75. Briere J, Weathers FW, Runtz M. Is dissociation a multidimensional construct? Data from the Multiscale Dissociation Inventory. J Traumatic Stress 2005; 18(3):221–31.
76. Hooper LM, Stockton P, Krupnick JL, et al. Development, use, and psychometric properties of the Trauma History Questionnaire. J Loss Trauma 2011;16(3): 258–83.

77. Najavits LM, Clark HW, DiClemente CC, et al. PTSD/Substance Use Disorder Comorbidity: Treatment Options and Public Health Needs. Curr Treat Options Psych 2020;7(4):544–58.
78. Najavits LM. Seeking safety: a treatment manual for PTSD and substance abuse. New York, NY: Guilford Publications; 2002.
79. Carletto S, Oliva F, Barnato M, et al. EMDR as Add-On Treatment for Psychiatric and Traumatic Symptoms in Patients with Substance Use Disorder. Front Psychol 2018;8:2333.
80. Kaysen D, Schumm J, Pedersen ER, et al. Cognitive Processing Therapy for veterans with comorbid PTSD and alcohol use disorders. Addict Behav 2014;39(2): 420–7.
81. Peirce JM, Schacht RL, Brooner RK. The Effects of Prolonged Exposure on Substance Use in Patients With Posttraumatic Stress Disorder and Substance Use Disorders. J Traumatic Stress 2020;33(4):465–76.
82. Roos C, Bowen S, Witkiewitz K. Approach coping and substance use outcomes following mindfulness-based relapse prevention among individuals with negative affect symptomatology. Mindfulness 2020;11(10):2397–410.
83. Vrana C, Killeen T, Brant V, et al. Rationale, design, and implementation of a clinical trial of a mindfulness-based relapse prevention protocol for the treatment of women with comorbid post traumatic stress disorder and substance use disorder. Contemp Clin Trials 2017;61:108–14.
84. Polusny MA, Erbes CR, Thuras P, et al. Mindfulness-Based Stress Reduction for Posttraumatic Stress Disorder Among Veterans: A Randomized Clinical Trial. JAMA 2015;314(5):456.
85. Berghoff CR, Tull MT. Third-wave behavioral therapies for the co-occurrence of PTSD and substance use disorders. In: Vujanavic AA, Back SE, editors. Posttraumatic stress and substance use disorders. New York, NY: Routledge; 2019.
86. Hermann BA, Meyer EC, Schnurr PP, et al. Acceptance and commitment therapy for co-occurring PTSD and substance use: A manual development study. J Contextual Behav Sci 2016;5(4):225–34.
87. Luoma JB, Kohlenberg BS, Hayes SC, et al. Slow and Steady Wins the Race: A Randomized Clinical Trial of Acceptance and Commitment Therapy Targeting Shame in Substance Use Disorders. J Consult Clin Psychol 2012;80(1):43–53.
88. Krejci J, Margolin J, Rowland M, et al. Integrated Group Treatment of Women's Substance Abuse and Trauma. J Groups Addict Recovery 2008;3(3–4):263–83.
89. Najavits LM. The problem of dropout from "gold standard" PTSD therapies. F1000prime Rep 2015;7:43.
90. Herman JL. Trauma and recovery: from domestic abuse to political terror. New York, NY: Basic Books; 1992.
91. Prochaska JO, DiClemente CC. Stages and processes of self-change of smoking: Toward an integrative model of change. J Consult Clin Psychol 1983;51(3): 390–5.
92. Cloitre M, Courtois CA, Ford JD, et al. The ISTSS expert consensus treatment guidelines for complex PTSD in adults. 2012. Available at: www.istss.org/ISTSS_Main/media/Documents/ISTSS-Expert-Concesnsus-Guidelines-for-Complex-PTSD-Updated-060315.pdf. Accessed January 10, 2020.
93. International Society for the Study of Trauma and Dissociation. Guidelines for treating dissociative identity disorder in adults, third revision: Summary version. J Trauma Dissociation 2011;12(2):188–212.
94. Dondanville KA, Fina BA, Straud CL, et al. Launching a Competency-Based Training Program in Evidence-Based Treatments for PTSD: Supporting

Veteran-Serving Mental Health Providers in Texas. Community Ment Health J 2021;57(5):910–9.

95. Harris R. Trauma-focused ACT: a practitioner's guide to working with mind, Body, and emotion using acceptance and commitment therapy. Oakland, CA: New Harbinger Publications; 2021.

96. Carlson EA. A Prospective Longitudinal Study of Attachment Disorganization/ Disorientation. Child Dev 1998;69(4):1107–28.

97. Lyons-Ruth K. Contributions of the mother–infant relationship to dissociative, borderline, and conduct symptoms in young adulthood. Infant Ment Health J 2008;29(3):203–18.

98. Gutheil TG, Simon RI. Between the Chair and the Door: Boundary Issues in the Therapeutic "Transition Zone. Harv Rev Psychiatry 1995;2(6):336–40.

99. Whitworth JD. The Role of Psychoeducation in Trauma Recovery: Recommendations for Content and Delivery. J Evidence-Informed Social Work 2016;13(5): 442–51.

100. Resick PA, Monson CM, Chard KM. Cognitive processing therapy for PTSD: a comprehensive manual. New York, NY: Guilford Press; 2017.

101. Foa E, Hembree EA, Rauch S, et al. Prolonged exposure therapy for PTSD: emotional processing of traumatic experiences - therapist guide. New York, NY: Oxford University Press; 2019.

102. Brem MJ, Shorey RC, Anderson S, et al. Dispositional Mindfulness, Shame, and Compulsive Sexual Behaviors Among Men in Residential Treatment for Substance Use Disorders. Mindfulness 2017;8(6):1552–8.

103. Talbot NL. Women sexually abused as children: The centrality of shame issues and treatment implications. Psychotherapy: Theor Res Pract Train 1996; 33(1):11.

104. Assed MM, Khafif TC, Belizario GO, et al. Facial Emotion Recognition in Maltreated Children: A Systematic Review. J Child Fam Stud 2020;29(5):1493–509.

105. Leiter MP, Maslach C. Interventions to prevent and alleviate burnout. In: Cooper C, editor. Current issues in work and Organizational Psychology. New York: Routledge; 2018. p. 32–50.

106. Huggard P, Law J, Newcombe D. A systematic review exploring the presence of Vicarious Trauma, Compassion Fatigue, and Secondary Traumatic Stress in Alcohol and Other Drug Clinicians. Australas J Disaster Trauma Stud 2017;21(2).

107. Dalenberg CJ. Countertransference and the treatment of trauma. Washington, DC: American Psychological Association; 2000.

108. Kluft RP. Countertransference in the treatment of multiple personality disorder. Countertransference in the treatment of PTSD. Published online 1994;122–50.

109. Salyers MP, Bonfils KA, Luther L, et al. The Relationship Between Professional Burnout and Quality and Safety in Healthcare: A Meta-Analysis. J Gen Intern Med 2017;32(4):475–82.

110. Willard-Grace R, Knox M, Huang B, et al. Burnout and Health Care Workforce Turnover. Ann Fam Med 2019;17(1):36–41.

111. Oser CB, Biebel EP, Pullen E, et al. Causes, Consequences, and Prevention of Burnout Among Substance Abuse Treatment Counselors: A Rural Versus Urban Comparison. J Psychoactive Drugs 2013;45(1):17–27.

112. McNulty TL, Oser CB, Aaron Johnson J, et al. Counselor Turnover in Substance Abuse Treatment Centers: An Organizational-Level Analysis. Sociological Inq 2007;77(2):166–93.

113. Gabbard GO. An overview of countertransference with borderline patients. J psychotherapy Pract Res 1993;2(1):7.

114. Silver D. Psychotherapy of the Characterologically Difficult Patient. Can J Psychiatry 1983;28(7):513–21.

115. Gutheil TG. Issues in civil sexual misconduct litigation. Physician Sex misconduct 1999;3–17.

116. Spero SJ, Cohen PL. Boundary violations and malpractice litigation. Psychiatr Times 2008;25(4).

117. Simon RI. The natural history of therapist sexual misconduct: Identification and prevention. Psychiatr Ann 1995;25(2):90–4.

118. Stein MB, Koverola C, Hanna C, et al. Hippocampal volume in women victimized by childhood sexual abuse. Psychol Med 1997;27(4):951–9. https://doi.org/10.1017/S0033291797005242.

119. Vythilingam M, Heim C, Newport J, et al. Childhood trauma associated with smaller hippocampal volume in women with major depression. Am J Psychiatry 2002;159(12):2072–80. https://doi.org/10.1176/appi.ajp.159.12.2072.

120. Driessen M, Herrmann J, Stahl K, et al. Magnetic resonance imaging volumes of the hippocampus and the amygdala in women with borderline personality disorder and early traumatization. Arch Gen Psychiatry 2000;57(12):1115–22. https://doi.org/10.1001/archpsyc.57.12.1115.

121. Smith ME. Bilateral hippocampal volume reduction in adults with post-traumatic stress disorder: A meta-analysis of structural MRI studies. Hippocampus 2005;15(6):798–807. https://doi.org/10.1002/hipo.20102.

122. Schuff N, Neylan TC, Fox-Bosetti S, et al. Abnormal N-acetylaspartate in hippocampus and anterior cingulate in posttraumatic stress disorder. Psychiatry Res 2008;162(2):147–57. https://doi.org/10.1016/j.pscychresns.2007.04.011.

123. Grace S, Rossetti MG, Allen N, et al. Sex differences in the neuroanatomy of alcohol dependence: hippocampus and amygdala subregions in a sample of 966 people from the ENIGMA Addiction Working Group. Transl Psychiatry 2021;11:156. https://doi.org/10.1038/s41398-021-01204-1.

124. Bittencourt AML, Bampi VF, Sommer RC, et al. Cortical thickness and subcortical volume abnormalities in male crack-cocaine users. Psychiatry Res Neuroimaging 2021;310:111232. https://doi.org/10.1016/j.pscychresns.2020.111232.

125. Nie L, Ghahremani DG, Mandelkern MA, et al. The relationship between duration of abstinence and gray-matter brain structure in chronic methamphetamine users. Am J Drug Alcohol Abuse 2021;47(1):65–73. https://doi.org/10.1080/00952990.2020.1778712.

126. Kasai K, Yamasue H, Gilbertson MW, et al. Evidence for acquired pregenual anterior cingulate gray matter loss from a twin study of combat-related posttraumatic stress disorder. Biol Psychiatry 2008;63(6):550–6. https://doi.org/10.1016/j.biopsych.2007.06.022.

127. Shin LM, McNally RJ, Kosslyn SM, et al. Regional cerebral blood flow during script-driven imagery in childhood sexual abuse-related PTSD: a PET investigation. Am J Psychiatry 1999;156(4):575–84. https://doi.org/10.1176/ajp.156.4.575.

128. Gold AL, Shin LM, Orr SP, et al. Decreased regional cerebral blood flow in medial prefrontal cortex during trauma-unrelated stressful imagery in Vietnam veterans with post-traumatic stress disorder. Psychol Med 2011;41(12):2563–72. https://doi.org/10.1017/S0033291711000730.

129. Liu X, Matochik JA, Cadet JL, et al. Smaller volume of prefrontal lobe in polysubstance abusers: a magnetic resonance imaging study. Neuropsychopharmacology 1998;18(4):243–52. https://doi.org/10.1016/S0893-133X(97)00143-7.

130. Volkow ND, Mullani N, Gould KL, et al. Cerebral blood flow in chronic cocaine users: a study with positron emission tomography. Br J Psychiatry 1988;152: 641–8. https://doi.org/10.1192/bjp.152.5.641.

131. Volkow ND, Hitzemann R, Wang GJ, et al. Long-term frontal brain metabolic changes in cocaine abusers. Synapse 1992;11(3):184–90. https://doi.org/10.1002/syn.890110303.

132. Kitayama N, Quinn S, Bremner JD. Smaller volume of anterior cingulate cortex in abuse-elated posttraumatic stress disorder. J Affect Disord 2006;90(2-3):171–4. https://doi.org/10.1016/j.jad.2005.11.006.

133. Woodward SH, Kaloupek DG, Streeter CC, et al. Decreased anterior cingulate volume in combat-related PTSD. Biol Psychiatry 2006;59(7):582–7. https://doi.org/10.1016/j.biopsych.2005.07.033.

134. Shin LM, Whalen PJ, Pitman RK, et al. An fMRI study of anterior cingulate function in posttraumatic stress disorder. Biol Psychiatry 2001;50(12):932–42. https://doi.org/10.1016/S0006-3223(01)01215-X.

135. Ersche KD, Barnes A, Simon Jones P, et al. Abnormal structure of frontostriatal brain systems is associated with aspects of impulsivity and compulsivity in cocaine dependence. Brain 2011;134(7):2013–24. https://doi.org/10.1093/brain/awr138.

136. Stark EA, Parsons CE, Van Hartevelt TJ, et al. Post-traumatic stress influences the brain even in the absence of symptoms: A systematic, quantitative meta-analysis of neuroimaging studies. Neurosci Biobehav Rev 2015;56:207–21. https://doi.org/10.1016/j.neubiorev.2015.07.007.

137. Lee MS, Anumagalla P, Pavuluri MN. Individuals with the post-traumatic stress disorder process emotions in subcortical regions irrespective of cognitive engagement: a meta-analysis of cognitive and emotional interface. Brain Imaging Behav 2021;15(2):941–57. https://doi.org/10.1007/s11682-020-00303-9.

138. Volkow ND, Wang GJ, Fowler JS, et al. Decreased striatal dopaminergic responsiveness in detoxified cocaine-dependent subjects. Nature 1997;386(6627): 830–3. https://doi.org/10.1038/386830a0.

139. Wang GJ, Volkow ND, Fowler JS, et al. Dopamine D2 receptor availability in opiate-dependent subjects before and after naloxone-precipitated withdrawal. Neuropsychopharmacology 1997;16(2):174–82. https://doi.org/10.1016/S0893-133X(96)00184-4.

140. Simmons AN, Paulus MP, Thorp SR, et al. Functional activation and neural networks in women with posttraumatic stress disorder related to intimate partner violence. Biol Psychiatry 2008;64(8):681–90. https://doi.org/10.1016/j.biopsych.2008.05.027.

141. Aupperle RL, Allard CB, Grimes EM, et al. Dorsolateral prefrontal cortex activation during emotional anticipation and neuropsychological performance in posttraumatic stress disorder. Arch Gen Psychiatry 2012;69(4):360–71. https://doi.org/10.1001/archgenpsychiatry.2011.1539.

142. Naqvi NH, Rudrauf D, Damasio H, et al. Damage to the insula disrupts addiction to cigarette smoking. Science 2007;315(5811):531–4. https://doi.org/10.1126/science.1135926.

143. Kilts CD, Schweitzer JB, Quinn CK, et al. Neural activity related to drug craving in cocaine addiction. Arch Gen Psychiatry 2001;58(4):334–41. https://doi.org/10.1001/archpsyc.58.4.334.

144. Sell LA, Morris J, Bearn J, et al. Activation of reward circuitry in human opiate addicts. Eur J Neurosci 1999;11(3):1042–8. https://doi.org/10.1046/j.1460-9568.1999.00522.x.

145. Lang AJ, Stein MB. An abbreviated PTSD checklist for use as a screening instrument in primary care. Behav Res Ther 2005;43(5):585–94. https://doi.org/10.1016/j.brat.2004.04.005.

146. Breslau N, Peterson EL, Kessler RC, et al. Short screening scale for DSM-IV posttraumatic stress disorder. Am J Psychiatry 1999;156(6):908–11. https://doi.org/10.1176/ajp.156.6.908.

147. Foa EB, McLean CP, Zang Y, et al. Psychometric properties of the posttraumatic diagnostic scale for DSM-5 (PDS-5). Psychol Assess 2016;28(10):1166–71. https://doi.org/10.1037/pas0000258.

Kratom: Substance of Abuse or Therapeutic Plant?

David A. Gorelick, MD, PhD, DLFAPA, FASAM

KEYWORDS

- Kratom • Mitragynine • 7-Hydroxymitragynine • Opioid receptor • Analgesia
- Biased agonist • Withdrawal

KEY POINTS

- An estimated 2.1 million US residents used kratom in 2020.
- Kratom has stimulant-like effects at low doses and opioid-like effects at higher doses.
- Daily, high-dose use can lead to physical dependence and kratom use disorder.
- Buprenorphine can be useful in treating kratom withdrawal and kratom use disorder.
- Kratom is proposed as having therapeutic benefits but this has not been evaluated in controlled clinical trials.

INTRODUCTION

Kratom (pronounced krah-tm) is the common term for the *Mitragyna speciosa* tree and products derived from it. *M speciosa* is native to Southeast Asia from Myanmar to the Philippines. The indigenous population has used kratom products, especially the leaves, for centuries as an herbal medicine, to increase energy and reduce fatigue and recreationally to enhance sociability and sexual desire.[1,2] The first documented use of kratom in the United States occurred around 2000.[3] Over the past two decades, use of processed and concentrated kratom products has expanded in North America and Western Europe, as a "legal high" and to self-medicate pain, opioid withdrawal, and other conditions.[2] Reports of medically serious toxicity and death due to kratom use and of users developing a kratom use disorder generated interest in legally restricting or banning kratom availability.

This article reviews current knowledge of the epidemiology and pharmacology of kratom and identifies gaps in our knowledge. The aim is to inform discussion on the benefits and harms of kratom and its appropriate legal status. We also review the relatively meager knowledge of the diagnosis and treatment of kratom-related disorders: intoxication/overdose, withdrawal, and kratom use disorder.

Department of Psychiatry, University of Maryland School of Medicine, PO Box 21247, MPRC—Tawes Building, Baltimore, MD 21228, USA
E-mail address: dgorelick@som.umaryland.edu

Psychiatr Clin N Am 45 (2022) 415–430
https://doi.org/10.1016/j.psc.2022.04.002
0193-953X/22/© 2022 Elsevier Inc. All rights reserved.

psych.theclinics.com

EPIDEMIOLOGY

The true prevalence of kratom use and misuse remains unclear. Kratom was only recently included in nationally representative, population-based epidemiologic surveys of psychoactive substance use. Data from the most recent surveys in Thailand (2015) and the United States (2020) are presented in **Table 1**. The prevalence of lifetime and current kratom use is about eight and three times greater, respectively, in Thailand than in the United States. Adults are at least twice as likely to use kratom as are adolescents in both Thailand[6] and the United States.[4] The 2020 US National Survey on Drug Use and Health (NSDUH) estimated that almost 5 million community-dwelling US residents used kratom in their lifetime, 2.1 million used during the past year, and 1 million used during the past month.[4] Past-month kratom use is most prevalent among those 26 years or older (0.4%) and least prevalent among adolescents (0.1%) (based on 2019 NSDUH).[7] Past-year kratom use is significantly less prevalent among women than men (adjusted odds ratio 0.70, 95% CI 0.51–0.97) and significantly less prevalent among non-Hispanic Blacks (adjusted odds ratio 0.27 [95% CI 0.15–0.47]) and Hispanics (adjusted odds ratio 0.39 [0.26–0.59]).[7]

Kratom users commonly use other psychoactive substances. The 2019 US NSDUH found current (past-year) kratom use significantly associated with the use of cannabis (adjusted odds ratio 4.57 [95% CI 3.29–6.35]), cocaine (adjusted odds ratio 1.69 [95% CI 1.06–2.69]), nonmedical use of prescription stimulants (adjusted odds ratio 2.10 [95% CI 1.44–3.05]), and prescription opioid use disorder (adjusted odds ratio 3.20 [95% CI 1.38–7.41]).[7] Opioid use, per se, was not associated with kratom use. Anonymous, online surveys of self-selected adult US current kratom users find that one-quarter to one-half are also current users of tobacco, alcohol, cannabis, or opioids (either illicit or prescribed), whereas less than 6% use cocaine or hallucinogens.[8,9]

PRECLINICAL PHARMACOLOGY

The kratom leaf contains at least 54 alkaloids as well as terpenes, flavonoids, and polyphenols.[10] Only two of these alkaloids have been well studied: mitragynine and 7-hydroxymitragynine. These two indole alkaloids comprise about two-thirds and 1%, respectively, of total alkaloids in the kratom leaf. The 7-hydroxymitragynine is also produced by the *in vivo* metabolism of mitragynine. A related indole alkaloid, mitragynine pseudoindoxyl, is not found in the plant but is an *in vivo* metabolite of mitragynine. Mitragynine and 7-hydroxymitragyine are considered to produce the major pharmacologic actions of kratom.[11,12]

Kratom extracts, mitragynine, and 7-hydroxymitragynine have a variety of opioid-like effects in animals, with almost all studies conducted in rodents.[13] The most consistently observed effects are analgesia, suppression of opioid withdrawal, and inhibition of gastrointestinal motility.

The analgesic effect of kratom extract and kratom alkaloids is blocked by pretreatment with mu-opioid receptor (mOR) antagonists[14] and does not occur in knock-out mice lacking the mOR,[15] suggesting an mOR receptor activation mechanism of action. The relative analgesic potency of kratom alkaloids versus conventional opioids is uncertain because few studies have compared the two using the same route of administration over a range of doses to establish equipotent doses. Oral mitragyine was about six times less potent than oral oxycodone in one rat study, that is, 100 mg/kg had the same analgesic effect as 6 mg/kg of oxycodone.[16]

Kratom extracts and mitragynine have inconsistent effects on locomotor activity in rodents, that is, neither consistently stimulant-like nor opioid-like.[17–19]

Table 1
Prevalence of kratom use in recent nationally representative, population-based epidemiologic surveys in Thailand and the United States

Country	Year	No. of Respondents	Respondent Age (years)	Product	Lifetime	Past Year	Past Month
United States[4]	2020	36,284	≥12	Kratom	1.9 (0.12)	0.8 (0.08)	0.4 (0.06)
Thailand[5]	2016	30,411	15–64	Kratom leaves	15.1 (14.7, 15.5)	2.1 (1.9, 2.3)	1.4 (1.3, 1.5)
"	"	"	"	Kratom cocktail	14.5 (14.1, 14.9)	0.7 (0.6, 0.8)	0.4 (0.3, 0.5)

Prevalence = % of community-dwelling population—(standard error) for the United States, (95% CI) for Thailand.
Overlap between use of kratom leaves and kratom cocktail not presented.
Kratom = any kratom product; kratom cocktail = water from boiled leaves + carbonated sugared beverage.

Receptor Mechanisms

The pharmacologic actions of mitragynine, 7-hydroxymitragynine, and mitragynine pseudoindoxyl are primarily due to their activation of mORs.[11,12,20,21] They act as partial agonists at the mOR, with less activity than does morphine, which is a full agonist. 7-Hydroxmitragynine has substantially more binding affinity and intrinsic activity (receptor activation) at the mOR than does mitragynine but less than does morphine (**Tables 2** and **3**). Unlike conventional opioid agonists such as morphine, mitragynine and 7-hydroxymitragynine are biased mOR agonists.[12] This means that they activate the G-protein-coupled intracellular pathway but produce little or no activation of the β-arrestin intracellular pathway. This differential activation may confer selectivity in producing beneficial effects such as analgesia (mediated by the G-protein-coupled pathway) while minimizing adverse effects such as respiratory depression or physical dependence (mediated by the β-arrestin pathway) (see the section below on therapeutic potential).

Mitragynine and 7-hydroxymitragyine act at other receptors as well. They are competitive antagonists at the kappa- and delta-opioid receptors, but with lesser potency than at the mOR (see **Tables 2** and **3**). Mitragynine binds to alpha 1-and alpha 2 adrenergic receptors, serotonin-1A and -2A receptors, and the dopamine D1 receptor.[22,23] The functional significance of such binding is unclear.

CLINICAL PHARMACOLOGY

Little is known about the pharmacodynamics and pharmacokinetics of kratom in humans. Almost all information comes from retrospective self-report surveys of self-selected or convenience samples of adult kratom users. We are aware of only three published studies of controlled kratom administration to humans (**Table 4**). Kratom increased pain tolerance and caused a variety of mild, transient signs and symptoms, such as tremor, nystagmus, pupil constriction, tongue numbness, lightheadedness, facial flushing, and nausea.[24–26] There were no clinically significant changes in vital signs.

A 2017 anonymous online survey of a self-selected sample of 2798 US adult kratom users were administered the Drug Effects Questionnaire, a standard instrument for self-rating subjective effects of psychoactive substances.[8] Respondents gave the

Table 2
Major kratom alkaloid binding affinity at opioid receptors (relative to mitragynine)

Alkaloid	Present in Kratom Leaf	μ-Opioid	δ-Opioid	κ-Opioid
Mitragynine	Yes	1	1	1
7-OH-mitragynine	Yes	5–20	11–80	2–10
Mitragynine pseudoindoxyl	No	300	300	10
Morphine	No	50–150	>50	10–30
Buprenorphine	No	200	>1000	700–1000

Notes: Receptor binding affinities measured in vitro with human or rodent opioid receptors. See sources for detailed methods.
Data from Todd DA, Kellogg JJ, Wallace ED, et al. Chemical composition and biological effects of kratom (Mitragyna peciose): In vitro studies with implications for efficacy and drug interactions. Sci Rep 2020;10:19158.; Obeng S, Wilkerson JL, Leon F, et al. Pharmacological comparison of mitragynine and 7-hydroxymitragynine: In vitro affinity and efficacy for μ-opioid and opioid-like behavioral effects on rats. J Pharmacol Exp Ther 2021;376:410-427; Varadi A, Marrone GF, Palmer TC, et al. Mitragynine/corynantheidine pseudoindoxyls as opioid analgesics with mu agonism and delta antagonism, which do not recruit β-arrestin-2. J Med Chem 2016;59:8381-8397.

highest ratings for their typical kratom experience to "good effects," "drug liking," "alert," "stimulated," "desire," "euphoric," and "sleepy." Ratings were much lower for "high," "bad effects," "sick," "dizzy," and "anxious."

Two human studies evaluated the pharmacokinetics of mitragynine after administration of liquid formulations of kratom (tea, decoction). The time to reach peak mitragynine blood concentration was 0.83 ± 0.35 hours[25] or 2.0 ± 0.8 hours.[26] In the study that varied the mitragynine dose (6–20 mg), there was a significant positive association between dose and peak mitragynine blood concentration.[25] In the study that

Table 3
Major kratom alkaloid intrinsic activity at opioid receptors (relative to mitragynine)

Alkaloid	Presence in Kratom Leaf	μ-Opioid	Δ-Opioid	κ-Opioid
Mitragynine	Yes	Partial agonist 1	Antagonist 1	Antagonist 1
7-Hydroxymitragynine	Yes	Partial agonist 4–8	Antagonist >6	Antagonist >1.5
Mitragynine pseudoindoxyl	No	Full agonist 120	Antagonist >65	Antagonist >130
Morphine	No	Full agonist 1.5–2.5	Partial agonist	

Notes: Receptor intrinsic activity measured in vitro with human or rodent opioid receptors. See sources for detailed methods.
Data from Todd DA, Kellogg JJ, Wallace ED, et al. Chemical composition and biological effects of kratom (Mitragyna peciose): In vitro studies with implications for efficacy and drug interactions. Sci Rep 2020;10:19158.; Obeng S, Wilkerson JL, Leon F, et al. Pharmacological comparison of mitragynine and 7-hydroxymitragynine: In vitro affinity and efficacy for μ-opioid and opioid-like behavioral effects on rats. J Pharmacol Exp Ther 2021;376:410-427; Varadi A, Marrone GF, Palmer TC, et al. Mitragynine/corynantheidine pseudoindoxyls as opioid analgesics with mu agonism and delta antagonism, which do not recruit β-arrestin-2. J Med Chem 2016;59:8381-8397.

Table 4
Human studies of controlled oral kratom administration

Location	N	Design	Preparation	Dose	Findings
Britain[24]	5	Open label	Mitragynine	50 mg 100 mg	↑heat tolerance Facial flushing, lightheadedness, tremor, nystagmus, "giddiness," nausea
"	"	"	Powdered leaves	0.65 g, 1.3 g	"
Thailand[25]	10	Open label	Tea	Mitragynine 6–20 mg	Slight, transient ↑HR, BP Tongue numbness
Malaysia[26]	26	Double-blind	Decoction	Mitragynine 1.6 mg/kg	↑pain tolerance No Δ BP No adverse effects

Notes: All study participants were healthy adult men. Participants in Thailand and Malaysia were regular (at least 6 mo) daily users of kratom.
Tea = fresh kratom leaves steeped in hot water.
Decoction = dried kratom leaves boiled in water for several hours
Abbreviations: BP, blood pressure; HR, heart rate.

administered the same mitragynine dose (1.6 mg/kg), there was a six-fold intersubject difference between the lowest and highest peak mitragynine concentrations.[26] The elimination half-life of mitragynine was 23.2 ± 16.1 hours.[25] No study evaluated the oral bioavailability of mitragynine or 7-hydroxymitragynine. This makes it impossible to confidently extrapolate to humans from the results of animal studies of kratom, especially given the substantial variability in mitragynine oral bioavailability across animal species.[27,28]

Routes of Administration

Kratom is almost always taken orally.[1,29] A 2016 anonymous online survey of a self-selected convenience sample of 8049 US adult kratom users found that at least 97% used kratom orally.[30] Intravenous use of kratom has been reported but is rare.[31]

Kratom is advertised online for inhalational use by electronic drug delivery device ("e-cigarette") or vaporizer. Mitragynine and 7-hydroxymitragynine have been detected in resins and liquids sold online for use in "e-cigarettes."[32] These findings suggest some kratom use by inhalation, at least in North America.

Formulations

Kratom is used in both liquid and solid oral formulations. In Southeast Asia, kratom users chew fresh leaves, ingest powdered dry leaves, or create a liquid formulation from leaves or leaf-extract.[1,29] Three common liquid kratom formulations are tea, decoction, and cocktail. Kratom tea is made by steeping leaves in hot water. Kratom decoction is made by boiling leaves in water for several hours. Kratom cocktail is a mixture of decoction with a flavored carbonated beverage (commonly cola) and often cough syrup or other beverage. This is done partly to hide the bitter taste of the decoction. Smoking of kratom leaves is rare.[33] In North America, kratom is commonly taken as lyophilized powdered leaf, often formulated in a capsule or tablet or dissolved in a liquid.[8,30] A 2016 anonymous online survey of a self-selected convenience sample of

8049 US adult kratom users found that 83.4% used powdered kratom (either as a solid [32.6%], mixed with food [2.2%], or dissolved in a beverage [48.6%]), 13% prepared kratom tea, and 0.5% drank already prepared kratom liquid.[30] A 2017 anonymous on-line survey of a self-selected sample of 2798 US adult kratom users found that only 0.4% smoked or injected kratom.[8] Most US kratom users buy their kratom online, and the remainder buys from "head shops," convenience stores, or other retail outlets.[34]

Processed kratom products available in North America and Europe may contain adulterants, although the data are very limited. 7-Hydroxymitragynine is often present in 3- to 4-fold higher concentration in processed kratom products in North America than it is in the fresh kratom leaf.[35] This finding suggests that some processed kratom products may be more potent than the natural kratom leaf. Kratom mixed with O-demethyltramadol, an active metabolite of the weak opioid analgesic medication tramadol, is marketed as "krypton" in Germany.[36] Phenylethylamine has been found in kratom products sold in New York State.[37]

Dosage and Patterns of Use

There are no US regulatory requirements for accurate labeling of kratom products, so it is impossible to know the actual doses of kratom alkaloids ingested by kratom users. In Southeast Asia, small surveys of convenience samples of kratom users suggest a range of dosages and use patterns, depending in part on the primary motivation for kratom use.[1,29,33,38] Lower doses are used for stimulant effect to enhance energy and reduce fatigue, especially among manual laborers. The commonest daily dose of liquid formulations (tea, decoction) is 2 to 3 glasses/d, containing an estimated 75 to 150 mg of mitragynine. Up to 40% of respondents report using more than 3 glasses/d, especially those self-medicating opioid withdrawal or opioid use disorder.

Anonymous online surveys of self-selected samples of US adult kratom users sug-gest that about three-quarters ingest 1 to 6 g/d of powder formulations.[8,30] Less than 10% ingest less than 1 g/d or more than 7 g/d. About two-thirds of adult kratom users use kratom daily; about 10% use less than weekly.[8,30]

ABUSE POTENTIAL
Preclinical

Kratom extracts and kratom alkaloids have inconsistent effects in rodent models of reward (**Table 5**), which are used to assess the abuse liability of compounds.[39] By comparison, conventional mOR agonists such as morphine are strongly rewarding in all four behavioral models tested. The rewarding effects of mitragynine (conditioned place preference)[40] and 7-hydroxymitragynine (self-administration)[41] are blocked by mOR antagonists, suggesting that they are mediated by activation of mOR.

Rats distinguish both mitragynine and 7-hydroxmitragyinine from saline but not from morphine,[20,42] suggesting that they generate internal sensations similar to those of a conventional opioid agonist. 7-Hydroxymitragynine is perceived as more morphine-like than is mitragynine.[20]

Repeated dosing of rodents with kratom extract or mitragynine daily for 4 to 14 days generates physical dependence, as evidenced by tolerance to analgesic effects, cross-tolerance with morphine,[14] and opioid-like withdrawal signs precipitated by administration of the mOR antagonist naloxone[18,43,44] The precipitated withdrawal syndrome is less intense than that generated after comparable chronic dosing with morphine. Spontaneous withdrawal signs are not observed or mild after the cessation of chronic kratom administration.

Table 5
Action of kratom and kratom alkaloids in rodent models of reward

Product/Alkaloid	Species	Self-Administration	Conditioned Place Preference	ICSS Threshold	Discrimination from Saline
Kratom extract	Mouse	?	–	?	?
Lyophilized kratom tea	Mouse	?	–	?	?
Mitryagynine	Rat	–	+	–	+
7-OH-mitragynine	Rat	+	?	+/–	+
Morphine	Rat, mouse	+	+	+	+

+ = rewarding effect, – = no effect, +/– = inconsistent effect, ? = no data.
Abbreviation: ICSS, intracranial self-stimulation.
Data from Obeng S, Wilkerson JL, Leon F, et al. Pharmacological comparison of mitragynine and 7-hydroxymitragynine: In vitro affinity and efficacy for μ-opioid and opioid-like behavioral effects on rats. J Pharmacol Exp Ther 2021;376:410-427, Japarin RA, Yusoff NH, Hassan Z, et al. Cross-reinstatement of mitragynine and morphine place preference in rats. Behav Brain Res 2021;399:113021.; Hemby SE, McIntosh S, Leon F, et al. Abuse liability and therapeutic potential of the Mitrogyna speciosa (kratom) alkaloids mitragynine and 7-hydroxymitragynine. Addict Biol 2018;24:874-885.; Behnood-Rod A, Chellian R, Wilson R, et al. Evaluation of the rewarding effects of mitragynine and 7-hydroxymitragynine in an intracranial self-stimulation procedure in male and female rats. Drug Alcohol Depend 2020;215:108235.; Yusoff NHM, Mansor SM, Muller CP, et al. Opioid receptors mediate the acquisition, but not the expression of mitragynine-induced conditioned place preference in rats. Behav Brain Res 2017;332:1-6.; Harun N, Hassan Z, Navaratnam V, et al. Discriminative stimulus properties of mitragynine (kratom) in rats. Psychopharmacol 2015;232:2227-2238.

Kratom methanolic extract (equivalent of 4.4 mg/kg mitragynine orally) does not acutely increase dopamine concentration in mouse brain nucleus accumbens.[45] Increasing nucleus accumbens dopamine concentration is an acute effect of almost all substances of abuse, including opioids.[46]

Clinical

Information about the abuse potential of kratom in humans comes mainly from two retrospective self-report surveys of self-selected samples of 3288 US adult kratom users conducted between 2016 and 2019.[8,9] These surveys suggest that 10% to 20% of regular kratom users develop a kratom use disorder. We are not aware of any human laboratory studies that assessed abuse potential using objective research methods.

A 2020 survey of a convenience sample of 69 US addiction medicine physicians found that 82.6% had encountered patients with what they considered kratom use disorder, one-quarter of whom had no lifetime history of opioid use disorder.[47]

Cross-sectional surveys of small convenience samples of adult regular kratom users in Southeast Asia find that many respondents report difficulty reducing or stopping their kratom use[33,48] but rarely find psychosocial impairment associated with kratom use.[29,49]

Tolerance to kratom's subjective and analgesic effects occurs after several weeks of regular use, based on the retrospective case reports,[50] but has not been systematically studied. Withdrawal signs and symptoms starting 12 to 48 hours after abrupt cessation of kratom use are retrospectively self-reported by 10% to 40% of US adult kratom users[8,30] and up to three-quarters of chronic daily kratom users in Southeast Asia.[51,52] There are published case reports of kratom withdrawal requiring medical treatment in US adults[53] and in neonates born to mothers who were chronic heavy kratom users.[54] Typical withdrawal symptoms resemble those occurring during opioid withdrawal, including irritability, anxiety, depression, sleep disturbance, lacrimation, rhinorrhea, muscle and bone pain, muscle spasm, diarrhea, and decreased appetite. The likelihood and severity of withdrawal are positively associated with duration, frequency, and intensity of kratom use. In one US online anonymous survey, respondents rated their past kratom withdrawal as mild (mean [SD] score of 8.8 [8.4] out of maximum 64) on a 16-item standardized rating instrument (Subjective Opiate Withdrawal Scale[55]).[8] In the one clinical trial that objectively evaluated kratom withdrawal, no withdrawal was observed (all scores 0.5 or lower out of a maximum 47) on an 11-item standardized rating instrument (Clinical Opiate Withdrawal Scale[56]) after 10 to 20 hours of abstinence.[26] However, this assessment period may have been too brief to allow kratom withdrawal to fully develop, given that self-reported withdrawal may take up to 48 hours to develop and the human elimination half-life of mitragynine is 23 hours (based on one study).[25]

ADVERSE EFFECTS

The three published clinical studies of oral kratom administration observed no long-lasting or clinically significant adverse effects or changes in vital signs in 41 adult men.[24–26] In the anonymous online surveys of self-selected US adult kratom users, the commonest adverse effects include dizziness, drowsiness, nausea, vomiting, constipation, and headache.[8,30,34] Most adverse effects are mild and self-limiting; few individuals seek medical attention. Respondents taking higher doses of kratom are more likely to report adverse effects.

At least 3859 cases of nonlethal adverse reactions associated with kratom use (but not necessarily caused by kratom) were reported to the US National Poison Data System between 2010 and 2019.[57,58] The number of cases reported annually increased more than 40-fold from 2010 (26) to 2019 (1218). Among the 1174 cases involving only kratom reported from 2011 to 2017, the commonest adverse reactions were agitation or irritability (22.9%), tachycardia (21.4%), nausea (14.6%), drowsiness or lethargy (14.3%), vomiting (13.2%), hypertension (10.1%), confusion (10.9%), and seizure (9.6%).[59] Life-threatening conditions were rare: coma (3.6%), cardiac arrest (0.4%), respiratory arrest (0.5%), and renal failure (0.5%). Kratom-associated cases reported to a major poison control center in Thailand from 2010 to 2017 had similar adverse reactions as those reported in the United States and the same common co-occurring substances (opiates, benzodiazepines).[60]

Small cross-sectional studies of adult kratom users in Southeast Asia find no significant association between long-term, frequent kratom use and clinically significant abnormalities in standard clinical laboratory tests,[61–63] blood concentrations of gonadal hormones,[64] electrocardiogram,[65,66] or echocardiogram.[67]

Chronic kratom use has been associated with at least 92 cases of liver toxicity published in the world-wide literature.[68,69] Presenting signs and symptoms typically start about 3 weeks after initiation of kratom use (range 1–8 weeks) and resolve within 1 month of stopping kratom use.

More than 300 deaths associated with kratom use have been reported in the world-wide medical literature through 2019, more than half in the United States and more than one-quarter in Thailand.[70–73] However, attributing causality to kratom alkaloids in a kratom-associated death can be difficult for several reasons. Other psychoactive substances are found along with kratom alkaloids in up to 95% of cases, most commonly opioids (including fentanyl), stimulants, alcohol, and benzodiazepines.[70,73] In cases where mitragynine is assayed quantitatively, there is no clear association between higher mitragynine concentrations and lethality.[74] Identification of mitragynine and 7-hydroxymitragynine can be problematic due to their instability over long periods at room or body temperature and the need for highly specific assays to distinguish them from their stereoisomers.[75] Many cases do not receive comprehensive toxicologic evaluation, and some novel psychoactive substances remain undetected because accurate assays are not available.

THERAPEUTIC POTENTIAL

Several therapeutic uses of kratom have been proposed, based largely on evidence from rodent studies or human self-report surveys (**Table 6**). Two small clinical studies (see **Table 4**) found that kratom had modest transient analgesic effects in human laboratory models of acute pain.[24,26] Neither the US Food and Drug Administration nor any other national regulatory authority has approved kratom or kratom alkaloids for the treatment of any medical or psychiatric condition.

Kratom alkaloids have been proposed as superior to conventional opioid agonists for the treatment of pain, opioid withdrawal, and opioid use disorder because of their selective actions at opioid receptors, biased agonism at the mOR,[12] and lessor potency in generating physical dependence and withdrawal at doses that produce analgesia in rodents.[18,43,44] Biased agonism at the mOR could, in principal, produce therapeutic effects such as analgesia at doses that do not produce unwanted effects such as physical dependence and respiratory depression. However, clinical trials with non-kratom compounds that have similar biased agonism at the mOR have not demonstrated fewer adverse effects at analgesic doses.[78]

LEGAL STATUS

Kratom, mitragynine, and 7-hydroxymitragynine are not controlled substances under UN international drug control treaties or the US Controlled Substances Act (CSA).[79] In

Table 6
Evidence for proposed therapeutic indications for kratom

| Indication | Types of Evidence | | | |
	Rodent Model[13]	Southeast Asia Self-Report Survey[38,76]	US Self-Report Online Survey[8,30,77]	Clinical Trial[24,26]
Analgesia	Yes	Yes	Yes	Yes
Fatigue	N/A	Yes	Yes	N/A
Opioid withdrawal	Yes	Yes	Yes	N/A
Opioid use disorder	Yes	Yes	Yes	N/A
Alcohol withdrawal	Yes	No	No	N/A
Alcohol use disorder	Yes	No	No	N/A
Stimulant use disorder	No	Yes	No	N/A
Anxiety	Yes	Yes	Yes	N/A
Depression	Yes	Yes	Yes	N/A
Psychosis	Yes	No	No	N/A

Southeast Asia self-report = use as herbal medicine by indigenous population in Southeast Asia.
US self-report = retrospective self-report in anonymous online surveys of self-selected US adult kratom users.
N/A = no relevant studies.

2016, the US Drug Enforcement Administration proposed placing kratom in schedule I of the CSA, which would effectively ban it. This proposal was withdrawn later that year after public protests, although kratom remains a "drug of concern."[80] Kratom is illegal in six US states (Alabama, Arkansas, Indiana, Rhode Island, Vermont, and Wisconsin) and several US cities.[81] Several states ban kratom sale to minors. Kratom is illegal in the United Kingdom and Ireland and illegal for human consumption in Canada.[79] Several dozen countries control kratom as a narcotic drug.

MANAGEMENT OF KRATOM-RELATED DISORDERS

Knowledge of kratom-related disorders comes chiefly from published case reports and small case series of patients who came to medical attention (most hospitalized). These patients represent the severe end of the diagnostic spectrum and are probably not representative of most patients with kratom-related disorders. There are currently no explicit diagnostic criteria or accepted clinical practice guidelines for kratom-related disorders. The standard drug screening tests do not detect kratom alkaloids, so they are not useful in identifying kratom-related disorders except by excluding the presence of other substances.[82]

Intoxication/Overdose

Patients with kratom intoxication/overdose typically present medically with an opioid-like toxidrome, including sedation, pupil constriction (miosis), respiratory depression, sweating, dry mouth, and nausea.[82,83] Kratom intoxication/overdose should be suspected in patients presenting with an opioid-like toxidrome in whom drug testing does not detect opioids. Treatment with naloxone, an mOR antagonist, is effective in most[83] but not all cases,[84] but has not been systematically studied.

Withdrawal

Kratom withdrawal should be suspected in patients with a typical opioid-like withdrawal syndrome (restlessness, irritability, pupil dilation [mydriasis], rhinorrhea, lacrimation, sweating) who report abrupt cessation of long-term daily kratom use within the prior 5 to 48 hours. Drug testing should be done to rule out concomitant opioid withdrawal. Kratom product doses less than 5 g daily are usually associated with mild withdrawal. Mild cases do well with several days of symptomatic treatment, such as tapering doses of an alpha-adrenergic agonist such as clonidine or lofexidine.[53] Kratom doses greater than 5 g daily are associated with more severe withdrawal. Severe cases in adults or neonates[54] need detoxification with tapering doses of an opioid agonist such as buprenorphine.

Kratom Use Disorder

Buprenorphine is the most widely used medication for treatment of kratom use disorder (diagnosed with criteria for opioid use disorder).[47,85–87] Outpatients using up to 92 g daily of kratom, with or without concomitant opioid use disorder, have been successfully treated with maintenance buprenorphine, whether initiated as treatment of severe kratom withdrawal or initiated before attempting kratom abstinence. Buprenorphine can be started 8 hours after the last kratom dose, at initial doses of 1 to 16 mg daily. Effective maintenance doses range from 4 to 24 mg daily, with no apparent correlation with daily kratom dose.[85] In a series of 28 outpatients in treatment for a mean of 11 months, 82% had urine samples negative for mitragyine at 8 and 12 weeks of treatment.[85] Buprenorphine can also be combined with contingency management treatment.[88] Methadone and naltrexone have been used in a few cases,[47] but naltrexone poses the risk of precipitating acute opioid withdrawal.[89]

DISCUSSION

The CSA lists eight criteria for whether psychoactive compounds should be controlled **(Box 1)**.[80] Current knowledge suggests that kratom meets several of these criteria. Kratom has reinforcing effects in some rodent models and is abused by some people, perhaps more so in processed and concentrated forms in North America and Europe than as the leaf in Southeast Asia. There is also clear evidence that some chronic heavy users develop physical (physiologic) dependence, as shown by tolerance and withdrawal, and psychic dependence (ie, a kratom use disorder in terms of the American Psychiatric Association Diagnostic and Statistical Manual of Mental Disorders 5th edition [DSM-5]). What remains unknown is the actual scope, duration and significance of kratom "abuse." Kratom use is associated with serious medical toxicity, including death, but the causal relationship with kratom itself, and thus the public health implications, remains unclear.

Were kratom to be scheduled under the CSA, "accepted medical use" would be a key factor in determining in which schedule it would be placed.[80] The evidence for the several proposed therapeutic applications for kratom comes from rodent studies and retrospective reports of human self-medication. Evidence from controlled clinical trials is lacking.

Given these substantial gaps in our knowledge of kratom epidemiology and pharmacology, the prudent course may be to delay regulatory action and keep kratom monitored as a "drug of concern" until better quality evidence is obtained. This avoids a scheduling decision that might limit the ability to conduct the necessary research. Future research should include large, population-based, epidemiologic surveys of kratom use and associated clinical variables and phase I (human laboratory studies) and phase II controlled clinical trials evaluating kratom's pharmacokinetics (especially oral bioavailability) and acute and chronic psychological and physiologic effects.

Box 1
Eight factors considered in placing a psychoactive substance under the US Controlled Substances Act

1. Actual or relative potential for abuse
    "Potential for abuse" (based on legislative intent):
    a. taking the drug creates a hazard to health or to community safety
    b. significant diversion of the drug from legitimate channels
    c. individuals take the drug on their own initiative, rather than on advice of a clinician

2. Scientific evidence of the drug's pharmacologic effect

3. State of current scientific knowledge regarding the substance

4. History and current pattern of abuse

5. Scope, duration, and significance of abuse

6. Is there risk to the public health?

7. Psychic or physiologic dependence liability

8. Is an immediate precursor already controlled?

Data from Drug Enforcement Administration. Drugs of Abuse, A DEA Resource Guide, 2020. Available at www.dea.gov. Accessed Feb. 2, 2022.

CLINICS CARE POINTS

- Kratom intoxication/overdose typically presents as an opioid-like toxidrome. Naloxone is usually effective in reversing acute signs and symptoms.

- Kratom withdrawal has opioid-like signs and symptoms. Mild cases can be treated symptomatically with tapering doses of an alpha-adrenergic agonist such as clonidine or lofexidine. More severe cases require buprenorphine tapering, with the initial dose adjusted to the severity of withdrawal.

- Kratom use disorder occurs in patients with daily, high-dose use. Treatment may require buprenorphine maintenance at doses up to 24 mg daily.

DISCLOSURE

The author has no conflicts of interest to disclose.

REFERENCES

1. Singh D, Narayanan S, Vicknasingam B. Traditional and non-traditional uses of Mitragynine (Kratom): A survey of the literature. Brain Res Bull 2016;126:41–9.
2. Kruegel AC, Grundmann O. The medicinal chemistry and neuropharmacology of kratom: A preliminary discussion of a promising medicinal plant and analysis of its potential for abuse. Neuropharmacology 2018;134:108–20.
3. Han C, Schmitt J, Gilliland KM. DARK Classics in Chemical Neuroscience: Kratom. ACS Chem Neurosci 2020;11:3870–80.
4. Center for Behavioral Health Statistics and Quality.. Results from the 2020 national survey on drug use and health: detailed tables. Rockville (MD): Substance Abuse and Mental Health Services Administration; 2021. Available at: https://www.samhsa.gov/data/. Accessed January 21, 2022.
5. Wonguppa R, Kanato M. The prevalence and associated factors of new psychoactive substance use: A 2016 Thailand national household survey. Addict Behav Rep 2018;7:111–5.
6. Angkurawaranon C, Jiraporncharoen W, Likhitsathian S, et al. Trends in the use of illicit substances in Thailand: Results from national household surveys. Drug Alcohol Rev 2018;37:658–63.
7. Palamar JJ. Past-year kratom use in the U.S.: Estimates from a nationally representative sample. Am J Prevent Med 2021;61(2):240–5.
8. Garcia-Romeu A, David J, Cox DJA, et al. Kratom (Mitragyna speciosa): User demographics, use patterns, and implications for the opioid epidemic. Drug Alcohol Depend 2020;208:107849.
9. Schimmel J, Amioka E, Rockhill K, et al. Prevalence and description of kratom (Mitragyna speciosa) use in the United States: a cross-sectional study. Addiction 2020;116:176–81.
10. Flores-Bocanegra L, Raja HA, Graf TN, et al. The chemistry of kratom [Mitragyna speciosa]: Updated characterization data and methods to elucidate indole and oxindole alkaloids. J Nat Prod 2020;83:2165–77.
11. Todd DA, Kellogg JJ, Wallace ED, et al. Chemical composition and biological effects of kratom (Mitragyna speciosa): In vitro studies with implications for efficacy and drug interactions. Sci Rep 2020;10:19158.
12. Zhou Y, Ramsey S, Provasi D, et al. Predicted mode of binding to and allosteric modulation of the μ-opioid receptor by kratom's alkaloids with reported antinociception in vivo. Biochem 2021;60:1420–9.

13. Prevete E, Kuypers KPC, Theunissen EL, et al. A systematic review of (pre)clinical studies on the therapeutic potential and safety profile of kratom in humans. Hum Psychopharmacol Clin Exp 2021;37:e2805.

14. Chin K-Y, Mark-Lee WF. A review on the antinociceptive effects of Mitragyna speciosa and its derivatives on animal model. Curr Drug Targets 2018;19:1359–65.

15. Bhowmik S, Galeta J, Havel V, et al. Site selective C-H functionalization of Mitragyna alkaloids reveals a molecular switch for tuning opioid receptor signaling efficacy. Nat Commun 2021;12:3858.

16. Carpenter JM, Criddle CA, Craig HK, et al. Comparative effects of Mitragyna speciosa extract, mitragynine, and opioid agonists on thermal nociception in rats. Fitoterapia 2016;109:87–90.

17. Gutridge AM, Robins MT, Cassell RJ, et al. G-protein-biased kratom-alkaloids and synthetic carfentanil-amid opioids as potential treatments for alcohol use disorder. Br J Pharmacol 2020;177:1497–513.

18. Wilson LL, Harris HM, Eans SO, et al. Lyophilized kratom tea as a therapeutic option for opioid dependence. Drug Alcohol Depend 2020;218:108310.

19. Suhaimi FW, Hassan Z, Mansor SM, et al. The effects of chronic mitragynine (Kratom) exposure on the EEG in rats. Neurosci Lett 2021;245:135632.

20. Obeng S, Wilkerson JL, Leon F, et al. Pharmacological comparison of mitragynine and 7-hydroxymitragynine: In vitro affinity and efficacy for μ-opioid and opioid-like behavioral effects on rats. J Pharmacol Exp Ther 2021;376:410–27.

21. Varadi A, Marrone GF, Palmer TC, et al. Mitragynine/corynantheidine pseudoindoxyls as opioid analgesics with mu agonism and delta antagonism, which do not recruit β-arrestin-2. J Med Chem 2016;59:8381–97.

22. Obeng S, Kamble SH, Reeves ME, et al. Investigation of the adrenergic and opioid binding affinities, metabolic stability, plasma protein binding properties, and functional effects of selected indole-based kratom alkaloids. J Med Chem 2020;65:433–9.

23. Stolt A-C, Schroder H, Neurath H, et al. Behavioral and neurochemical charactierization of kratom (Mitragyna speciosa) extract. Psychopharmacol 2014;231: 13–25.

24. Grewal KS. The effect of mitragynine on man. Br J Med Psychol 1932;12(1): 41–58.

25. Trakulsrichai S, Sathirakul K, Auparakkitanon J, et al. Pharmacokinetics of mitragynine in man. Drug Des. Develop Ther 2015;9:2421–9.

26. Vicknasingam B, Chooi WT, Rahim AA, et al. Kratom and pain tolerance: A randomized, placebo-controlled, double-blind study. Yale J Biol Med 2020;93: 229–38.

27. Avery BA, Boddu SP, Sharma A, et al. Comparative pharmacokinetics of mitragynine after oral administration of Mitragyna speciosa (kratom) leaf extracts in rats. Planta Med 2019;85(4):340–6.

28. Maxwell EA, King TL, Kambie SH, et al. Pharmacokinetics and safety of mitragynine in beagle dogs. Planta Med 2020;86(17):1278–85.

29. Singh D, Narayanan S, Vicknasingam B, et al. Changing trends in the use of kratom (Mitragyna speciosa) in Southeast Asia. Hum Psychopharmacol Clin Exp 2017;32:e2582.

30. Grundmann O. Patterns of kratom use and health impact in the US—Results from an online survey. Drug Alcohol Depend 2017;176:63–70.

31. Lydecker A, Zuckerman MD, Hack JB, et al. Intravenous kratom use in a patient with opioid dependence. J Toxicol Pharmacol 2017;1:003.

32. Pearce MR, Smith ME, Poklis JL. The analysis of commercially available products recommended for use in electronic cigarettes. Rapid Commun Mass Spectrom 2020;34(17):e771.

33. Ahmad K, Aziz Z. Mitragyna speciosa use in the northern states of Malaysia: A cross-sectional study. J Ethnopharmacol 2012;2012(141):446–50.

34. Coe MA, Pillitteri JL, Sembower MA, et al. Kratom as a substitute for opioids: Results from an online survey. Drug Alcohol Depend 2019;202:24–32.

35. Lydecker AG, Sharma A, McCurdy CR, et al. Suspected adulteration of commercial kratom products with 7-hydroxymitragynine. J Med Toxicol 2016;12:341–9.

36. Phillip AA, Meyer MR, Wissenbach DK, et al. Monitoring of kratom or Krypton intake in urine using GC-MS in clinical and forensic toxicology. Analy Bioanalytic Chem 2011;400:127–35.

37. Nacca N, Schult RF, Lingyun LI, et al. Kratom adulterated with phenylethylamine and associated intracerebral hemorrhage: Linking toxicologists and public health officials to identify dangerous adulterants. J Med Toxicol 2020;16:71–4.

38. Saref A, Suraya S, Singh D, et al. Self-reported prevalence and severity of opioid and kratom (Mitragyna speciosa korth.) side effects. J Ethnopharmacol 2019;38: 111876.

39. García-Pardo MP, Roger-Sánchez C, de la Rubia Ortí E, et al. Animal models of drug addiction. Addictiones 2017;29(4):278–92.

40. Yusoff NHM, Mansor SM, Muller CP, et al. Opioid receptors mediate the acquisition, but not the expression of mitragynine-induced conditioned place preference in rats. Behav Brain Res 2017;332:1–6.

41. Hemby SE, McIntosh S, Leon F, et al. Abuse liability and therapeutic potential of the Mitrogyna speciosa (kratom) alkaloids mitragynine and 7-hydroxymitragynine. Addict Biol 2018;24:874–85.

42. Harun N, Hassan Z, Navaratnam V, et al. Discriminative stimulus properties of mitragynine (kratom) in rats. Psychopharmacol 2015;232:2227–38.

43. Harun N, Johari IS, Manor SM, et al. Assessing physiological dependence and withdrawal potential of mitragynine using schedule-controlled behavior in rats. Psychopharmacol 2020;237:855–67.

44. Wilson LL, Chakraborty S, Eans SO, et al. Kratom alkaloids, natural and semisynthetic, show less physical dependence and ameliorate opioid withdrawal. Cell Mol Neurobiol 2021;41(5):1131–43.

45. Vijeepallam K, Pandy V, Murugan DD, et al. Methanolic extract of Mitragyna speciosa Korth leaf inhibits ethanol seeking behavior in mice: involvement of antidopaminergic mechanism. Metabol Brain Dis 2019;34:1713–22.

46. Gardner EL. Introduction: Addiction and brain reward and anti-reward pathways. Adv Psychosom Med 2011;30:22–60.

47. Stanciu C, Ahmed S, Hybki B, et al. Pharmacotherapy for management of 'kratom use disorder': A systematic literature review with survey of experts. WMJ 2021; 120(1):54–61.

48. Saingam D, Assanangkomchai S, Geater AF, et al. Pattern and consequences of kratom (Mitragyna speciosa Korth.) use among male villagers in southern Thailand: A qualitative study. Int J Drug Policy 2013;24:351–8.

49. Singh D, Muller CP, Vicknasingam BK, et al. Social functioning of kratom (Mitragyna speciosa) users in Malaysia. J Psychoactive Drugs 2015;47(2):125–31.

50. Alsarraf E, Myers J, Culbreth S, et al. Kratom from head to toe—Case reviews of adverse events and toxicities. Curr Emerg Hosp Med Rep 2019;7:141–68.

51. Singh D, Narayanan S, Vicknasingam BK, et al. Severity of pain and sleep problems during kratom (Mitragyna speciosa Korth.) cessation among regular kratom users. J Psychoactive Drugs 2018;50(3):266–74.
52. Singh D, Narayanan S, Muller CP, et al. Severity of kratom (Mitragyna speciosa Korth.) psychological withdrawal symptoms. J Psychoactive Drugs 2018;50(5): 445–50.
53. Stanciu C, Gnanasegaram SA, Ahmed S, et al. Kratom withdrawal: A systematic review with case series. J Psychoactive Drugs 2019;51(1):12–8.
54. Wright ME, Ginsberg C, Parkison AM, et al. Outcomes of mothers and newborns to prenatal exposure to kratom: a systematic review. J Perinatol 2021;41:1236–43.
55. Handelsman L, Cochrane KJ, Aronson MJ, et al. Two new rating scales for opiate withdrawal. Am J Drug Alcohol Abuse 1987;13:293–308.
56. Wesson DR, Ling W. The Clinical Opiate Withdrawal Scale (COWS). J Psychoactive Drugs 2003;35:253–9.
57. Anwar M, Law R, Schier J. Kratom (Mitragyna speciosa) exposures reported to poison center—United States, 2010-2015. MMWR Morb Mort Wkly Rep 2016; 65(29):748–9.
58. Graves JM, Dilley JA, Terpak L, et al. Kratom exposures among older adults reported to U.S. poison centers, 2014-2019. J Am Geriatr Soc 2021;69:2176–84.
59. Post S, Spiller HA, Chounthirath T, et al. Kratom exposures reported to United States poison control centers: 2011-2017. Clin Toxicol 2019;57(10):847–54.
60. Davidson C, Cao D, King T, et al. A comparative analysis of kratom exposure cases in Thailand and the United States from 2010-2017. Am Drug Alcohol Abuse 2021;47(1):74–83.
61. Abdullah MFILB, Tan KL, Isa SM, et al. Lipid profile of regular kratom (Mitrygyna speciosa Korth.) users in the community setting. PLoS One 2020;15(6): e0234630.
62. La-up A, Saengow U, Aramrattana A. High serum high-density lipoprotein and low serum triglycerides in Kratom users: A study of Kratom users in Thailand. Heliyon 2021;7:e06931, 907–910.
63. Singh D, Muller CP, Murugaiyah V, et al. Evaluating the hematological and clinical-chemistry parameters of kratom (Mitragyna speciosa) users in Malaysia. J Ethnopharmacol 2018;214:187–206.
64. Singh D, Murugaiyah V, Hamid SBS, et al. Assessment of gonadotropins and testosterone hormone levels in regular Mitragyna speciosa (Korth.) users. J Ethnopharmacol 2018;221:30–6.
65. Abdullah MFILB, Singh D. The adverse cardiovascular effects and cardiotoxicity of kratom (Mitragyna speciosa Korth): A comprehensive review. Front Pharmacol 2021;12:726003.
66. Abdullah MFIL, Tan KL, Narayanan S, et al. Is kratom (Mitragyna speciosa Korth.) use associated with ECG abnormalities? Electrocardiogram comparisons between regular kratom users and controls. Clin Toxicol (Philadelphia) 2021;59(5): 400–8.
67. Abdullah MFILB, Singh D. Assessment of cardiovascular functioning among regular kratom (Mitragyna speciosa Korth) users: A case series. Front Pharmacol 2021;12:723567.
68. Ballotin VR, Bigarella LG, de Mello Brandao AB, et al. Herb-induced liver injury: Systematic review and meta-analysis. World J Clin Cases 2021;9(20):5490–513.
69. Schimmel J, Dart RC. Kratom (Mitragyna speciosa) liver injury: A comprehensive review. Drugs 2020;80:263–83.

70. Corkery JM, Streete P, Claridge H, et al. Characteristics of deaths associated with kratom use. J Psychopharmacol 2019;33(9):1102–23.
71. Eggleston W, Stoppacher R, Suen K, et al. Kratom use and toxicities in the United States. Pharmacotherapy 2019;39(7):775–7.
72. Mata DC, Anders KM. Case series: Mitragynine blood and tissue concentrations in fatalities from 2017 to 2018 in Orange County, CA, USA. Forens Chem 2019;7: 100205.
73. Olsen EO, O'Donnell J, Matteson CL, et al. Unintentional drug overdose deaths with kratom—27 states, July 2016-December 2017. MMWR Morb Mort Wkly Rep 2019;68(14):326–7.
74. Schmitt J, Bingham K, Knight KD. Kratom-associated fatalities in Northern Nevada—what mitragynine level is fatal? Am J Forensic Med Pathol 2021;42(4): 341–9.
75. Papsun DM, Chan-Hosokawa A, Friederich L, et al. The trouble with kratom: Analytical and interpretive issues involving mitragynine. J Analyt Toxicol 2019; 43(8):615–29.
76. Singh D, Narayanan S, Muller CP, et al. Motives for using kratom (Mitragyna speciosa Korth.) among regular users in Malaysia. J Ethnopharmacol 2019;233: 34–40.
77. Bath R, Bucholz T, Buros AF, et al. Self-reported health diagnoses and demographic correlates with kratom use: Results from an online survey. J Addict Med 2020;14:244–52.
78. Tan HS, Habib AS. Oliceridine: A novel drug for the management of moderate to severe acute pain—A review of current evidence. J Pain Manag 2021;14:969–79.
79. Wikipedia. Mitragyna speciosa. Available at: https://en.wikipedia.org/wiki/Mitragyna_speciosa#United_States. Accessed February 2, 2022.
80. Drug Enforcement Administration. Drugs of Abuse, A DEA Resource Guide, 2020. Available at: www.dea.gov. Accessed February 2, 2022.
81. Coonan E, Tatum W. Kratom: The safe legal high? Epilepsy Behav 2021;117: 107882.
82. Groff D, Stuckey H, Philpott C, et al. Kratom use disorder: a primer for primary care physicians. J Addict Dis 2021. https://doi.org/10.1080/10550887.2021. 1950263.
83. Reinert JP, Colunga K, Etuk A, et al. Management of overdoses of salvia, kratom, and psilocybin mushrooms: a literature review. Expert Rev Clin Pharmacol 2020; 13:847–56.
84. Shekar SP, Rojas EE, D'Angelo CC, et al. Legally lethal kratom: A herbal supplement with overdose potential. J Psychoactive Drugs 2019;51:28–30.
85. Broyan VR, Brar JK, Allgaier Student T, et al. Long-term buprenorphine treatment for kratom use disorder: A case series. Subst Abus 2022;43(1):763–6.
86. Lei L, Butz A, Valentino N. Management of kratom dependence with buprenorphine/naloxone in a veteran population. Substance Abuse 2021;22:1–11.
87. Weiss MD, Douglas HE. Treatment of kratom withdrawal and dependence with buprenorphine/naloxone: A case series and systematic literature review. J Addict Med 2021;15:167–72.
88. Kalin S, Dakhlalla S, Bhardwaj S. Treatment for kratom abuse in a contingency-management-based MAT setting: A case series. J Opioid Manag 2020;16(5): 391–4.
89. Jensen AN, Truong Q-N, Jameson M, et al. Kratom-induced transaminitis with subsequent precipitated opioid withdrawal following naltrexone. Ment Health Clin 2021;11(3):220–4.

Important Drug-Drug Interactions for the Addiction Psychiatrist

Neil Sandson, MD[a,b]

KEYWORDS

• Interaction • Inhibitor • Inducer • Cytochrome • P-glycoprotein • Metabolism

KEY POINTS

• It is important to consider drug-drug interactions with respect to illicit drugs and alcohol.
• Drug-drug interactions can occur through both metabolic and nonmetabolic mechanisms.
• Recognizing the recurring patterns and themes of drug-drug interactions will allow clinicians to assimilate this complicated body of information.

The misuse of drugs and alcohol poses obvious health risks to afflicted individuals. When addressing these health risks, the overarching concerns generally relate to the direct effects that various substances can have on the functioning of multiple organ systems: cardiac, pulmonary, central nervous system (CNS), and others. What is not always evident, but potentially equally or even more dire, are the risks arising from drug-drug interactions (DDIs) involving these drugs, whether with each other or with prescribed medications. In this review, the author first provides some basics that will enable the reader to fruitfully approach the broad topic of DDIs. After that, the author examines DDIs involving many of these drugs, as well as many of the medications that are used in the treatment of individuals afflicted with substance use disorders.

As with traditional (psycho)pharmacology, the 2 major forms of DDIs are pharmacodynamic interactions and pharmacokinetic interactions. Pharmacodynamic interactions represent the synergy or antagonism of each drug's effects at target receptors. For example, the synergistic anticholinergic activity of amitriptyline combined with benztropine can produce constipation, heat stroke, urinary retention, and other related difficulties.[1] Another familiar example would be a central serotonin syndrome resulting from the combination of a monoamine oxidase inhibitor with a selective serotonin reuptake inhibitor (SSRI).[2,3] By way of contrast, in pharmacokinetic DDIs, one agent affects the movement of another agent through the body, resulting

a Department of Psychiatry, University of Maryland, 126 East Aylesbury Road, Timonium, MD, USA; b VA Maryland Health Care System, 10 North Greene St, Baltimore, MD 21201, USA
E-mail address: neil.sandson@gmail.com

Psychiatr Clin N Am 45 (2022) 431–450
https://doi.org/10.1016/j.psc.2022.05.004
0193-953X/22/Published by Elsevier Inc.

in alterations in drug absorption, metabolism, distribution, and excretion, which usually impacts blood levels but can also lead to sequestration of drugs into or away from physiologic subdomains, like the CNS.

Pharmacodynamic DDIs are usually intuitively straightforward. If one has a basic sense of a drug's mechanism of action and corresponding receptor occupancies, these interactions can often be predicted and, with traditional psychopharmacology, it is hoped, avoided. Pharmacokinetic DDIs are much more difficult to anticipate. Knowing how a drug/medication accomplished its intended effects rarely confers meaningful knowledge of its kinetic parameters, or the ways that these parameters will interact with those of another drug to potentially increase or decrease blood levels. Hence, most of the challenge involved in anticipating and avoiding DDIs rests in the pharmacokinetic domain, which is predominantly concerned with metabolic alterations.

In approaching the topic of DDIs involving use of illicit substances and misuse of prescribed medications, it quickly became clear that there is one paradigm that is common in the treatment of substance use disorders, but otherwise almost unheard of in psychopharmacology, namely, deliberate pharmacodynamic antagonism. In traditional psychopharmacology, standard augmentation strategies typically represent contrived mobilization of pharmacodynamic synergies, such as the combination of an SSRI like citalopram with a noradrenergic/dopamine reuptake inhibitor like bupropion.[4] However, in the treatment of opioid overdoses with naloxone,[5] or the use of disulfiram in the treatment of alcohol use disorder,[6] and other examples that the author examines, the deliberate and otherwise unusual mobilization of pharmacodynamic antagonism is seen. Aside from the occasional need to reverse the effects of anesthetic agents, the other area of medicine in which we would commonly encounter therapeutic applications of pharmacodynamic antagonism is toxicology, which is telling in itself.

PHARMACOKINETICS BASICS

In exploring the topic of pharmacokinetic DDIs, the most frequently involved component is the cytochrome P450 system. The P450 system is a family of mostly hepatic enzymes that perform oxidative (phase I) metabolism, which is typically, but not always, the most consequential step in metabolic clearance. Specific P450 enzymes are identified by number-letter-number sequences, analogous to a family-genus-species taxonomic ranking. The major P450 enzymes are as follows: 1A2, 2B6, 2C9, 2C19, 2D6, 2E1, and 3A4. P450 substrates are drugs whose metabolism is catalyzed by one or more of these specific P450 enzymes. P450 inhibitors impair the ability of specific P450 enzymes to catalyze the metabolism of their substrates, whether via competitive (essentially avidly bound cosubstrates) or noncompetitive means, thus producing increased blood levels of those substrates. Conversely, P450 inducers cause the liver to increase the production of specific P450 enzymes, leading to increased metabolic efficiency and a subsequent decrease of substrate blood levels. Enzymatic inhibition often produces meaningful increases in substrate blood levels within a few days, whereas induction usually requires 2 or more weeks to exert a clinically meaningful effect on drug metabolism (the main exception to this is induction of 1A2 and 2E1 via tobacco smoking, which takes just a few days).[7] All P450 enzymes are inducible, with the exception of 2D6.

Although the P450 system is the mainstay of metabolic drug clearance, phase II metabolism plays an important role as a capstone for drug clearance, and for some drugs it is actually the primary metabolic pathway. Just as P450 is the main phase I oxidative enzyme family, the main phase II enzyme family is the uridine 5′-diphosphate glucuronosyltransferases (UGTs). Much like the P450 system, specific UGT enzymes are also identified by a number-letter-number scheme (1A1, 1A4, 2B7, 2B15, and so forth), and each enzyme has a unique array of substrates, inhibitors, and inducers. Because this topic is already complex enough, and the role of UGTs will be relatively minimal for the drugs examined, when there is a phase II contribution to a drug's metabolism, the author refers to it in those general terms and does not delve into specifics.

The final pharmacokinetic system that the author explores is the P-glycoprotein transporter. Although P450 and UGT relate to drug metabolism, P-glycoprotein relates to the other modalities of pharmacokinetic drug handling: absorption, distribution, and excretion. The P-glycoprotein transporter is an ATP-dependent, extruding pump, which acts to decrease bioavailability of compounds that are substrates of this pump. P-glycoprotein resides in the plasma membrane of enterocytes that line the gut lumen, where it can decrease absorption and increase excretion of P-glycoprotein substrates. It is also found in the capillaries of the blood-brain barrier, where it acts as one of the main influences that prevents various substances that should diffuse down their concentration gradients from gaining meaningful access to the CNS. Like P450 and UGT metabolic systems, there are P-glycoprotein substrates, inhibitors, and inducers. P-glycoprotein inhibitors, as they decrease the activity of this extruding transporter, will increase bioavailability, and potentially blood levels, of P-glycoprotein substrates. Conversely, P-glycoprotein inducers will increase the magnitude of extrusion of substrates, leading to less absorption, more excretion, and potentially a decrease in substrate levels.

The pharmacodynamics of illicit substances is more intuitively straightforward, so the author covers this aspect in a more cursory fashion and instead focuses more on pharmacokinetics. As the metabolic pathways and inhibitory and induction profiles of various illicit drugs are examined, it will be useful to have a database of similar information regarding drugs with which they might interact. Toward that end, the author provides several (deliberately incomplete) tables that will facilitate the determination of meaningful and significant DDIs involving illicit drugs.

In addition, the author has a few illustrative vignettes depicting validated DDIs scattered throughout the following exploration of potential interactions.

Illicit Substances, Misused Prescribed Medications, and Alcohol

Tobacco
Pharmacodynamics. Tobacco acts as a potent agonist at nicotinic acetylcholine receptors, leading to adrenergic and secondarily dopaminergic effects.[8,9] As might be expected, this leads to general stimulant effects and euphoria, which accounts for the high potential for addiction, but no notable DDIs.

Pharmacokinetics. When smoked, tobacco acts as a uniquely rapid (about 3 days vs 2–3 weeks) enzymatic inducer of P450 1A2 and 2E1,[7] which would be expected to produce significant decreases in the blood levels of coadministered 1A2 and 2E1 substrates, such as caffeine, clozapine, and olanzapine (**Table 1**; see **Table 6** for details).

Ethanol
Pharmacodynamics. Alcohol is a general CNS depressant. As such, it can synergize with other CNS depressants (opioids, benzodiazepines, and others) to produce potentially lethal consequences, such as cardiopulmonary arrest.

Pharmacokinetics. Ethanol is metabolized to acetaldehyde primarily by alcohol dehydrogenase and secondarily by catalase and P450 2E1; acetaldehyde is then further

Table 1 P450 1A2 substrates, inhibitors, and inducers	
Substrates	Acetaminophen
	Caffeine
	Clozapine
	Cyclobenzaprine
	Duloxetine
	Fluvoxamine
	Mirtazapine
	Olanzapine
	Phencyclidine (PCP)
	Propranolol
	R-warfarin
	Typical antipsychotics
Inhibitors	Caffeine
	Cannabidiol (CBD)
	Ciprofloxacin (and some other quinolones)
	Ethanol
	Ethinylestradiol
	Fluvoxamine
	Grapefruit juice
	Tetrahydrocannabinol (THC)
Inducers	Carbamazepine
	Modafinil
	Pentobarbital
	Phenobarbital
	Rifampin
	Ritonavir
	Secobarbital
	Tetrahydrocannabinol (THC) (smoked)
	Tobacco smoking

metabolized by aldehyde dehydrogenase to acetate.[10,11] Ethanol acts as an inhibitor of P450 1A2, 2D6, and intestinal 3A4, leading to potential increases in coadministered substrates of those enzymes, such as olanzapine, tricyclic antidepressants, and quetiapine[12,13] (see **Tables 1**, **5**, and **7** for details). In addition, chronic ethanol use acts as an inducer of P450 2E1.[14] Ethanol autoinduction may be expected to lead to lower blood levels per quantity consumed over time, but this is unlikely to be a clinically significant mitigating factor preventing adverse sequelae of alcohol toxicity. Ethanol's 2E1 induction profile may be expected to lead to a potential decrease in coadministered 2E1 substrates, such as acetaminophen (see **Table 6**). However, this property of ethanol plays into a specific dangerous clinical scenario: an acetaminophen overdose in a chronic active drinker. Induction of 2E1 via chronic ethanol use will shunt acetaminophen metabolism down pathways that lead to increased production of the hepatotoxic *N*-acetyl-*p*-benzoquinone metabolite, making it that much more critical to promptly enough administer *N*-acetylcysteine (Mucomyst) to counter the even greater than normal hepatotoxic potential of an acetaminophen overdose cooccurring with chronic active ethanol use.[14,15] Discussion of the ethanol-disulfiram DDI occurs in the section dealing with treatments for substance use disorders.

Cannabis
Pharmacodynamics. Cannabis has mixed sympathetic and parasympathetic autonomic nervous system activity, leading to a mixed picture of sedation and/or anxiety,

increased heart rate and blood pressure, euphoria, nausea/vomiting, incoordination, confusion, and so forth.[16] Cannabis contains dozens of pharmacologically active compounds, but the 3 best studied are delta-9-tetrahydrocannabinol (THC), cannabidiol (CBD), and cannabinol (CBN). THC is the most psychoactive of the three, producing euphoria by triggering increased release of dopamine in the ventral tegmental area.[17] Because cannabis has such a wide range of varied pharmacodynamic activities, it is very difficult to characterize pharmacodynamic DDIs in a systematic manner. Perhaps the most reliable statement that can be made is that it can certainly act in concert with other drugs that derange CNS function to produce additive sedation, confusion, poor judgment, poor coordination and reaction time, and other gross indicators of intact CNS functioning.

Pharmacokinetics. THC is a substrate of P450 2C9 and 3A4, and it is an inhibitor of P450 1A2, 2B6, 2C9, 2C19, and 2D6,[18–22] as well as some UGT enzymes, so it can be expected to potentially increase the levels of substrates of those enzymes, such as methadone, phenytoin, and tricyclic antidepressants, if both drugs are being stably coadministered (see **Table 1**; **Tables 2–5**, and see **Table 8** for further details). THC is an inducer of P450 1A2, so, much like smoked tobacco, this can lead to decreases in the blood levels of coadministered substrates of that enzyme[22] (see **Table 1** for details). THC also has some limited UGT induction capabilities, but these are unlikely to become clinically significant. In addition, THC is an inhibitor of the function of the P-glycoprotein transporter,[23] and as such, it can be expected to increase the bioavailability of P-glycoprotein substrates (see **Table 9** for details). CBD is a substrate of P450 2C19 and 3A4, and an inhibitor of P450 1A2, 2B6, 2C9, 2C19, 2D6, and 3A4, as well as some UGT enzymes,[18–22,24] so it can be expected to increase the blood levels of stably coadministered substrates of those enzymes, such as carbamazepine, glipizide, olanzapine, and zolpidem (see **Tables 1–5, 7**, and **8** for further details). As such, THC and CBD can both be considered as essentially metabolic pan-

| Table 2 | |
P450 2B6 substrates, inhibitors, and inducers	
Substrates	Bupropion
	Cyclophosphamide (prodrug)
	Ifosfamide (prodrug)
	Ketamine
	Methadone
	Phencyclidine (PCP)
	Tamoxifen (prodrug)
Inhibitors	Cannabidiol (CBD)
	Fluoxetine
	Fluvoxamine
	Paroxetine
	Phencyclidine (PCP)
	Ritonavir
	Sertraline
	Tetrahydrocannabinol (THC)
Inducers	Carbamazepine
	Phenobarbital
	Phenytoin
	Rifampin
	Ritonavir

Table 3 P450 2C9 substrates, inhibitors, and inducers	
Substrates	Fluvastatin Glipizide Glyburide Ketamine NSAIDs Phenobarbital (major) Phenytoin S-warfarin Tetrahydrocannabinol (THC)
Inhibitors	Cannabidiol (CBD) Clopidogrel Fluconazole Fluoxetine Fluvastatin Fluvoxamine Isoniazid Modafinil Ritonavir Sulfamethoxazole Tetrahydrocannabinol (THC) Valproate
Inducers	Carbamazepine Pentobarbital Phenobarbital Phenytoin Rifampin Ritonavir Secobarbital

inhibitors, although THC exerts both inhibitory and inductive effects with regard to 1A2 substrates, so it is difficult to predict which, if either, effect will predominate ahead of time. Typically, this sort of determination is made empirically, after the fact, and on a highly individual basis.

Vignette A 56-year-old woman with generalized anxiety and atrial fibrillation has been stably maintained on warfarin, 5 mg/d, producing an international normalized ratio (INR) of 2.4. Her college-aged children were having academic and social difficulties, leading to an exacerbation of her anxiety and insomnia. She took the advice of a friend and went to dispensary, where she was given CBD, 50 mg/d. Two weeks later, she accidentally bumped her elbow on a door frame, and she quickly developed a massive bruise at the point of impact. She astutely reported immediately to check her INR, and it had increased to 6.7. She experienced an improvement in anxiety with the CBD and wanted to continue taking it. A decrease in warfarin dosage to 2.5 mg/d led to a decrease of the INR to 2.8.

In this case, CBD inhibited 2C9 and 1A2, both of which led to a significant increase in warfarin levels and thus INR. Decrease in the warfarin dosing compensated for this effect.

Cocaine
Pharmacodynamics. Cocaine is a potent monoaminergic (serotonin, norepinephrine, epinephrine, and dopamine) reuptake inhibitor,[25,26] and as such, acts as a powerful

Table 4 P450 2C19 substrates, inhibitors, and inducers	
Substrates	Cannabidiol (CBD) Citalopram Clozapine Cyclophosphamide (prodrug) Diazepam Escitalopram Ifosfamide (prodrug) Phencyclidine (PCP) Phenytoin
Inhibitors	Cannabidiol (CBD) (Es)omeprazole Ethinylestradiol Fluoxetine Fluvoxamine Modafinil Oxcarbazepine Ritonavir Tetrahydrocannabinol (THC) Topiramate
Inducers	Carbamazepine Pentobarbital Phenobarbital Phenytoin Rifampin Ritonavir

stimulant and euphoriant. Of course, it can synergize with other stimulants to produce, for instance, lowering of the seizure threshold, psychosis, and/or cardiac arrhythmias or ischemia arising from acute increased metabolic requirements combined with coronary artery vasoconstriction.

Pharmacokinetics. About 30% to 50% of cocaine is metabolized by butyrylcholinesterase into ecgonine methyl ester; 30% to 40% is metabolized by tissue esterase and spontaneous conversion into benzoylecgonine, and the remainder is converted into norcocaine by P450 3A4.[24,27,28] Norcocaine produces oxidative stress and is thus hepatotoxic. There has been some investigation as to whether use of 3A4 inhibitors decreases cocaine-induced hepatoxicity, but this remains only conjectural.[24] Cocaine also acts as an inhibitor of P450 2D6,[29–31] and as such, it can be expected to increase the blood levels of coadministered 2D6 substrates, such as beta-blockers and tricyclic antidepressants (see **Table 5**).

Opioids
Pharmacodynamics. All opioids act as mu-receptor agonists, and several have significant binding to other opioid receptors as well. As such, opioids act as nonspecific CNS depressants with the capacity to synergize with other CNS depressants (such as ethanol or benzodiazepines) to suppress cardiopulmonary function, possibly with fatal consequences.

Codeine
  Pharmacokinetics Codeine is mostly a prodrug, relying on metabolism via P450 2D6 to undergo transformation from a relatively ineffective analgesic into morphine.[32,33] If

Table 5
P450 2D6 substrates and inhibitors

Substrates	Amphetamine
	Aripiprazole
	Beta-blockers
	Codeine (prodrug)
	Dextromethorphan
	Hydrocodone (prodrug)
	Methamphetamine
	Mirtazapine
	Oxycodone
	Paroxetine
	Risperidone
	Tamoxifen (prodrug)
	Tramadol (prodrug)
	Tricyclic antidepressants
	Typical antipsychotics
Inhibitors	Bupropion
	Cannabidiol (CBD)
	Cocaine
	Diphenhydramine
	Ethanol
	Fluphenazine
	Fluoxetine
	Haloperidol
	Methadone
	Paroxetine
	Perphenazine
	Quinidine
	Risperidone
	Ritonavir
	Tetrahydrocannabinol (THC)
	Tricyclic antidepressants

codeine is administered to a 2D6 poor metabolizer, or to someone who is being coadministered a meaningful 2D6 inhibitor, such as bupropion, fluoxetine, or ritonavir (see **Table 5** for details), then it is unlikely to be an effective analgesic drug.

Fentanyl

Pharmacokinetics Fentanyl is a substrate primarily of P450 3A4.[34] As such, coadministered inhibitors of 3A4, such as ciprofloxacin, protease inhibitors, and verapamil, can be expected to increase fentanyl levels, whereas inducers of 3A4, such as carbamazepine and phenytoin, would be expected to lower fentanyl levels (see **Table 7** for further details). In addition, fentanyl is an inhibitor of the P-glycoprotein transporter.[35] As such, if it is consistently used, it is likely to increase the blood levels of coadministered P-glycoprotein substrates, such as carbamazepine, digoxin, and quetiapine (see **Table 9** for details).

Heroin

Pharmacokinetics Heroin is transformed by various esterases into 6-monoacetylmorphine and morphine[36] (see later discussion for morphine pharmacokinetics).

Hydrocodone

Pharmacokinetics Much like codeine, hydrocodone is a prodrug that relies on transformation via P450 2D6 into an active analgesic metabolite, hydromorphone.[37] If hydrocodone is administered to a 2D6 poor metabolizer, or to someone who is being coadministered a meaningful 2D6 inhibitor, such as bupropion, fluoxetine, or ritonavir (see **Table 5** for details), then it is unlikely to be an effective analgesic drug.

Morphine

Pharmacokinetics Morphine is a substrate of UGT enzymes and the P-glycoprotein transporter.[35,38] As such, coadministered inhibitors of these systems, such as fluoxetine, omeprazole, and sertraline, can be expected to increase morphine levels, whereas inducers of these systems, such as carbamazepine, phenytoin, and prazosin, would be expected to lower morphine levels (see **Tables 8** and **9** for details).

Oxycodone

Pharmacokinetics Oxycodone is a substrate of 3A4 > 2D6.[39] As such, coadministered inhibitors of these enzymes, such as ciprofloxacin, fluoxetine, and verapamil, can be expected to increase oxycodone levels, whereas inducers of 3A4, such as carbamazepine and phenytoin, would be expected to lower oxycodone levels (see **Tables 5** and **7** for details).

Benzodiazepines

Pharmacodynamics. Benzodiazepines all facilitate the binding of gamma-aminobutyric acid (GABA) to inhibitory GABA receptors. As such, benzodiazepines act as nonspecific CNS depressants with the capacity to synergize with other CNS depressants (such as ethanol or opioids) to suppress cardiopulmonary function, possibly with fatal consequences. These properties are true for all benzodiazepines. In later discussion, the author focuses on the pharmacokinetic differences between various specific benzodiazepines.

Alprazolam

Pharmacokinetics Alprazolam is a specific P450 3A4 substrate.[40] As such, coadministered inhibitors of 3A4, such as protease inhibitors and verapamil, can be expected to increase alprazolam levels, whereas inducers of 3A4, such as carbamazepine and phenytoin, would be expected to lower alprazolam levels (see **Table 7** for details).

Vignette A 32-year-old gardener has been taking alprazolam, 1 mg 3 times a day for panic disorder, and enjoys the benefit from this regimen. In the course of his work, he was stuck with a thorn in the nail bed of his right index finger and developed a case of onychomycosis. His primary care provider prescribed itraconazole, initially dosed at 200 mg twice a day for 1 week. Three days after starting the itraconazole, he was so tired he could not get out of bed and had to take the day off and was so unsteady and uncoordinated that he did not feel it was safe for him to drive. He contacted his primary care provider, who consulted a pharmacist, leading to the suggestion to decrease alprazolam dosing in half while taking itraconazole, which corrected the problem.

In this case, itraconazole inhibited 3A4, leading to a significant increase in alprazolam levels. Decreasing the alprazolam dosage while taking the itraconazole remedied the problem.

Chlordiazepoxide/Clonazepam

Pharmacokinetics The metabolism of these benzodiazepines is quite varied and involves many different enzyme systems, as well as many different P450 enzymes. As such, these drugs are susceptible to metabolite accumulation if metabolic clearance is impaired by poor hepatic function or some other acute or chronic processes, but these drugs are not particularly susceptible to DDIs per se.

Diazepam
Pharmacokinetics Diazepam is a substrate of P450 2C19 > 3A4.[41] As such, coadministered inhibitors of these enzymes, such as omeprazole and fluoxetine, can be expected to increase diazepam levels, whereas inducers of these enzymes, such as carbamazepine and phenytoin, would be expected to lower diazepam levels (see **Tables 4** and **7** for details).

Lorazepam/xazepam
Pharmacokinetics Lorazepam and oxazepam are handled primarily by UGT enzymes.[42] They tend to not be particularly susceptible to pharmacokinetic DDIs nor to metabolite accumulation even in physiologically vulnerable individuals, which is why these are the benzodiazepines of choice for alcohol detoxification in the context of hepatic encephalopathy.

Barbiturates
Pharmacodynamics. In a manner similar but not identical to benzodiazepines, barbiturates act to enhance the activity of GABA, thus acting as CNS depressants. As such, they can act synergistically with other CNS depressants (benzodiazepines, ethanol, and/or opioids) to produce potentially fatal suppression of cardiopulmonary activity. The pharmacokinetics of specific barbiturates are examined in later discussion.

Phenobarbital
Pharmacokinetics Phenobarbital is a substrate primarily of P450 2C9, with secondary contributions from 2C19 and 2E1.[43,44] As such, coadministered inhibitors of 2C9, such as clopidogrel, fluoxetine, and valproate, can be expected to increase phenobarbital levels, while inducers of 2C9, such as carbamazepine and phenytoin, would be expected to lower phenobarbital levels (see **Table 3** for details). Phenobarbital is a pan-inducer of P450 and UGT enzymes,[45,46] and accordingly, ongoing and consistent use of phenobarbital can be expected to decrease the blood levels of a host of coadministered drugs that have meaningful components of phase I and/or phase II metabolism (see **Tables 1–4**; **Tables 6–8** for details).

Secobarbital
Pharmacokinetics Secobarbital is an inducer of P450 1A2 and 2C9.[46] Accordingly, the ongoing and consistent use of secobarbital can be expected to decrease the blood levels of coadministered 1A2 and 2C9 substrates, such as olanzapine and phenytoin (see **Tables 1** and **3** for details).

Amobarbital
Pharmacokinetics Although amobarbital is among the more misused barbiturates, its pharmacokinetic properties are only poorly understood. It appears to be a pan-inducer in animals, but it is unclear whether that is the case in humans as well.[47]

Table 6
P450 2E1 substrates, inhibitors, and inducers

Substrates	Acetaminophen
	Ethanol
Inhibitors	Disulfiram
	Isoniazid
Inducers	Ethanol
	Isoniazid
	Obesity
	Tobacco smoking

Table 7
P450 3A4 substrates, inhibitors, and inducers

Substrates	Alprazolam
	Aripiprazole
	Atorvastatin
	Azole antifungals
	Buprenorphine
	Buspirone
	Calcium-channel blockers
	Cannabidiol (CBD)
	Carbamazepine
	Citalopram
	Cocaine
	Cortisol
	Cyclosporine
	Diazepam
	Escitalopram
	Ethinylestradiol
	Fentanyl
	Ketamine
	Lurasidone
	Methadone
	Mirtazapine
	Nonnucleoside reverse transcriptase inhibitors
	Oxycodone
	Phencyclidine (PCP)
	Phosphodiesterase Inhibitors
	Pimozide
	Prednisone
	Protease inhibitors
	Quetiapine
	Risperidone
	Tetrahydrocannabinol (THC)
	Simvastatin
	Sirolimus
	Tacrolimus
	Testosterone
	Trazodone
	Zolpidem
Inhibitors	Azole antifungals
	Cannabidiol (CBD)
	Ciprofloxacin
	Clarithromycin
	Delavirdine
	Diltiazem
	Efavirenz
	Erythromycin
	Ethanol
	Fluoxetine
	Fluvoxamine
	Grapefruit juice
	Phencyclidine (PCP)
	Protease inhibitors
	Verapamil

(continued on next page)

Table 7 (continued)	
Inducers	Carbamazepine
	Modafinil
	Oxcarbazepine
	Pentobarbital
	Phenobarbital
	Phenytoin
	Rifampin
	Ritonavir
	St. John's wort

Pentobarbital

Pharmacokinetics Pentobarbital is an inducer of P450 1A2, 2C9, 2C19, and 3A4.[46] Accordingly, the ongoing and consistent use of pentobarbital can be expected to decrease the blood levels of coadministered substrates of these enzymes (see **Tables 1, 3, 4,** and **7** for details).

Methamphetamine/amphetamine

Pharmacodynamics. In a manner somewhat similar to cocaine, these drugs act to both increase presynaptic release and inhibit synaptic reuptake of monoamines (serotonin, norepinephrine, epinephrine, and dopamine). As such, they act as stimulants and euphoriants. Of course, these stimulants can synergize with other similarly acting drugs to produce, for instance, lowering of the seizure threshold and cardiac arrhythmias or

Table 8 Uridine 5′-diphosphate glucuronosyltransferase substrates, inhibitors, and inducers	
Substrates	Buprenorphine
	Hydromorphone
	Lamotrigine
	Lorazepam
	Morphine (partial prodrug)
	NSAIDs
	Oxazepam
	Valproate
Inhibitors	Cannabidiol (CBD)
	Methadone
	NSAIDs
	Probenecid
	Tacrolimus
	Tetrahydrocannabinol (THC)
	Trimethoprim
	Valproate
Inducers	Carbamazepine
	Ethinylestradiol
	Oxcarbazepine
	Phenobarbital
	Phenytoin
	Rifampin
	Ritonavir
	Tetrahydrocannabinol (THC)
	Tobacco smoking

ischemia arising from acute increased metabolic requirements combined with coronary artery vasoconstriction.

Pharmacokinetics. Amphetamine and methamphetamine are both substrates of P450 2D6, and so inhibitors of this enzyme, such as bupropion, fluoxetine, and ritonavir, can be expected to increase amphetamine blood levels[48–50] (see **Table 5** for details). Methamphetamine is also a possible substrate of the P-glycoprotein transporter,[51] and as such, levels of methamphetamine may be higher or lower than expected in the presence of coadministered P-glycoprotein inhibitors (such as omeprazole and paroxetine) or inducers (such as aspirin, prazosin, and trazodone), respectively (**Table 9**).

Ketamine

Pharmacodynamics. Ketamine acts as an *N*-methyl-D-aspartate (NMDA) receptor antagonist. It also acts at opioid, muscarinic, and other voltage-gated channel receptors, which is how it functions as a dissociative anesthetic.[52] Use of ketamine can produce CNS depression, confusion, dissociation, hallucinations, and euphoria, and it can act synergistically with other CNS depressants to magnify those symptoms. Curiously, ketamine is less apt to produce suppression of cardiopulmonary function than other CNS depressants.

Pharmacokinetics. Ketamine is primarily a substrate of P450 2B6 and 3A4, with 2C9 making a secondary contribution to its metabolism.[53–55] As such, coadministered inhibitors of 2B6 and/or 3A4, such as fluoxetine and verapamil, can be expected to increase ketamine levels, whereas inducers of 2B6 and/or 3A4, such as carbamazepine and phenytoin, would be expected to lower ketamine levels (see **Tables 2** and **7** for details). In addition, ketamine is a substrate of the P-glycoprotein transporter,[56] so coadministration with P-glycoprotein inhibitors, such as omeprazole and sertraline, would be expected to increase ketamine levels, whereas coadministered P-glycoprotein inducers, such as aspirin and prazosin, would be expected to lower ketamine levels (see **Table 9** for details).

Phencyclidine

Pharmacodynamics. Like ketamine, phencyclidine (PCP) is an NMDA-receptor antagonist. In addition, it binds to some opioid receptors, and it has stimulant capabilities, as it inhibits reuptake of serotonin, norepinephrine, and dopamine, and increases neuronal intracellular production of both dopamine and norepinephrine through stimulation of the activity of tyrosine hydroxylase.[57,58] It can act synergistically with other CNS depressants to exacerbate confusion, behavioral dyscontrol, or dissociation, or with stimulants to produce seizures, hallucinations, and increases in cardiac demand.

Pharmacokinetics. PCP is a meaningful substrate of both P450 1A2 and 3A4,[59] although PCP also undergoes non-P450 mechanisms of metabolic clearance.[60] As such, coadministered inhibitors of 1A2 and/or 3A4, such as fluvoxamine and protease inhibitors, may be expected to increase PCP levels, whereas inducers of 1A2 and/or 3A4, such as carbamazepine and phenytoin, would be expected to lower PCP levels (see **Tables 1** and **7** for details). In addition, PCP is an inhibitor of P450 2B6 and 3A4,[59,61] and if taken with regularity, it would be expected to increase the levels of coadministered 2B6 and/or 3A4 substrates, such as carbamazepine, methadone, and quetiapine (see **Tables 2** and **7** for details).

Table 9 P-glycoprotein substrates, inhibitors, and inducers	
Substrates	Antihistamines (nonsedating only) Carbamazepine Cyclosporine Digoxin Ketamine Loperamide Methadone Methamphetamine (possible) Morphine Ondansetron Phenytoin Quetiapine Risperidone Ritonavir Tacrolimus Tricyclic antidepressants
Inhibitors	Atorvastatin Buprenorphine Clarithromycin Diltiazem Disulfiram Erythromycin Fentanyl Grapefruit juice Green tea Itraconazole Ketoconazole Methadone Omeprazole Phenothiazines (and some other typical antipsychotics) Quinidine Ritonavir Simvastatin SSRIs (except for citalopram/escitalopram) Tetrahydrocannabinol (THC) Tricyclic antidepressants Verapamil
Inducers	Aspirin Prazosin Rifampin Ritonavir St. John's wort Trazodone

Therapeutic Agents for Substance Use Disorders

Acamprosate

Pharmacodynamics. Acamprosate acts as an NMDA-receptor "modulator."[62] It is hypothesized that this mechanism acts to diminish cravings for ethanol.

Pharmacokinetics. The clearance of acamprosate is fundamentally renal. There are no known relevant DDIs.

Buprenorphine

Pharmacodynamics. Buprenorphine acts as a partial opioid agonist with very avid binding to opioid receptors,[63] by which mechanisms it acts to both manage acute opioid withdrawal and, when used as maintenance therapy, reduce craving for opioids.

Pharmacokinetics. Buprenorphine is primarily a substrate of P450 3A4, with some UGT enzymes making a secondary contribution to its metabolic clearance.[47,64] As such, coadministered inhibitors of 3A4, such as ciprofloxacin, protease inhibitors, and verapamil, may be expected to increase buprenorphine levels, whereas inducers of 3A4, such as carbamazepine and phenytoin, would be expected to lower buprenorphine levels (see **Table 7** for details). In addition, buprenorphine acts as an inhibitor of the functioning of the P-glycoprotein transporter.[23] Accordingly, if buprenorphine is being used in a maintenance fashion, then it would be likely to increase the blood levels of coadministered P-glycoprotein substrates, such as carbamazepine and quetiapine (see **Table 9** for details).

Disulfiram

Pharmacodynamics. As mentioned in the section on ethanol, ethanol is metabolized by multiple mechanisms to acetaldehyde. Acetaldehyde is in turn metabolized into acetate by aldehyde dehydrogenase.[10,11] Disulfiram acts as an inhibitor of the action of aldehyde dehydrogenase, leading to an accumulation of acetaldehyde that would generally not occur in the course of standard, unimpeded metabolism of ethanol. This accumulation of acetaldehyde produces an array of very unpleasant symptoms, including diaphoresis, flushing, throbbing headache, tachypnea, nausea, vomiting, dizziness, blurry vision, fatigue/malaise, syncope, and tachycardia/palpitations.[6] Although rare, this reaction has even proven fatal to physiologically vulnerable individuals. Obviously, the use of disulfiram is as a deterrent to ethanol consumption, and ideally this reaction should never occur.

Pharmacokinetics. Disulfiram is an inhibitor of both P450 2E1 and also of the P-glycoprotein transporter.[65,66] Seldom, if ever, does the inhibition of 2E1 prove clinically relevant. However, if disulfiram is used as a maintenance treatment, then it may be expected to potentially increase the levels of coadministered P-glycoprotein substrates, such as morphine, phenytoin, and quetiapine (see **Table 9** for details).

Methadone

Pharmacodynamics. Methadone acts as mu-receptor agonist, and it binds to other opioid receptors as well. As such, methadone acts as a nonspecific CNS depressant with the capacity to synergize with other CNS depressants (such as ethanol or benzodiazepines) to suppress cardiopulmonary function, possibly with fatal consequences.

Pharmacokinetics. Methadone is a substrate of P450 2B6 > 3A4, as well as the P-glycoprotein transporter.[23,47,67,68] As such, coadministered inhibitors of 2B6, 3A4, and P-glycoprotein, such as fluoxetine and omeprazole, may be expected to increase methadone levels, whereas inducers of 2B6, 3A4, and P-glycoprotein, such as carbamazepine, phenytoin, and trazodone, would be expected to lower methadone levels (see **Tables 2, 7,** and **9** for details). In addition, methadone acts as an inhibitor of P450 2D6, some UGT enzymes,[69] and the P-glycoprotein transporter. Accordingly, methadone may be expected to increase the levels of coadministered substrates of 2D6 and P-glycoprotein, and some UGT substrates, such as carbamazepine, quetiapine, and tricyclic antidepressants (see **Tables 5, 8,** and **9**).

Vignette. A 42-year-old man has been successfully maintained on methadone, 120 mg/d for treatment of opioid dependence, as well as divalproex sodium, 1500 mg/d (level = 89 μg/mL) for treatment of a seizure disorder. For unclear reasons, he has experienced more breakthrough seizures. With a careful eye on potential phenytoin-valproate DDIs, his neurologist added phenytoin, 300 mg twice a day (level = 16 μg/mL). Within 2 weeks of starting the phenytoin, the patient complained of anxiety, restlessness, diaphoresis, nausea, and diarrhea. Consultation with the Opioid Agonist Treatment Program led to a dialogue with the neurologist and the selection of a different anticonvulsant.

In this case, the addition of phenytoin led to the induction of 2B6 and 3A4 and subsequent significant decrease in methadone levels, producing an emerging opioid withdrawal syndrome. If the neurologist insisted on remaining on phenytoin, then the methadone dosage could have been increased to compensate for this issue.

Naloxone
Pharmacodynamics. Naloxone acts as an antagonist of mu, kappa, delta, and sigma opioid receptors.[5] It is most often used to rapidly reverse the effects of suspected opioid intoxication. For not well-understood reasons, it also acts to diminish the anticonvulsant effects of phenytoin.[5]

Pharmacokinetics. Naloxone is a UGT substrate, but this seldom, if ever, yields any meaningful DDIs.

Naltrexone
Pharmacodynamics. Similar to naloxone, naltrexone is a strong antagonist of the mu-opioid receptor and a weaker antagonist of kappa and delta opioid receptors.[70] There has been lore about adverse DDIs with dextromethorphan, disulfiram, and several other drugs, but none of these has ever been meaningfully substantiated.

Pharmacokinetics. There appear to be no meaningful pharmacokinetic DDIs.

Varenicline
Pharmacodynamics. Varenicline acts as a selective partial agonist of the alpha-4, beta-2 nicotinic acetylcholine receptor, by which action it diminishes nicotine craving.[71]

Pharmacokinetics. Clearance is accomplished through UGT enzymes and renally. There are no likely meaningful DDIs.

CLINICS CARE POINTS

- In assessing the potential for meaningful drug-drug interactions, the first and most important step is to identify the drugs of concern if their levels are increased or decreased. Attention will often appropriately be drawn to agents with a low therapeutic index (ED50/LD50), like digoxin, lithium, methadone, and tricyclic antidepressants. Once these agents of concern have been identified, then identification of potential inhibitors and inducers can follow.

- Be aware that drug-drug interactions need not be unidirectional, but rather they can be reciprocal. A given drug can have its metabolism inhibited or induced by other drugs, and this drug can simultaneously act as an inhibitor or inducer of the metabolism of those drugs or still different drugs in a regimen.

- If there was ever an area of medicine in which it would truly be said that "an ounce of prevention is worth a pound of cure," that would be drug-drug interactions. Drug-drug interaction "victories" are boring, because one anticipated a potential problem and made choices to avoid it in the first place, rather than responding to it after having caused it to arise. When it comes to drug-drug interactions, boring is good.

DISCLOSURE

The author has no financial conflicts of interest to disclose.

REFERENCES

1. Cogentin package insert. West Point, PA: Merck; 1996.
2. Nardil package insert. New York, NY: Pfizer; 2003.
3. Parnate package insert. Research Triangle Park, NC: Glaxo-SmithKline; 2001.
4. Rush J, Fava M, Wisniewski SR, et al. Sequenced treatment alternatives to relieve depression (STAR*D): rationale and design. Control Clin Trials 2004;25(1): 119–42.
5. Frey HH, Schicht S. Interaction of mu-opioid antagonistic drugs with antiepileptics. Pharmacol Toxicol 1996;78(4):264–8.
6. Lipsky JJ, Shen ML, Naylor S. In vivo inhibition of aldehyde dehydrogenase by disulfiram. Chem Biol Interact 2001;130-132(1–3):93–102.
7. Zevin S, Benowitz NL. Drug interactions with tobacco smoking. an update. Clin Pharmacokinet 1999;36(6):425–38.
8. Mansvelder HD, McGehee DS. Cellular and synaptic mechanisms of nicotine addiction. J Neurobiol 2002;53(4):606–17.
9. Haass M, Kübler W. Nicotine and sympathetic neurotransmission. Cardiovasc Drugs Ther 1997;10(6):657–65.
10. Lu Y, Cederbaum AI. CYP2E1 and oxidative liver injury by alcohol. Free Radic Biol Med 2008;44(5):723–38.
11. Zakhari S. Overview: how is alcohol metabolized by the body? Alcohol Res Health 2006;29(4):245–54.
12. Gazzaz M, Kinzig M, Schaeffeler E, et al. Drinking ethanol has few acute effects on CYP2C9, CYP2C19, NAT2, and P-Glycoprotein activities but somewhat inhibits CYP1A2, CYP2D6, and intestinal CYP3A: so what? Clin Pharmacol Ther 2018;104(6):1249–59.
13. Mitchell MC, Hoyumpa AM, Schenker S, et al. Inhibition of caffeine elimination by short-term ethanol administration. J Lab Clin Med 1983;101(6):826–34.
14. Manyike PT, Kharasch ED, Kalhorn TF, et al. Contribution of CYP2E1 and CYP3A to acetaminophen reactive metabolite formation. Clin Pharmacol Ther 2000;67(3): 275–82.
15. Thummel KE, Slattery JT, Ro H, et al. Ethanol and production of the hepatotoxic metabolite of acetaminophen in healthy adults. Clin Pharmacol Ther 2000;67(6): 591–9.
16. Kariyanna PT, Wengrofsky P, Jayarangaiah A, et al. Marijuana and cardiac arrhythmias: a scoping study. Int J Clin Res Trials 2019;4(1):132.
17. Ameri A. The effects of cannabinoids on the brain. Prog Neurobiol 1999;58(4): 315–48.
18. Arellano AL, Papaseit E, Romaguera A, et al. Neuropsychiatric and general interactions of natural and synthetic cannabinoids with drugs of abuse and medicines. CNS Neurol Disord Drug Targets 2017;16(5):554–66.
19. Bornheim LM, Everhart ET, Li J, et al. Characterization of cannabidiol-mediated cytochrome P450 inactivation. Biochem Pharmacol 1993;45(6):1323–31.

20. Qian Y, Gurley BJ, Markowitz JS. The potential for pharmacokinetic interactions between cannabis products and conventional medications. J Clin Psychopharmacol 2019;39(5):462–71.
21. Alsherbiny MA, Li CG. Medicinal cannabis-potential drug interactions. Medicines (Basel) 2018;6(1):3.
22. Vázquez M, Guevara N, Maldonado C, et al. Potential pharmacokinetic drug-drug interactions between cannabinoids and drugs used for chronic pain. Biomed Res Int 2020;2020:3902740.
23. Tournier N, Chevillard L, Megarbane B, et al. Interaction of drugs of abuse and maintenance treatments with human P-glycoprotein (ABCB1) and breast cancer resistance protein (ABCG2). Int J Neuropsychopharmacol 2010;13(7):905–15.
24. Pellinen P, Honkakoski P, Stenbäck F, et al. Cocaine N-demethylation and the metabolism-related hepatotoxicity can be prevented by cytochrome P450 3A inhibitors. Eur J Pharmacol 1994;270(1):35–43.
25. Schindler CW, Goldberg SR. Accelerating cocaine metabolism as an approach to the treatment of cocaine abuse and toxicity. Future Med Chem 2012;4(2):163–75.
26. Gallelli L, Gratteri S, Siniscalchi A, et al. Drug-drug interactions in cocaine-users and their clinical implications. Curr Drug Abuse Rev 2017;10(1):25–30.
27. Kolbrich EA, Barnes AJ, Gorelick DA, et al. Major and minor metabolites of cocaine in human plasma following controlled subcutaneous cocaine administration. J Anal Toxicol 2006;30(8):501–10.
28. LeDuc BW, Sinclair PR, Shuster L, et al. Norcocaine and N-hydroxynorcocaine formation in human liver microsomes: role of cytochrome P-450 3A4. Pharmacology 1993;46(5):294–300.
29. Shen H, He MM, Liu H, et al. Comparative metabolic capabilities and inhibitory profiles of CYP2D6.1, CYP2D6.10, and CYP2D6.17. Drug Metab Dispos 2007; 35(8):1292–300.
30. Ramamoorthy Y, Yu A, Suh N, et al. Reduced (+/-)-3,4-methylenedioxymethamphetamine ("Ecstasy") metabolism with cytochrome P450 2D6 inhibitors and pharmacogenetic variants in vitro. Biochem Pharmacol 2002;63(12):2111–9.
31. Tyndale RF, Sunahara R, Inaba T, et al. Neuronal cytochrome P450IID1 (debrisoquine/sparteine-type): potent inhibition of activity by (-)-cocaine and nucleotide sequence identity to human hepatic P450 gene CYP2D6. Mol Pharmacol 1991; 40(1):63–8.
32. Dayer P, Desmeules J, Leemann T, et al. Bioactivation of the narcotic drug codeine in human liver is mediated by the polymorphic monooxygenase catalyzing debrisoquine 4-hydroxylation (cytochrome P-450 dbl/bufl). Biochem Biophys Res Commun 1988;152(1):411–6.
33. Gasche Y, Daali Y, Fathi M, et al. Codeine intoxication associated with ultrarapid CYP2D6 metabolism. N Engl J Med 2004;351(27):2827–31.
34. Ziesenitz VC, König SK, Mahlke NS, et al. Pharmacokinetic interaction of intravenous fentanyl with ketoconazole. J Clin Pharmacol 2015;55(6):708–17.
35. Wandel C, Kim R, Wood M, et al. Interaction of morphine, fentanyl, sufentanil, alfentanil, and loperamide with the efflux drug transporter P-glycoprotein. Anesthesiology 2002;96(4):913–20.
36. Kamendulis LM, Brzezinski MR, Pindel EV, et al. Metabolism of cocaine and heroin is catalyzed by the same human liver carboxylesterases. J Pharmacol Exp Ther 1996;279(2):713–7.
37. Otton SV, Schadel M, Cheung SW, et al. CYP2D6 phenotype determines the metabolic conversion of hydrocodone to hydromorphone. Clin Pharmacol Ther 1993;54(5):463–72.

38. Ofoegbu A, Ettienne EB. Pharmacogenomics and Morphine. J Clin Pharmacol 2021;61(9):1149–55.
39. Söderberg-Löfdal KC, Andersson ML, Gustafsson LL. Cytochrome P450-mediated changes in oxycodone pharmacokinetics/pharmacodynamics and their clinical implications. Drugs 2013;73(6):533–43.
40. Dresser GK, Spence JD, Bailey DG. Pharmacokinetic-pharmacodynamic consequences and clinical relevance of cytochrome P450 3A4 inhibition. Clin Pharmacokinet 2000;38(1):41–57.
41. Ono S, Hatanaka T, Miyazawa S, et al. Human liver microsomal diazepam metabolism using cDNA-expressed cytochrome P450s: role of CYP2B6, 2C19 and the 3A subfamily. Xenobiotica 1996;26(11):1155–66.
42. Docci L, Umehara K, Krähenbühl S, et al. Construction and verification of physiologically based pharmacokinetic models for four drugs majorly cleared by glucuronidation: lorazepam, oxazepam, naloxone, and zidovudine. AAPS J 2020; 22(6):128.
43. Goto S, Seo T, Murata T, et al. Population estimation of the effects of cytochrome P450 2C9 and 2C19 polymorphisms on phenobarbital clearance in Japanese. Ther Drug Monit 2007;29(1):118–21.
44. Pacifici GM. Clinical pharmacology of phenobarbital in neonates: effects, metabolism and pharmacokinetics. Curr Pediatr Rev 2016;12(1):48–54.
45. Sabers A. Pharmacokinetic interactions between contraceptives and antiepileptic drugs. Seizure 2008;17(2):141–4.
46. Hakkola J, Hukkanen J, Turpeinen M, et al. Inhibition and induction of CYP enzymes in humans: an update. Arch Toxicol 2020;94(11):3671–722.
47. Ferrari A, Rosario-Coccia CP, Bertolini A, et al. Methadone–metabolism, pharmacokinetics and interactions. Pharmacol Res 2004;50(6):551–9.
48. Lin LY, DiStefano EW, Schmitz DA, et al. Oxidation of methamphetamine and methylenedioxymethamphetamine by CYP2D6. Drug Metab Dispos 1997;25(9): 1059–64.
49. de la Torre R, Yubero-Lahoz S, Pardo-Lozano R, et al. MDMA, methamphetamine, and CYP2D6 pharmacogenetics: what is clinically relevant? Front Genet 2012; 3:235.
50. Hales G, Roth N, Smith D. Possible fatal interaction between protease inhibitors and methamphetamine. Antivir Ther 2000;5(1):19.
51. Mann H, Ladenheim B, Hirata H, et al. Differential toxic effects of methamphetamine (METH) and methylenedioxymethamphetamine (MDMA) in multidrug-resistant (mdr1a) knockout mice. Brain Res 1997;769(2):340–6.
52. Sinner B, Graf BM. Ketamine. Handb Exp Pharmacol 2008;182:313–33.
53. Dinis-Oliveira RJ. Metabolism and metabolomics of ketamine: a toxicological approach. Forensic Sci Res 2017;2(1):2–10.
54. Hijazi Y, Boulieu R. Contribution of CYP3A4, CYP2B6, and CYP2C9 isoforms to N-demethylation of ketamine in human liver microsomes. Drug Metab Dispos 2002;30(7):853–8.
55. Peltoniemi MA, Saari TI, Hagelberg NM, et al. Exposure to oral S-ketamine is unaffected by itraconazole but greatly increased by ticlopidine. Clin Pharmacol Ther 2011;90(2):296–302.
56. Ganguly S, Panetta JC, Roberts JK, et al. Ketamine pharmacokinetics and pharmacodynamics are altered by p-glycoprotein and breast cancer resistance protein efflux transporters in mice. Drug Metab Dispos 2018;46(7):1014–22.
57. Javitt DC, Zukin SR. Recent advances in the phencyclidine model of schizophrenia. Am J Psychiatry 1991;148(10):1301–8.

58. Bey T, Patel A. Phencyclidine intoxication and adverse effects: a clinical and pharmacological review of an illicit drug. Cal J Emerg Med 2007;8(1):9–14.

59. Laurenzana EM, Owens SM. Metabolism of phencyclidine by human liver microsomes. Drug Metab Dispos 1997;25(5):557–63.

60. Kammerer RC, Schmitz DA, Hwa JJ, et al. Induction of phencyclidine metabolism by phencyclidine, ketamine, ethanol, phenobarbital and isosafrole. Biochem Pharmacol 1984;33(4):599–604.

61. Shebley M, Kent UM, Ballou DP, et al. Mechanistic analysis of the inactivation of cytochrome P450 2B6 by phencyclidine: effects on substrate binding, electron transfer, and uncoupling. Drug Metab Dispos 2009;37(4):745–52.

62. Kalk NJ, Lingford-Hughes AR. The clinical pharmacology of acamprosate. Br J Clin Pharmacol 2014;77(2):315–23.

63. Zoorob R, Kowalchuk A, de Grubb MM. Buprenorphine therapy for opioid use disorder. Am Fam Physician 2018;97(5):313–20.

64. Rouguieg K, Picard N, Sauvage FL, et al. Contribution of the different UDP-glucuronosyltransferase (UGT) isoforms to buprenorphine and norbuprenorphine metabolism and relationship with the main UGT polymorphisms in a bank of human liver microsomes. Drug Metab Dispos 2010;38(1):40–5.

65. Kharasch ED, Hankins DC, Jubert C, et al. Lack of single-dose disulfiram effects on cytochrome P-450 2C9, 2C19, 2D6, and 3A4 activities: evidence for specificity toward P-450 2E1. Drug Metab Dispos 1999;27(6):717–23.

66. Loo TW, Bartlett MC, Clarke DM. Disulfiram metabolites permanently inactivate the human multidrug resistance P-glycoprotein. Mol Pharm 2004;1(6):426–33.

67. Kharasch ED, Regina KJ, Blood J, et al. Methadone pharmacogenetics: CYP2B6 polymorphisms determine plasma concentrations, clearance, and metabolism. Anesthesiology 2015;123(5):1142–53.

68. Kharasch ED. Current concepts in methadone metabolism and transport. Clin Pharmacol Drug Dev 2017;6(2):125–34.

69. Gelston EA, Coller JK, Lopatko OV, et al. Methadone inhibits CYP2D6 and UGT2B7/2B4 in vivo: a study using codeine in methadone- and buprenorphine-maintained subjects. Br J Clin Pharmacol 2012;73(5):786–94.

70. Liu JC, Ma JD, Morello CM, et al. Naltrexone metabolism and concomitant drug concentrations in chronic pain patients. J Anal Toxicol 2014;38(4):212–7.

71. Obach RS, Reed-Hagen AE, Krueger SS, et al. Metabolism and disposition of varenicline, a selective alpha4beta2 acetylcholine receptor partial agonist, in vivo and in vitro. Drug Metab Dispos 2006;34(1):121–30.

Nicotine Addiction

A Burning Issue in Addiction Psychiatry

George Kolodner, MD, DLFAPA, FASAM[a],*,
Carlo C. DiClemente, PhD, ABPP[b,1],
Michael M. Miller, MD, DLFAPA, DFASAM[c,d,2]

KEYWORDS

• Nicotine • Addiction • Tobacco • Cigarettes • NRT • SUD • Addiction treatment
• Recovery support services

KEY POINTS

• Nicotine use is of significant importance, not just an incidental issue, when it is used along with other substances by persons with substance use disorders (SUDs).

• Addressing nicotine addiction is given relatively low priority by both the addiction treatment field and the recovery support community.

• Effective treatment of nicotine addiction is available and can be delivered without endangering overall SUD treatment outcomes.

INTRODUCTION

How does one account for the deadliest of the substance use disorders (SUDs)—nicotine addiction—still being given the least attention by many clinicians in the addiction treatment community?

Why did the documentation of the damaging effect of nicotine addiction have much less impact on reducing tobacco use in the SUD patient population than it did in the general population?

The authors wish to thank Lori Karan, William White, Neil Grunberg, Annie Kleykamp, and Joel Guydish for their generous contributions to the content of this article and also Lisa Ilium for formatting the references.

Note on terminology: In this article, the term "nicotine addiction" is used rather than the term "tobacco use disorder" because non-tobacco nicotine delivery devices (ie, electronic cigarettes) emerged after the new substance use disorders (SUDs) nomenclature was established in DSM-5.

[a] Georgetown University School of Medicine, Washington, DC, USA; [b] University of Maryland Baltimore County, Baltimore, MD, USA; [c] University of Wisconsin School of Medicine and Public Health, Madison, WI, USA; [d] Medical College of Wisconsin, Wauwatosa, WI, USA

[1] Present address: 9728 Starling Road; Ellicott City, MD 21042.

[2] Present address: 22 Settler Hill Cir, Madison, WI 53717.

* Corresponding author. 3204 Klingle Road Northwest, Washington, DC 20008.

E-mail address: georgekolodner@gmail.com

One way to start to answer these questions is by asking you, the reader, if you are unfamiliar with any of the following statements about the problems associated with nicotine addiction in the United States?

Nicotine addiction kills as many people *every year* (approximately 480,000) as COVID-19 did in 2021 (476,433).[1] In addition, secondhand tobacco smoke annually kills 50,000 nonsmokers—15,000 more than annual deaths from alcohol impaired driving.[1]

Even with the huge surges in opioid and other drug overdose deaths, nicotine addiction kills more than twice as many people as do all other SUDs combined.

More people in recovery from alcohol use disorder die of nicotine addiction-related illnesses than from any other cause.[2]

The leading cause of death among persons with an alcohol use disorder is not alcohol-related injuries and illnesses—it is medical complications (cardiovascular and pulmonary) of nicotine addiction.[3]

SUD treatment programs rarely include nicotine addiction in their treatment plans.

Effective medications have been approved by the FDA for nicotine addiction but are not consistently offered to patients in SUD treatment programs.

Addiction rehabilitation programs do not permit the continued addictive use of other substances but make an exception for nicotine with patients as well as staff.

How about any of these more hopeful statements?

Two-thirds of tobacco smokers want to quit their use,[4] and many have made multiple actual attempts at quitting. An average of 6 attempts is necessary to achieve stable abstinence, which has been achieved by more than 60% of smokers.[5–7]

Addiction treatment programs that treat nicotine on the same basis as other substances have found either improvement or no decrease in long-term abstinence for all other addictive substances.[8,9]

Stopping tobacco smoking leads to reduced symptoms of depressed mood and anxiety in people with or without psychiatric diagnoses.[10]

The pioneers of addiction treatment in America in the late nineteenth and early twentieth centuries were quite clear about the danger posed to overall SUD recovery by continued nicotine addiction.[11] How and why did this awareness change? In an era when clinicians aspire to practice evidence-based medicine, how is it that they commonly hold nonevidenced-based beliefs and biases such as the following:

1. Patients with SUD are not interested in stopping their use of nicotine.
2. Overall SUD recovery outcomes would be reduced by including nicotine in the treatment plan for abstinence.

This article argues that beliefs and biases such as these contribute significantly to the low priority currently being given to nicotine addiction by many addiction treatment professionals. The persistent segregation of nicotine addiction away from the treatment of all other SUDs persists despite a growing scientific literature supporting the availability of effective treatment options for nicotine addiction. This article builds on these efforts by examining some of the persistent obstacles to change and by making suggestions for ways in which they can be addressed.

A further argument will be made that treatment outcomes for nicotine addiction and cooccurring SUDs could be improved by fully integrating nicotine addiction interventions into the mainstream of addiction treatment programs. This would involve applying clinical interventions regarded as being effective for other SUDs and in which the addiction treatment workforce is already skilled.

The focus of the article is at a clinical level. Because of space limitations, the important policy level of change will only be briefly addressed. Readers interested in learning more broadly about nicotine addiction would benefit from reading a recent review by Prochaska and Benowitz.[12] For a review of treatment, the recent JAMA review by Rigotti and colleagues is recommended.[13]

SELECTED ASPECTS OF NICOTINE ADDICTION
People Exposed to Nicotine Are Highly Likely to Progress to Problematic Use

"Social" tobacco use is much less common than addicted use—the opposite of what occurs with alcohol use. This is consistent with the extensive distribution of nicotine receptors throughout the nervous system. Furthermore, because the most common route of administration is inhalation, thus providing access to the brain even more rapidly than by injection, the addictive potential of nicotine is maximized.

Nicotine Enhances the Rewarding Effect of Other Substances

Although individuals with SUD frequently use more than one substance at a time, this association is particularly common with the use of nicotine. The neurobiological explanation for this clinical finding may be an amplification effect by nicotine on other substances. Recent studies have found that the impact of cocaine on mice was increased if nicotine was given to the animals *before* the cocaine. This did not occur if the nicotine was given *after* the cocaine. The action of histone deacetylase on chromatin is inhibited by nicotine, which allows the cocaine to remain active for a longer period of time.[14–16] In addition, extensive research documents the synergistic interaction between alcohol and nicotine.[17]

Substance Use Disorder Patients Often Downplay the Importance of Their Nicotine Use

Patients focus primarily on the problems created by their "drug of choice." Clinicians are usually able to convince patients to abstain as well from what they regard as a "nonproblem" drug, such as alcohol in a patient with a cocaine use disorder, cannabis for a patient with an alcohol use disorder, and benzodiazepines for a patient with an opioid use disorder. By contrast, when clinicians suggest that nicotine be included in the abstinence treatment plan, the common patient response is "I'm not ready to do that right now." Frequently, there is no follow-up, and many addiction treatment programs fail to explore nicotine use by patients at all.

Strikingly, although the prevalence of tobacco use has fallen to 14% in the general population, rates of use in the SUD population range from 30% to 70% and in some subpopulations reach 90%.[18]

The Contribution of Nicotine Withdrawal Symptoms to Unsuccessful Quit Attempts is Underappreciated

The nicotine withdrawal syndrome is very uncomfortable for most nicotine users but it is not as physiologically debilitating and dangerous as the withdrawal syndromes for most other addictive substances. The intensity of physical and psychological withdrawal symptoms, however, result in an inability of the individual to establish and sustain abstinence. What also distinguishes nicotine from other classes of addictive drugs is the persistence of cravings for years after last use. Over time, these cravings erode determination, especially for those who attempt to quit without the use of symptom-relieving medications. (See "Using Medications More Effectively" section below on medication.)

Most People with Nicotine Addiction Recognize Nicotine to be a Problem for Them and Want to Quit Their Use

In the language of the Transtheoretical Model of the Stages of Change, many people with nicotine addiction would be considered to be in Precontemplation because they are "not seriously considering modifying addictive behavior" in the next 6 months.[19] This disinclination, however, is often due to feelings of hopelessness and helplessness because of past unsuccessful quit attempts. In contrast to people with other SUDs, denying that nicotine is a problem is less frequently the obstacle. Up to 80% of them have not only expressed a desire to quit but have actually made multiple attempts to do so.[8] They might, in fact, be better be described as being in the contemplation or preparation rather than the Precontemplation stages of change. This difference has significant clinical implications as will be discussed in section "Enhancing Psychosocial Interventions."

WHAT IS ALREADY BEING DONE
Outside of the Addiction Treatment Field

Most of the progress being made in reducing the addictive use of nicotine is attributable to the work of behavioral health experts outside of the traditional addiction treatment field. In the United States and the developed world, efforts to intervene have created a wealth of services, strategies, and products that have been successful in reducing initiation of nicotine use and promoting abstinence. A broad array of effective interventions has been developed, largely by psychologists and others, under a framework of "smoking cessation"—language that is not used in addiction treatment toward other SUDs. These interventions range from telephone Quitlines (1–800-QuitNow) to websites, from Screening, Brief Intervention, and Referral to Treatment (SBIRT)[20] to individual and group treatments, as well as support services and mutual help programs. Resources include the following:

a. For clinicians, state-of-the-art smoking cessation treatment protocols can be found at "RX for Change" [https://rxforchange.ucsf.edu/]
b. For smokers and vapers, useful support and suggestions are available at "BecomeAnEX" [https://www.becomeanex.org/]
c. Guidelines for addressing nicotine addiction have been developed by many medical groups such as the American College of Chest Physicians [https://foundation.chestnet.org/wp-content/uploads/2021/06/Tobacco_Dependence_Treatment_Toolkit_CHEST_Foundation.pdf]. Substantial resources have also been developed by public education and advocacy organizations such as the American Lung Association [https://www.lung.org/quit-smoking] and the American Cancer Society [https://www.cancer.org/cancer/cancer-causes/tobacco-and-cancer.html].

A series of groundbreaking reports from the US Surgeons General from 1964 to 2020, documenting the toxic and addictive properties of tobacco, have had a powerful effect in preventing and reducing tobacco use in the general adult and adolescent populations. In addition, significant and successful policy initiatives have increased cessation on a population basis and deterred initiation, especially among youth. These include the following:

a. Laws protecting exposure to secondhand smoke and restrictions on where and when individuals can smoke
b. Tax increases that discourage use, especially among youth
c. Restrictions on advertising, media, and depiction in movies

d. Regulations on commercial tobacco-containing products (prohibition of menthol and other flavorings in cigarettes, small cigars, and cut/smokeless tobacco) and on the quantity of nicotine in tobacco products

Within the Addiction Treatment Field

The American Society of Addiction Medicine (ASAM)—the largest professional society in America that focuses on addiction—has long assumed a leadership role regarding nicotine addiction. Beginning with the pioneering efforts of the late John Slade and Richard Hurt and in the mid-1980s, ASAM pressed for increased attention from clinicians and action from policy makers. More details are available in a recently compiled book titled *Treat Addiction Save Lives: The History of ASAM* [*In Press*]. In 2022, in collaboration with the Smoking Cessation Leadership Center of UCSF [*https:// smokingcessationleadership.ucsf.edu/*], ASAM issued the guidance "Integrating Tobacco Cessation Interventions in Addiction Treatment" [*https://www.asam.org/ quality-care/clinical-guidelines/tobacco*].

Two examples of policy change at a state level to bring nicotine addiction treatment into traditional addiction treatment have occurred recently. In New York State, the Office of Alcohol and Addiction Services adopted regulations that required residential addiction treatment programs to integrate nicotine addiction into diagnostic evaluations at intake and into individualized treatment plans. In 2021, the California Society of Addiction Medicine helped to craft a law that required SUD treatment programs in that state to integrate into their care plans the treatment of nicotine addiction [https:// a24.asmdc.org/press-releases/20210901-governor-newsom-signs-bill-integrate-tobacco-treatment-substance-use].

ADDRESSING OBSTACLES TO CHANGE
Addiction Treatment Field

Studies are minimal that would explain the exception usually made for nicotine by SUD rehabilitation programs to the standard requirement for abstinence from the addictive use of all substances during treatment. This section is, therefore, based on the personal observations of the authors.

The reluctance of SUD patients to discontinue nicotine use is frequently reinforced by the recommendation from their 12-step supporters that doing so would be dangerous to their recovery efforts (see "12-Step Mutual Help Community" section below). Clinicians are likely to defer to this combination of forces if they do not know of the well-done studies documenting better treatment outcome for all substances when nicotine use is also stopped.[21] Other studies indicate that continued addictive nicotine use is associated with increased SUD relapse risk.[22] One of the goals of this article is to increase awareness of these studies.

In addition, clinicians sometimes lack confidence in dealing effectively with nicotine addiction, despite the reality that the interventions with which they are already familiar about other SUDs, such as motivational interviewing and CBT, are fully applicable to nicotine addiction. Furthermore, lack of experience with the medication protocols described in "Using Medications More Effectively" section below leaves them unaware of how effective these medications can be.

Vignette 1

A 52-year-old woman, who was admitted to an intensive outpatient addiction treatment program for an alcohol use disorder, smoked her first cigarette in 20 years during a smoking break in that program's daily treatment schedule.

This particularly unfortunate consequence of the nicotine exception is familiar to many clinicians who work in outpatient and inpatient rehabilitation programs. Breaks during the treatment schedule are important opportunities for patients to have informal social interactions with each other. Because these times are used by many patients to smoke cigarettes, nonsmokers wanting to be included socially are at risk to begin or resume their nicotine use during these breaks. Staff smoking—particularly staff smoking with patients—further increases the difficulty for patients who are attempting to abstain from smoking.[23]

Most states have adopted indoor Clean Air Acts, which prohibit smoking in public indoor facilities. Although some states initially enacted such laws with specific exceptions for addiction and psychiatric treatment facilities, such exceptions are now rare. The Joint Commission, which accredits many health-care organizations, has standards that address tobacco use among patients. Some organizations find that the goal of tobacco-free grounds is still difficult to implement and enforce. A recent study, however, indicated that tobacco-free grounds in SUD programs in California demonstrated more use of nicotine replacement therapy (NRT) and a significant decrease in smoking prevalence by patients.[24]

Optimally, these types of initiatives are linked to a comprehensive approach to patients' use of nicotine. This could include screening, identification of high-risk use situations, referral for counseling, access to nicotine replacement and other appropriate medications, eliminating "smoking" breaks in the daily schedule, and enforcement of policies regarding smoking. Efforts to help staff to quit smoking could also be included.[25]

If total smoke-free efforts are not feasible, creating welcoming spaces comparable to "smoking areas" with alternative activities and smoke-free opportunities for socialization for those trying to become or remain abstinent would support those efforts.

12-Step Mutual Help Community

Vignette 2

A 55-year-old man, who was 10 years in recovery from an alcohol use disorder, decided to enter a nicotine addiction treatment program because he had returned to smoking cigarettes after having a lobe of his lung removed due to cancer. He followed through on this decision despite being warned by his sponsor that stopping his tobacco use could jeopardize his alcohol recovery.

Why do so many of the members of the 12-step recovery community advise delaying addressing tobacco use despite the fact that it was responsible for the death of the cofounders of Alcoholics Anonymous as well as other pioneers of the recovery movement?

One source of the widely held belief that addressing nicotine addiction presents a threat to alcohol recovery can be found at the end of "The Family Afterward" chapter in "The Big Book" of Alcoholics Anonymous.[26] That section describes a man who, although successfully abstaining from alcohol, continued heavy use of tobacco and coffee:

"His wife believed that 'there is something rather sinful about these commodities, so she nagged, and her intolerance finally threw him into a fit of anger. He got drunk.'" The vignette concludes that the man had to "painfully admit" that he was wrong and "Though he is now a most effective member of Alcoholics Anonymous, he still smokes and drinks coffee, but neither his wife nor anyone else stands in judgment. She sees that she was wrong to make a burning issue out of such a matter when his more serious ailments were being rapidly cured."

Written by AA cofounder Bill Wilson,[27] this anecdote is still influential with AA members. Tobacco use was equated with coffee and was considered as not germane to the person's efforts to stop drinking. Wilson's own life provides a contrast to his assertion that nicotine addiction was not a "burning issue." His cigarette use resulted in severe Chronic Obstructive Pulmonary Disease (COPD). He also suffered from major depression, which he was able to relieve by taking long walks. When his COPD became too severe for him to exercise, he lapsed back into a painful depression that lasted to the end of his life.[28] He was not alone; other pioneers such as AA co-founder Dr Bob Smith and Marty Mann, the founder of the National Council on Alcoholism, died of medical consequences of their nicotine addiction.

Although indoor smoking bans have eliminated smoke-filled 12-step meetings, outdoor smoking is common during meeting breaks. Suggestions that "sobriety dates" be determined by the last use of nicotine are unpopular and can be met with hostility.

The critical element of support from mutual help organizations has largely been missing for people struggling with nicotine addiction, meetings of Nicotine Anonymous being less available than those for other substances.

Health Insurance Coverage

Why do insurance companies exclude coverage for psychological interventions for nicotine addiction despite their willingness to pay for treatment later for the extensive medical consequences of tobacco use?

The cost for effective treatment of SUDs is usually beyond the means of the typical patient, making third party coverage essential. Insurance coverage has lagged for all SUDs—a problem addressed by the Mental Health Parity and Addiction Equity Act.[29] Regarding nicotine addiction, however, the payers continue to refuse to provide the coverage for "tobacco use disorder" that is afforded to other SUDs. Brief counseling interventions are sometimes reimbursed but not more substantial counseling or psychoeducational group activities that are necessary for better treatment outcomes.

Almost all plans include coverage for prescription medications but not for over-the-counter patches, lozenges, and gum. Initially, however, even medication coverage was resisted by some health insurance companies. When bupropion was granted an FDA indication for smoking cessation in the late 1990s,[30] it was marketed for that purpose as "Zyban." Some insurance companies not only refused to pay for Zyban but also required any clinician prescribing brand name "Wellbutrin" to certify that it was being used for depression and not for "smoking cessation."

Broader access to NRT is limited because the inhaler and nasal spray are only available by prescription. However, the requirement to self-pay for over-the-counter products can create financial obstacles. In some states, fortunately, the cost is covered by Medicaid or state-subsidized programs.

MORE THAT CAN BE DONE CLINICALLY

Some clinical interventions that are basic to the treatment of other SUDs have not been consistently applied to the treatment of nicotine addiction. Applying the following interventions could improve treatment outcomes.

Enhancing Psychosocial Interventions

Focusing on patient feelings of resignation regarding addressing their addiction to nicotine

When a patient is in Precontemplation because of discouragement about past failed quit attempts, a different treatment strategy would be in order than if the patient doubted that nicotine was a problem. For example, the clinician could point out that multiple quit attempts are the norm and that as the number of quit attempts increases, the probability of success at achieving and sustaining abstinence from nicotine use also increases. Furthermore, if previous attempts were not well organized and did not incorporate the proper use of medication, appropriate instructions from the clinician can increase the likelihood of a successful attempt.

Understanding the underlying obstacle as being resignation rather than "denial" may help clinicians to be more hopeful about the prognosis of these patients. As a result, they would be more likely to incorporate interventions addressing nicotine addiction into their regular repertoire of addiction treatment interventions.

Intensifying patient ambivalence about their nicotine use

Within the motivational interviewing approach, a clinical intervention that intensifies the ambivalence that characterizes the Contemplation stage of change can facilitate progression to the Preparation stage. Patients often downplay the importance of their nicotine addiction by focusing on the danger that accompanied being intoxicated by alcohol or obtaining illegal drugs. A useful way to address this tendency is to ask a patient "What is the wildest thing you have done to get a cigarette or a vape?" (Lori Karan, Personal Communication, 2022). The sometimes-startling answer can elevate patients' awareness of the significant role that nicotine has assumed in their lives.

Using more intensive levels of treatment

Increased intensity and structure of psychosocial interventions have been essential to improving outcomes in traditional SUD treatment. A chapter in the current edition of the ASAM Criteria[31] reviews what these traditional levels of addiction treatment might look like if the addiction treatment delivery system were reengineered to address nicotine addiction. Residential treatment (ASAM Criteria Level 3) is rarely available for nicotine addiction and intensive outpatient and partial hospitalization (ASAM Criteria Level 3) are nonexistent.[32] Providing a remedy for this vacuum, however, would require a change in insurance coverage as mentioned in "Health Insurance Coverage" section above.

Using Medications More Effectively

Medications are available to substantially reduce or eliminate nicotine withdrawal symptoms, including craving. Most people with nicotine addiction, however, attempt to quit without using any medications, thereby decreasing the likelihood of success. Many patients have not had positive experiences using medications and are, therefore, highly skeptical that their withdrawal symptoms can be adequately relieved. They tend, at the same time, to be accepting of exaggerated reports about the side effects of medication or the prospect of medication causing nicotine toxicity. In addition, some patients try to use the gum or lozenges without proper instructions and get discouraged with the disappointing results.

Anticipation of the expected discomfort of withdrawal is a significant deterrent to patients' willingness to address their nicotine addiction. Patients who are informed about the effectiveness and safety of properly dosed medications and then personally witness the relative comfort of well-medicated patients may be more willing to use these medications.

Some considerations are as follows:

a. *Dosing.* These medications are often used in inadequate doses. Regarding the nicotine patch, for example, 1 mg of patch is approximately equivalent in nicotine content to one cigarette. Therefore, if a patient is smoking 1 1/2 packs per day, the appropriate initial patch strength would be to use 2 patches—one of 21 mg and one of 14 mg. These initial doses can be adjusted higher or lower depending on the patient response.

Medication combinations. Many clinicians continue to use only a single medication despite randomized studies demonstrating the effectiveness of using a combination of longer-acting and shorter-acting medications[33–37] as well as by recommendations in a recent JAMA review.[13] One example of this approach, developed at the Mayo Clinic (Dr Taylor Hays, Personal Communication, 2022), suggests that patients using more than 10 cigarettes daily take varenicline for 2 weeks and then use a patch daily, beginning on the evening before the first day of stopping cigarette use. If cravings persist, a short-acting agent such as gum or lozenges can be added. Variations include omitting varenicline, just using the patch and short-term agents. However, if outcomes have been poor, bupropion and varenicline can be given concurrently.

b. *Proper use of oral products.* Patients need education about oral NRT. Nicotine is a nitrogen-containing molecule with a basic pH. For optimum absorption across the membranes of the oral mucosa, the oral cavity must not be an acidic pH environment because the nicotine will ionize and not cross the membranes. Patients need to be educated on avoiding acidic products such as carbonated beverages, fruit juices, tea, and dairy products immediately before using the gum or a lozenge.

Patients also need to keep nicotine-containing saliva in their mouth for 30 seconds, to "feel the tingling," and allow for oral absorption. If they swallow the nicotine-containing saliva, instead of the nicotine being absorbed and reaching the bloodstream then the brain, it will enter the stomach where hydrochloric acid will completely ionize it—but often not without some gastric irritation and dyspepsia from the nicotine itself.

c. *Duration of use.* Medications tend to be discontinued prematurely. Package inserts for patches recommend tapering doses at a rate that might not match individual differences. Furthermore, the common practice in SUD treatment of using medications for months or years for relapse prevention is not done in the treatment of nicotine addiction. Although gum and lozenges are used as needed for extended periods of time, varenicline is rarely used for more than several months. Interestingly, the one study looking at longer term use of varenicline found improved outcomes.[38] A substantial change in this clinical practice would probably require changing the FDA packaging, which is not worded in the same way as it is for longer term use in OUD and AUD.

Expanding Newer Interventions

Effective SUD treatment using virtual technology has become routine since regulatory barriers were lowered during the Spring of 2020 because of the COVID-19 epidemic. For nicotine addiction, treatment outcomes equivalent to in-person settings have been achieved by using telehealth interventions that incorporated contingency management.[39] Devices to measure breath carbon monoxide remotely are available and can be used effectively to motivate current smokers as well as to provide accountability for those in treatment.

MORE THAT CAN BE DONE IN THE MUTUAL HELP COMMUNITY

1. Within the 12-step recovery community, signs of a change in culture are emerging. Written largely by people in long-term personal recovery, "A Time to Lead: The Case for Integrating Treatment of Tobacco Use Disorder in the Treatment of Other Substance Use and Mental Health Disorders"[40] is a comprehensive analysis and a "call to action" for members of the mutual help community, as well as for professional organizations.

2. Non-12-step recovery support programs, such as Self-Management and Recovery Training (SMART) Recovery, explicitly include nicotine in the array of other

addictive substances and have specific interventions described on their websites [https://www.smartrecovery.org/addiction-recovery/stop-smoking; https://www. smartrecovery.org/tips-to-quit-smoking]

3. A large recovery community in Iran, "Congress 60," initially limited its focus to opioid addiction. When the founder—a heavy cigarette smoker—experienced a near fatal heart attack, he stopped using cigarettes and has been working with some success to convince all members of his organization to follow suit.[41]

ELECTRONIC CIGARETTES

This topic is included, despite the limited consensus that surrounds it, because it has already assumed a significant role in the issue of nicotine addiction and will likely play an even larger role in the future. E-cigarettes, also known as electronic nicotine delivery systems or "vapes," arrived in the United States in 2007 and were promoted by manufacturers, with no evidence, as a possible tool to exit from nicotine addiction. There is considerable controversy about whether e-cigarettes are in fact helpful or whether they will exacerbate the problem of nicotine addiction. Differences in their use by youth, with no history of tobacco use, versus by older cigarette smokers, who are already addicted to nicotine, further complicate the debate.

Supporters argue that e-cigarettes:

1. Lack the toxic products from tobacco combustion, making them safer than cigarettes
2. Have a potential for helping people abstain entirely from tobacco use (an approach explicitly endorsed by the National Health Service in the United Kingdom)

Critics, including the regular reports of AMA Council on Science and Public Health on e-cigarettes, argue that e-cigarettes:

1. Contain toxic chemicals of unknown kind and quantity in the vaping fluid and the long-term health effects of these are unknown
2. Are introducing young people to nicotine, leading to addiction and transition to tobacco use
3. Are often used in combination with cigarettes instead of as an alternative.

One response to patients who ask about the advisability of shifting from tobacco cigarettes to e-cigarettes would be to emphasize the importance of making a total shift while being clear that the safety of the e-cigarettes has not been established.

Adolescents who vape are 3 times more likely to initiate cigarette smoking than do adolescents who do not vape.[42] A familiar tension point around underage use has developed between regulators and manufacturers. With adolescents and young adults providing an eager market, manufacturers strive to satisfy those demands. A nicotine delivery system has been designed which is as addictive or perhaps more addictive than cigarettes. Some brands of e-cigarettes deliver high-nicotine content in chemical forms that maximize delivery deep into the lungs where the nicotine is readily carried by the pulmonary vascular circuit to the brain. By adding flavorings and reducing the harshness of the inhaled aerosol, manufacturers have succeeded in making e-cigarette use very popular with teenagers and young adults.

Their success has led to a dramatic increase in vaping by high school students. Fortunately, the sharp increases seen between 2017 and 2019 leveled off in 2020 and decreased significantly in all grades in 2021, according to the NIDA-sponsored Monitoring the Future survey. Nevertheless, vaping continues to be the predominant method of nicotine consumption among young people—more teens vape than smoke.[43] A recent study found that for adolescents, stopping the use of e-cigarettes is even more difficult than stopping traditional cigarettes.[44]

Interventions by government regulators in response to this use have included restricting the flavorings for nondisposable devices. E-cigarette manufacturers responded by finding loopholes that allow them to maintain the popular flavorings in disposable devices.

The trend for workplaces and schools to establish "tobacco-free" grounds creates an incentive for the clandestine use of e-cigarettes.[45] Devices are designed to not resemble cigarettes but rather to look like objects such as flash drives, watches, or pens and to emit small amounts of visible material—mostly water vapor.[46] They are small enough to be hidden in a sleeve or concealed within the palm of the hand and brought out in a way that avoids detection. Videos are available online with instructions about how youthful users can hide vapor by swallowing or exhaling it surreptitiously.

The complexity of this issue is illustrated by a recent authorization decision by the FDA to allow the marketing of a few e-cigarette products [https://www.fda.gov/news-events/press-announcements/fda-permits-marketing-e-cigarette-products-marking-first-authorization-its-kind-agency]. Although not declaring the product to be safe, they judged that the products "could benefit addicted adult smokers who switch to these products" without unduly endangering youth.

Because of how rapidly this field is changing, research data is limited, and references are quickly outdated. For a summary of the most recent developments, readers are referred to these websites:

- NIDA [https://www.drugabuse.gov/publications/research-reports/tobacco-nicotine-e-cigarettes/what-are-electronic-cigarettes]
- CDC: https://www.cdc.gov/tobacco/basic_information/e-cigarettes/about-e-cigarettes.html
- NIOSH [https://www.cdc.gov/niosh/topics/tobacco/electronicnicotinedeliverysystems.html].

SUMMARY

SUD patients with nicotine addiction discourage clinicians from addressing their nicotine use for at least 2 reasons. First, they are in, or have returned to, a Precontemplative stage of change because, discouraged by their previous unsuccessful attempts to stop using nicotine, they are resigned to the idea that no effective treatment exists. Second, they accept warnings of other members of the recovery community that to stop their use of nicotine would jeopardize their overall recovery.

Addiction clinicians tend to focus their therapeutic efforts in directions where they believe they can make a difference. They would perhaps be more perseverant in addressing nicotine addiction if they were more aware of the evidence that contradicts the inaccurate cultural beliefs within the recovery community. Furthermore, clinicians would achieve better treatment outcomes if their motivational strategy was directed toward patient discouragement, and they used a more aggressive protocol with medications. Support by the insurance community of higher-intensity treatment would lead to even better clinical results.

The recent emergence of e-cigarettes has complicated the issue of nicotine addiction and reinforced the importance of increasing professional attention to this problem.

CLINICS CARE POINTS

- Part of any treatment plan for SUD patients with cooccurring nicotine addiction should include a concrete plan for when and how the nicotine addiction will be addressed.
- Inaccurate beliefs in the recovery community about the danger of addressing nicotine addiction need to be energetically addressed.
- Efforts to motivate patients to address their nicotine addiction should be directed toward patient discouragement about unsuccessfulpast abstinence attempts.
- Better outcomes could be achieved by:
  ○ Using psychosocial interventions that have been effective in the treatment of other SUDs.
  ○ Using medications in adequate doses and in combinations for withdrawal management, as well as continuing their use for months or years if necessary for relapse prevention.
- Better treatment outcomes could increase the likelihood that addiction medicine specialists would address nicotine addiction.

DISCLOSURE

The authors have no commercial relationships related to the content of this article.

REFERENCES

1. National Center for Chronic Disease Prevention and Health Promotion (US) Office on Smoking and Health. The health consequences of smoking—50 Years of progress: a report of the Surgeon general. Atlanta (GA): Centers for Disease Control and Prevention (US); 2014.
2. Hurt RD, Offord KP, Croghan IT, et al. Mortality following inpatient addictions treatment. Role of tobacco use in a community-based cohort. JAMA 1996;275(14): 1097–103.
3. Bandiera FC, Anteneh B, Le T, et al. Tobacco-related mortality among persons with mental health and Substance Abuse problems. PLoS One 2015;10(3). https://doi.org/10.1371/journal.pone.0120581.
4. Babb S, Malarcher A, Schauer G, et al. Quitting Smoking Among Adults - United States, 2000-2015. MMWR Morb Mortal Wkly Rep 2017;65(52):1457–64.
5. Chaiton M, Diemert L, Cohen JE, et al. Estimating the number of quit attempts it takes to quit smoking successfully in a longitudinal cohort of smokers. BMJ open 2016;6(6):e011045.
6. Hughes JR, Solomon LJ, Naud S, et al. Natural history of attempts to stop smoking. Nicotine Tob Res 2014;16(9):1190–8.
7. Creamer MR, Wang TW, Babb S, et al. Tobacco Product Use and Cessation Indicators Among Adults - United States, 2018. MMWR Morb Mortal Wkly Rep 2019;68(45):1013–9.
8. Prochaska JJ, Delucchi K, Hall SM. A meta-analysis of smoking cessation interventions with individuals in substance abuse treatment or recovery. J Consult Clin Psychol 2004;72(6):1144–56.
9. Thurgood SL, McNeill A, Clark-Carter D, et al. A Systematic Review of Smoking Cessation Interventions for Adults in Substance Abuse Treatment or Recovery. Nicotine Tob Res 2016;18(5):993–1001.
10. Taylor G, McNeill A, Girling A, et al. Change in mental health after smoking cessation: systematic review and meta-analysis. BMJ 2014;348:g1151 [published correction appears in BMJ. 2014;348:g2216].

11. White W. Slaying the dragon: the history of addiction treatment and recovery in America. 2nd edition. Bloomington: Chestnut Health Systems; 2014.

12. Prochaska JJ, Benowitz NL. Current advances in research in treatment and recovery: Nicotine addiction. Sci Adv 2019;5(10):eaay9763.

13. Rigotti NA, Kruse GR, Livingstone-Banks J, et al. Treatment of Tobacco Smoking: A Review. JAMA 2022;327(6):566–77.

14. Kandel E. Investigating the Paradigm that Nicotine Boosts the Effects of Cocaine (66/80) [Video]. YouTube. 2017. Available at: https://www.youtube.com/watch?v=Yz34-3H6TJo&t=16s. Accessed February 20, 2022.

15. Levine A, Huang Y, Drisaldi B, et al. Molecular mechanism for a gateway drug: epigenetic changes initiated by nicotine prime gene expression by cocaine. Sci Transl Med 2011;3(107):107ra109.

16. Kandel ER, Kandel DB. Shattuck Lecture. A molecular basis for nicotine as a gateway drug. N Engl J Med 2014;371(10):932–43.

17. Morel C, Montgomery S, Han MH. Nicotine and alcohol: the role of midbrain dopaminergic neurons in drug reinforcement. Eur J Neurosci 2019;50(3):2180–200.

18. Chou SP, Goldstein RB, Smith SM, et al. The Epidemiology of DSM-5 Nicotine Use Disorder: Results from the National Epidemiologic Survey on Alcohol and Related Conditions-III. J Clin Psychiatry 2016;77(10):1404–12.

19. DiClemente CC. Addiction and change: how addictions develop and addicted people recover. 2nd edition. New York: The Guilford Press; 2018.

20. Screening, Brief Intervention, and Referral to Treatment (SBIRT): An Efficacious Public Health Approach to Substance Use Prevention and Treatment. In: Ciminni D, Martin J, editors. Screening, brief intervention, and referral to treatment for substance use: a practitioner's guide. Washington, DC: American Psychological Association; 2020.

21. Schroeder SA, Clark B, Cheng C, et al. Helping Smokers Quit: The Smoking Cessation Leadership Center Engages Behavioral Health by Challenging Old Myths and Traditions. J Psychoactive Drugs 2018;50(2):151–8.

22. Weinberger AH, Platt J, Esan H, et al. Cigarette Smoking Is Associated With Increased Risk of Substance Use Disorder Relapse: A Nationally Representative, Prospective Longitudinal Investigation. J Clin Psychiatry 2017;78(2):e152–60.

23. Guydish J, Le T, Hosakote S, et al. Tobacco use among substance use disorder (SUD) treatment staff is associated with tobacco-related services received by clients. J Subst Abuse Treat 2022;132. https://doi.org/10.1016/j.jsat.2021.108496.

24. McCuistian C, Kapiteni K, Le T, et al. Reducing tobacco use in substance use treatment: An intervention to promote tobacco-free grounds. J Subst Abuse Treat 2022;135:108640.

25. Marynak K, VanFrank B, Tetlow S, et al. Tobacco Cessation Interventions and Smoke-Free Policies in Mental Health and Substance Abuse Treatment Facilities - United States, 2016. MMWR Morb Mortal Wkly Rep 2018;67(18):519–23.

26. Anonymous. Alcoholics anonymous: the Big book. 4th edition. New York: Alcoholics Anonymous World Services, Inc; 2001.

27. Schaberg W. The writing of the Big book. Las Vegas: Central Recovery Press; 2020.

28. Cheever S. My name is Bill: Bill Wilson: his life and the creation of Alcoholics anonymous. New York: Simon & Schuster; 2004.

29. Centers for Medicare and Medicaid Services. The Mental Health Parity and Addiction Equity Act (MHPAEA). Available at: https://www.cms.gov/CCIIO/

Programs-and-Initiatives/Other-Insurance-Protections/mhpaea_factsheet. Accessed January 29, 2022.

30. Hurt RD, Sachs DP, Glover ED, et al. A comparison of sustained-release bupropion and placebo for smoking cessation. N Engl J Med 1997;337(17):1195–202.

31. Mee-Lee D. The ASAM Criteria : treatment for addictive, substance-related, and Co-occurring conditions. 3rd edition. Chevy Chase (MD): American Society of Addiction Medicine; 2013.

32. Williams JM, Steinberg ML, Kenefake AN, et al. An Argument for Change in Tobacco Treatment Options Guided by the ASAM Criteria for Patient Placement. J Addict Med 2016;10(5):291–9.

33. Lindson N, Chepkin SC, Ye W, et al. Different doses, durations and modes of delivery of nicotine replacement therapy for smoking cessation. Cochrane Database Syst Rev 2019;4:CD013308.

34. Steinberg MB, Greenhaus S, Schmelzer AC, et al. Triple-combination pharmacotherapy for medically ill smokers: a randomized trial. Ann Intern Med 2009;150(7): 447–54.

35. Koegelenberg CFN, Noor F, Bateman ED, et al. Efficacy of Varenicline Combined With Nicotine Replacement Therapy vs Varenicline Alone for Smoking Cessation. A Randomized Clinical Trial. JAMA 2014;312(2):155–61.

36. Jon O, Ebbert JO, Dorothy K, et al. Combination Varenicline and Bupropion SR forTobacco-Dependence Treatment in Cigarette Smokers. A Randomized Trial. JAMA 2014;311(2):155–63.

37. Baker TB, Piper ME, Smith SS, et al. Effects of Combined Varenicline With Nicotine Patch and of Extended Treatment Duration on Smoking Cessation: A Randomized Clinical Trial. JAMA 2021;326(15):1485–93.

38. Evins AE, Cather C, Pratt SA, et al. Maintenance treatment with varenicline for smoking cessation in patients with schizophrenia and bipolar disorder: a randomized clinical trial. JAMA 2014;311(2):145–54.

39. Kurti AN, Tang K, Bolivar HA, et al. Smartphone-based financial incentives to promote smoking cessation during pregnancy: A pilot study. Prev Med 2020;140: 106201.

40. Wrich JT, Macmaster D. The Case for integrating treatment of tobacco use disorder in the treatment of other substance use and mental health disorders. 2nd ed 2008. Available at: https://archive.hshsl.umaryland.edu/bitstream/handle/10713/14004/A%20TIME%20TO%20LEAD%20SECOND%20EDITION%20FINAL%20PDF%20%20NOVEMBER%201%202018._%20%283%29.pdf?sequence=1&isAllowed=y. Accessed January 29, 2022.

41. White WL, Daneshmand R, Funk R, et al. A Pilot Study of Smoking Cessation within an Iranian Addiction Recovery Community. Alcohol Treat Q 2016;34(1): 15–29.

42. Chaffee BW, Watkins SL, Glantz SA. Electronic Cigarette Use and Progression from Experimentation to Established Smoking. Pediatrics 2018;141.

43. National Institute on Drug Abuse. Monitoring the Future. December 15, 2021. Available at: https://nida.nih.gov/drug-topics/trends-statistics/monitoring-future. Accessed January 23, 2022.

44. Miech R, Leventhal AM, O'Malley PM, et al. Failed Attempts to Quit Combustible Cigarettes and e-Cigarettes Among US Adolescents. JAMA 2022;327(12): 1179–81.

45. Russell AM, Yang M, Barry AE, et al. Stealth Vaping Among College Students on Four Geographically Distinct Tobacco-Free College Campuses: Prevalence and Practices. Nicotine Tob Res 2022;24(3):342–8.
46. Edwards E. Vaping illness epidemic shows no sign of slowing. 2019. Available at: https://www.nbcnews.com/health/vaping/vaping-illness-epidemic-shows-no-sign-slowing-n1064546. Accessed January 5, 2022.

Substance Use Disorders in Postacute and Long-Term Care Settings

Abhilash Desai, MD[a,b,*], George Grossberg, MD[a,b]

KEYWORDS

- Alcohol • Benzodiazepines • Opioid • Cannabis • Tobacco • Older • Elderly
- Addiction

KEY POINTS

- Primary care providers can initiate several practical medication misuse and substance use disorder (SUD) prevention strategies in their routine care such as avoiding prescription of opioids for chronic noncancer pain in patients at higher-than-usual risk of opioid use disorder.
- Screening for SUD using brief easy-to-use screening tools is recommended for all new admissions to postacute and long-term care (PALTC) settings to improve earlier diagnosis and treatment.
- Food and Drug Administration–approved pharmacologic interventions when appropriate can greatly reduce mortality, relapse rates, and improve well-being of individuals with SUD living in PALTC settings.
- Staff education and early identification and treatment of co-occurring mental health conditions and pain are essential for successful outcomes.

INTRODUCTION

Substance use disorder (SUD) is a psychiatric disorder, diagnosed using the Diagnostic and Statistical Manual 5th Edition (DSM 5) criteria, and involves the compulsive use of addictive substances (refer to **Box 1**) despite negative physical, social, and mental health consequences.[1] SUD is a serious, disabling, chronic, and relapsing disorder. SUDs are among the fastest growing disorders in community dwelling older population.[2–6] In older adults and postacute and long-term care (PALTC) populations,

[a] Division of Geriatric Psychiatry, Department of Psychiatry & Behavioral Neuroscience, Saint Louis University School of Medicine, 1438 South Grand Boulevard, Saint Louis, MO 63104, USA; [b] Department of Psychiatry and Behavioral Sciences, University of Washington School of Medicine, UW Boise Psychiatry Residency, BVAMC Wellness Center B. 116, 500 W. Fort street, Boise, ID 83702, USA
* Corresponding author. 413 North Allumbaugh Street, #101, Boise, ID 83704.
E-mail address: dr.abhilashdesai@icloud.com

Psychiatr Clin N Am 45 (2022) 467–482
https://doi.org/10.1016/j.psc.2022.05.005
0193-953X/22/© 2022 Elsevier Inc. All rights reserved.

Box 1
Substance use disorders based on DSM 5

- Alcohol use disorder (AUD)

- Cannabis use disorder (CUD)

- Hallucinogen use disorder (phencyclidine, ketamine, mescaline, 3,4-methylenedioxymethamphetamine [MDMA], psilocybin, lysergic acid diethylamide [LSD])

- Inhalant use disorder (includes solvents [eg, paint thinners, gasoline], aerosol sprays, nitrites, gases [eg, chloroform, nitrous oxide])

- Nicotine use disorder (includes tobacco use disorder)

- Opioid use disorder (OUD) (includes prescription opioids, illicit opioids including heroin)

- Sedative, hypnotic, or anxiolytic use disorder (eg, benzodiazepines, barbiturates, Z-drugs [eszopiclone, zaleplon, zolpidem])

- Stimulant use disorder (eg, methamphetamine, cocaine)

- Other (or unknown) substance use disorder (includes but not limited to—gabapentinoids [gabapentin, pregabalin], anabolic steroids, anti-Parkinsonian medications, nitrous oxide, betel nut, kava)

Data from Ref.[1]

SUD carries higher risk of serious disability, mortality (eg, overdose deaths), emergency department visits, and hospitalization compared with younger cohorts.[2,3] Medication misuse (MM) represents a broad clinical syndrome of using addictive substances (refer to **Box 2**) without a prescription or in doses and frequencies greater than prescribed and for purposes other than its intended medical use.[4] MM is not a clinical diagnosis, but it is important to note its presence in the medical record, as it can cause serious negative events (eg, falls and injury, delirium, overdose death) and may develop into SUD. Co-occurrence of 2 or more SUDs and SUD co-occurring with MM (eg, a patient with opioid use disorder [OUD] with misuse of prescription stimulants and a patient with alcohol use disorder [AUD] with misuse of prescription benzodiazepines [BZD]) is prevalent in younger as well as older populations.[4–10] Although caffeine is highly addictive and excessive use in older adults can have serious negative effects (eg, insomnia, anxiety), the DSM 5 does not list caffeine use disorder as a diagnosis.[1,11]

Box 2
Commonly misused prescription drugs

- Opioids (eg, hydrocodone, oxycodone, morphine, fentanyl, tramadol)

- Benzodiazepines (eg, lorazepam, diazepam, alprazolam)

- Z-drugs (zolpidem, zaleplon, eszopiclone)

- Stimulants (eg, methylphenidate)

- Miscellaneous (any medication that has sedating properties [eg, gabapentin, pregabalin, quetiapine, diphenhydramine, muscle relaxants])

Data from Ref.[4]

The PALTC population includes patients admitted to inpatient rehabilitation facilities and skilled nursing facilities for rehabilitative care after acute hospitalization (typically for a few weeks), residents living in long-term care and assisted living communities (typically for the rest of their lives) and continuous care retirement communities, as well as individuals receiving home care, hospice care, and care through PACE programs (program for all-inclusive care of the elderly).[12,13] PALTC populations typically have multiple serious medical conditions and functional disabilities. In addition, co-occurring mental health conditions (especially dementia, delirium, depression, psychotic symptoms, anxiety, insomnia), chronic noncancer pain, and inappropriate polypharmacy are prevalent in this population.[12–14]

Research to date has neglected PALTC population regarding prevalence and care of SUD.[3] Preliminary research indicates that PALTC facilities are seeing an increase in residents with SUDs.[15–17] In a study involving Veterans Administration Nursing Homes, residents with SUD were more likely to have dementia, serious mental illness, depressive disorders, and posttraumatic stress disorder compared with residents without SUD.[15] In nursing homes in Norway, the staff generally did not know how much alcohol the residents consumed because alcohol was often brought by family or friends.[16] Homeless veterans admitted to nursing homes are more likely to have a diagnosis of SUD compared with stably housed veterans.[17] Most of the PALTC populations with SUD and MM are older adults but in the last decade, PALTC settings have seen a growing influx of younger nontraditional patients who have mental health conditions and are in the PALTC settings because of consequences of SUD. This younger cohort typically has a variety of complex medical and psychiatric comorbidities and disabilities (eg, cardiac infections from intravenous drug abuse requiring long-term intravenous antibiotics). In our clinical experience, younger patients with SUD often find admission to PALTC boring, and this may cause them to seek substances to cope with this. Patients with SUD admitted for rehabilitation (postacute care) after an acute hospitalization generally stay for only a short time (a few weeks typically) and may not be ready or committed to begin addressing their SUD. They may still crave substances they are addicted to (illicit [eg, cannabis, methamphetamine] or legal [eg, alcohol, cannabis in states where it is legal]) and look for opportunities to obtain and use them.

Based on the rapidly growing prevalence of SUDs in older populations, aging of the cohort with early onset SUD (in their 20s and 30s), aging of the baby-boomers (who as a cohort have had higher prevalence of use of illicit drugs compared with previous cohorts), preliminary research regarding SUD in PALTC settings, and our clinical experience over more than 2 decades of working in PALTC settings, the SUDs and MM are prevalent in PALTC population and are underdiagnosed and undertreated[2–10,15–17] (**Tables 1** and **2**). Onset of SUD in PALTC populations may begin early in life with the pattern persisting into older age or the onset may be later in life (late onset) as a maladaptive coping mechanism to social (eg, grief), health, and other stressful circumstances.

Primary care providers (PCPs [physicians, nurse practitioners, physician assistants]) working in PALTC settings can and should play a key role in the prevention and treatment of SUDs; this includes prevention strategies, routine screening, brief intervention, substance withdrawal management, and treatment with Food and Drug Administration (FDA)-approved medications (when available) and psychosocial interventions that are strength-based, age- and culture-appropriate, and individually tailored.[2–10,18–24] This clinical review identifies several practical evidence-based strategies that PCPs can incorporate in their daily practice to improve the lives of the PALTC population with SUD.

Table 1 Substance use disorders and medication misuse in postacute and long-term care populations		
PALTC Populations	**SUD and MM Concerns**	**Clinical Pearls**
Older adults with advanced dementia in long-term care	Low prevalence of active SUD and MM	Some patients with dementia may still want to drink alcohol because it gives them pleasure and contributes to better quality of life and efforts to control the amount of alcohol consumed may be appropriate
Older adults without advanced dementia in long-term care	Low prevalence of active SUD but medication misuse (especially opioids, benzodiazepines) may be prevalent, especially in those with past history of medication misuse and or SUD	Except in hospice settings, very gradually tapering and discontinuing either opioids or benzodiazepines is recommended for those taking both concurrently to reduce risk of overdose death
Older adults in postacute settings	Prevalence of SUD and MM may be closer to the prevalence in older community-dwelling adults	Those with preexisting active SUD before hospitalization may experience significant ongoing withdrawal symptoms and craving during their postacute stay
Younger population (age <65 y) in long-term care	Higher prevalence of active SUD and MM compared with older adults in long-term care	Co-occurring mental health disorders (eg, depression, anxiety, PTSD, personality disorders) is more prevalent in this population
Younger population in postacute settings	Prevalence of SUD and MM may be closer to the prevalence in community dwelling adults	Active use of substances (eg, cannabis, methamphetamine) may need to be looked into in those with history of SUD and MM before admission

Data from Refs.[2–10]

Prevention of Substance Use Disorder and Medication Misuse in Postacute and Long-Term Care Settings

PCPs can play a key role in routinely implementing a host of practical prevention strategies identified by research on SUD and MM in older adults (refer to **Box 3**).[2–10,18–27] Other prevention strategies specifically for OUD and opioid misuse in PALTC populations include the following:

- All patients who come from the hospital on opioids for acute pain should be assessed for pain control

| Table 2 Prevalence of substance use disorders | | |
Substance Use Disorder and Medication Misuse	Lifetime Prevalence in Community-Dwelling Adults	Other Relevant Information
Any drug use disorder (not including alcohol, nicotine)	9%–10%	Lifetime drug use disorder was associated with comorbid anxiety disorders
Alcohol use disorder (AUD)	20%–30%	Alcohol is recognized by CDC as the third leading cause of preventable death
Cannabis use disorder (CUD)	1%–3%	Older adults are the fastest growing cohort of cannabis users of any age group and represent 17% of nonmedical cannabis users and 30% of medical cannabis users
Hallucinogen use disorder	Unknown	In 2010, an estimated 32 million people reported lifetime use of LSD, psilocybin, mescaline, or peyote
Inhalant use disorder	Rare	Inhalant use is primarily seen in adolescents although some cases persist into adulthood
Nicotine use disorder (NUD)	20%–30%	Most common SUD in PALTC populations
Opioid use disorder (OUD)	0.5%–1%	Heroin use disorder doubled in prevalence (from 0.03% to 0.06%) from 2001–2002 to 2012–2013.
Opioid medication misuse (OM)	8%–11%	Data collected from 2006–2013 found that 35% of adults older than 50 y reported OM in the past 30 d
Sedative hypnotic use disorder (eg, benzodiazepines, Z drugs)	0.1%–0.2%	It often co-occurs with other SUDs (eg, cannabis, opioids, cocaine, methamphetamine)
Benzodiazepine misuse (BZDM)	1%–3%	0.6% in older adults and concomitant misuse of opioids, stimulant is strongly associated with BZDM
Stimulant use disorder (eg, methamphetamine, cocaine)	0.01%–0.03%	2.3% of older adults screened positive for cocaine in emergency department settings in one study
Prescription stimulant misuse (PSM) (eg, methylphenidate, dextroamphetamine)	1%–2%	PSM often co-occurs with other SUD (eg, opioids) and other misuse (eg, BZD)
Other substances use disorder and misuse (eg, gabapentin, pregabalin)	0.1%–0.2%	Pregabalin has a higher misuse potential than gabapentin

Data from Refs.[2–10]

- PCP should prescribe a stop-date for opioid use to prevent excessive use of opioids
- Medical directors of PALTC settings (eg, nursing home) may need to provide guidance to other providers who have high opioid prescription rate for treatment of chronic noncancer pain.

Box 3
Prevention of substance use disorder in postacute long-term care populations

Key goals of prevention
- Prevent medication misuse
- Prevent development of SUD
- Prevent overdose death
- Prevent progression of SUD to more severe stages
- Prevent relapse
- Prevent complications due to SUD

Key examples of prevention strategies that PCPs can support and implement

Universal Prevention Strategies (applicable to the entire PALTC population)
- Use of the American Geriatrics Society (AGS) Beers criteria, STOPP/START criteria, and other similar tools to avoid inappropriate prescribing and implement rational deprescribing for opioids, benzodiazepines, and Z-drugs
- Routine, periodic drug evaluation, and optimization of treatment of physical and mental health conditions and geriatric syndromes (eg, frailty, sarcopenia)
- Routine periodic (at least annual) screening for SUD

Selective Prevention Strategies (applicable to PALTC population at higher-than-average risk of SUD)
- Staff education on SUD to eliminate stigma and improve early detection of SUD
- Avoid LTOT for treatment of chronic noncancer pain, especially in individuals at risk of developing OUD
- Avoiding concomitant use of benzodiazepines and opioids
- Prescribe naloxone when opioids are prescribed
- Routinely checking PDMP before prescribing controlled substances
- For patients currently on opioids for chronic noncancer pain, offer the option to safely taper off opioids and discuss alternative nonopioid treatments

Indicated Prevention Strategies (applicable to individuals with current SUD)
- Prescribe medications approved by the FDA to treat SUD
- Collaborative care with guidance from consultant psychiatrists to manage complex cases

Abbreviation: PDMP, prescription drug monitoring program.

Data from Refs.[2–10,18–27]

Team Approach to Screening, Assessment, and Management of Substance Use Disorder in Postacute and Long-Term Care Settings

SUD is a complex disorder that is best managed via a team approach[2,3,20] (**Box 4**). No screening tool for SUD has been validated in PALTC POPULATIONS. Screening tools the authors recommend (**Box 5**) are based on studies in older adults.[28–30] These 3 screening tools are simple, take only a few minutes, and thus practical in PALTC settings compared with other tools used in older adults. SUD and MM should be considered in the differential diagnosis for all new admissions to PALTC experiencing delirium, falls, and or agitation. SUD and MM should also be considered as a potential cause of poor response to treatment of common physical and mental health conditions in patients with current or past history of SUD. Once screening is positive, a focused assessment by the PCP is necessary to accurately diagnose SUD based on DSM 5 criteria (**Box 6**).[2,3,20] It is important to recognize that the DSM 5 criteria often miss SUD in older adults due to one of the criteria being occupational impairment.[2] In patients suspected to have SUD (eg, past history of heroin addiction, current behaviors indicating SUD), use of biomarkers when available (eg, elevated gamma glutamyl transferase and carbohydrate deficient transferrin in the serum of patients with history of heavy alcohol use; presence of ethyl glucuronide in the urine [a direct metabolite of

---

Box 4
Team approach to prevention, diagnosis, and treatment of substance use disorders in postacute long-term care settings

Admitting nurse—uses a screening tool (refer to **Box 5**) and reports a positive screen to the admitting PCP.

Admitting PCP—reviews the positive screen results with the patient in a respectful, empathic, and nonjudgmental manner; addresses stigma; informs social worker about the positive screen; completes assessment for SUD diagnosis; provides brief intervention; and initiates appropriate treatment including referral to consultant psychiatrist or local addiction centers/programs.

Social worker—provides patient education, addresses stigma, and works toward bolstering social support, connection to local and online resources, and when appropriate, helps establish psychosocial treatment interventions (eg, cognitive behavioral therapy).

Nurse—provides patient education and support, monitors for ongoing substance use and misuse and for withdrawal symptoms, informs the PCP the results

PCP—provides ongoing patient education and support, monitors for ongoing substance use and withdrawal symptoms and complications, collaborates care with consultant psychiatrist in complex cases

Consultant pharmacist—provides guidance to PCP regarding substance—prescription drug interactions, drug-drug interactions between drugs prescribed by PCP to treat SUDs and other current drug therapies

Consultant psychiatrist—provides guidance to PCP in complex cases, provides staff and PCP education on evidence-based treatments for SUD

Peer recovery support specialists—provides education and social support to the patient and their family, encourages adherence to treatment, provides praise for small successes, and helps problem solve challenges (eg, coping with craving triggered by new adversity)

Data from Refs.[2,3,14]

---

alcohol that can be detected in the urine for up to 72 hours after alcohol consumption]) and a confirmatory drug test may be needed if the presumptive drug screen for SUD is negative. Positive screen is not sufficient to diagnose SUD. After the diagnosis of SUD, the PCP helps the team institute a plan for the management of SUD using evidence-based psychosocial and pharmacologic interventions[2–6,10,20] (**Box 7**, **Table 3**). Some patients who are ambivalent about accepting treatment may benefit from motivational interviewing via consultation with recovery coaches or addiction counselors (via tele-health if necessary).

Box 5
Screening tools for substance use disorder in postacute long-term care settings

NIDA (National Institute for Drug Abuse) Quick Screen—excellent screening tool for common addictive substances (alcohol, tobacco, prescription drugs, illicit drugs); typically takes 1 to 2 minutes to complete

AUDIT-C—excellent screening tool for alcohol use disorder, generally takes less than a minute to complete

ORT (Opioid Risk Tool)—excellent screening tool to screen for individuals at higher-than-usual risk of opioid misuse and opioid use disorder; recommended to be done before prescribing opioids; typically takes 1 to 2 minutes

Data from Refs.[28–30]

> **Box 6**
> **Assessment of patients in postacute long-term care settings after they screen positive**
>
> - Use DSM 5 criteria to diagnose SUD but be aware that these criteria may miss SUD in older adults
>
> - Inquire about use of other substances of addiction and misuse of prescription drugs
>
> - Clinically relevant details of substance use (eg, snorting, intravenous injection, amount, duration)
>
> - Inquire about precipitating factors and stressors contributing to SUD
>
> - Request permission and obtain collateral history of knowledgeable family/friend, previous PCP, and previous medical records
>
> - Screen for comorbid depression, anxiety, insomnia, neurocognitive conditions, suicidal ideas, and trauma-related and other psychiatric conditions
>
> - Prescribe baseline blood and urine tests as appropriate to clarify severity of SUD
>
> - Inform the findings of the assessment to the patient and care team
>
> *Data from* Refs.[2,3,20]

Staff need to be vigilant about the possibility that some visitors of residents with SUD may bring in alcohol and/or illicit drugs. PCPs are strongly encouraged to seek additional training in diagnosis, prevention, and treatment of SUDs. Nurses, nursing assistants, social workers, and rehabilitation therapists (eg, physical therapists, occupational therapists, speech therapists) should also receive targeted training on SUDs.

Treatment

Goal of treatment typically is safe withdrawal from the substance and total abstinence.[20] The PCP should recommend complete abstinence for all patients with SUD. Abstinence may not be an appropriate goal for some individuals living in PALTC settings. Even a modest reduction (eg, 20%) of substance use should also be considered a successful outcome. Treatment of SUD involves psychosocial interventions, substance withdrawal management, and pharmacologic interventions.[20] Traditional SUD treatment centers and programs are typically not an option for PALTC population due to challenges with transportation and other logistical concerns, functional and medical needs, and cognitive challenges.[2,3,20] Many patients with SUD may not perceive need for formal treatment at addiction centers but may be open to 1 or 2 interventions (eg, initiation of buprenorphine for OUD and individual addiction counseling via telemedicine) at the facility. Treatment needs to be person-centered and individualized. PALTC facilities may not have resources to care for some patients with severe SUD, and finding other treatment facilities that are willing to take these residents can be very challenging. To overcome this, the authors urge PCPs working in PALTC to routinely seek telemedicine consultation with consultant psychiatrists and to build partnerships with local addiction centers. PALTC owners should financially support PCPs in these efforts. Referral to an addiction center when feasible for comprehensive, multidisciplinary, multimodal evidence-based treatments is recommended for complex cases of SUD (eg, co-occurring OUD and AUD, OUD [with intravenous heroin] and BZD use disorder).

Psychosocial interventions

All patients diagnosed with SUD can benefit from one or more strength-based, age- and culture-appropriate, individually tailored psychosocial interventions (see

---

Box 7
Psychosocial interventions for substance use disorder

Education—most important psychosocial intervention; needs to be done at the time of positive screen and on an ongoing basis; needs to be done with patient as well as their support system (including family, friends); includes providing information pamphlets from reputable organizations and information on local and online resources for treatment of addiction

Motivational interviewing (MI)—MI is the key intervention to address denial or reluctance on the part of the patient to accept diagnosis of SUD and treatment

Individual counseling/psychotherapy (eg, cognitive behavioral therapy, relaxation training, strategies to cope with cravings and stress)—should be offered to all patients with relatively preserved cognitive function; this may need to be via telehealth; may need to accommodate hearing and vision deficits; may need to be modified based on cognitive function, cultural expectations, and medical comorbidity (eg, frailty); may need to be brief (20–25 minutes rather than 45–50 minutes)

Group therapy—should be offered to patients able and willing to go to local addiction centers/programs for more intensive treatment; group therapy is often a part of intensive outpatient addiction treatment

Mutual aid support groups (eg, Narcotic Anonymous, Alcoholic Anonymous, Self-Management and Recovery Training, Celebrate Recovery; they support abstinence, foster new social connections, a sense of belonging, and healthy lifestyles)—should be offered to all patients able and open to support groups and patients who have had positive experience in the past with support groups

Contingency management (a form of behavior therapy where desired behaviors [eg, abstinence] are systematically reinforced and reinforcements are withdrawn for undesired behavior)—should be considered in some patients with guidance from consultant psychiatrist or another addiction specialist.

Data from Refs.[2–10,20]

Box 7).[2–10,20] All team members should consistently reinforce the understanding to patients and their families that SUD is a medical condition and not a moral defect and that there are serious risks associated with untreated SUDs (eg, overdose death). For older PALTC patients, the team members should proactively address ageism—the false belief that older adults do not develop SUD or do not benefit from its treatment. Some higher functioning residents with SUD may be appropriate candidates for individual counseling and group psychotherapy and should be supported if they wish to access these services in the community or via telehealth. Many residents with SUD may feel that they do not have a purpose, and helping them find a reason to get up in the morning, engage in the difficult work of recovery and meaningful activities (eg, starting regular Alcohol Anonymous meetings at the facility, mentoring students, gardening) can make a huge difference.

Substance Withdrawal Management

Mild withdrawal symptoms can be safely managed in PALTC settings, with the guidance of consultant psychiatrist or a medical professional with addiction medicine training in complex cases.[4–7,10,20] Moderate to severe opioid, alcohol, BZD and stimulant withdrawal symptoms are best managed in hospital settings or addiction programs because of high risk of complications (eg, delirium tremens and seizures in the case of alcohol withdrawal). Withdrawal from other substances (eg, cannabis, nicotine) can generally be safely managed in PALTC settings.

Pharmacotherapy for Substance Use Disorders

Several medications have been approved by the FDA for the treatment of SUD (see **Table 3**).[5,6,10,20] Although prescribing a drug to help a patient not use another drug seems counterintuitive for many of us who practice geriatric and long-term care medicine, treatment of SUD with FDA-approved drugs generally has more benefits than risks even in this vulnerable population and should be considered as part of best practices. These medications have not been studied in PALTC populations, and thus, starting low and escalating the dose slowly if needed and closer monitoring for adverse effects is recommended. Besides the FDA-approved medications for AUD, in select cases, gabapentin may be considered as off-label use in patients with AUD for treatment of protracted alcohol withdrawal symptoms and for relapse prevention.[5,23] Buprenorphine is a potent opioid, and although the risk of adverse effects and overdose death is lower than other opioids, it is still a high-risk medication and should be used with the same precautions that are required with other opioids (eg, close monitoring for adverse effects, avoiding concomitant use of BZD).[6] The authors recommend against the use of methadone as first-line agent for treatment of OUD in PALTC populations due to higher risks of adverse effects compared with buprenorphine and higher risks of adverse drug-drug interactions due to prolongation of QTc interval by methadone.[6] However, there may be certain situations where it may be appropriate (eg, patient with heroin addiction and past history of good response to methadone). Methadone for OUD can only be prescribed in federally designated opioid treatment programs (OTPs) by qualified medical professionals and require daily visits for supervised methadone administration; this poses a considerable barrier for PALTC population because of their functional limitations, frailty, and difficulty obtaining daily transportation. On the other hand, patients on methadone treatment of their OUD may get admitted to PALTC settings. Although the PCP will not be prescribing or managing methadone maintenance treatment in such cases, they need to be aware of the unique risks associated with methadone use and work collaboratively with the OTP team that is prescribing methadone. Involvement of consultant pharmacist and consultant psychiatrist can help the PCP navigate the challenges of using buprenorphine and methadone in PALTC population. Disulfiram and topiramate are also options for treatment of AUD but should in general be avoided in PALTC population due to significant risk of adverse events.[5]

Buprenorphine, methadone, naltrexone, and disulfiram are metabolized by the liver, and hence, their use in PALTC residents with liver disease should be done with extreme caution and very low doses may need to be used.[5,6] Acamprosate and gabapentin are excreted primarily through the kidneys, and hence, their use in PALTC residents (in whom prevalence of chronic kidney disease is high) should be done with caution and very low doses may be adequate.[5] Acamprosate is contraindicated in patients with severe renal impairment.

Case 1: alcohol use disorder

Ms VL is a 78-year-old woman, recently admitted to a nursing home for rehabilitation after hospitalization for hip fracture surgery. Ms VL drank half a gallon of vodka a week and had developed alcohol-induced liver disease with ascites. She was started on sertraline, 50 mg, daily for anxiety and depression. After assessment, the PCP gave a diagnosis of AUD, and Ms VL agreed to a trial of naltrexone to address her cravings and prevent relapse. Ms VL was told of the need to avoid opioids, as naltrexone is an opioid-antagonist, and she reported that her pain was mild and agreed to the plan. Ms VL declined referral to mutual-aid support groups and addiction counseling.

Table 3 Pharmacotherapy for substance use disorders		
Substance	Medications Approved by the FDA	Clinical Pearls
Nicotine	Bupropion Varenicline Nicotine transdermal patch	Quit rates for bupropion are about half that of varenicline Quit rates for nicotine patch as similar to those of bupropion
Alcohol	Naltrexone Acamprosate Disulfiram	Naltrexone can be taken even if the person continues to drink, as naltrexone may reduce the amount of drinking
Opioids	Naltrexone Buprenorphine Methadone Lofexidine (for withdrawal symptom management)	Clonidine may be used instead of lofexidine, as it is cheaper

Data from Refs.[5,6,10,20]

Teaching points: AUD is prevalent in PALTC populations, and naltrexone may play a significant role in managing cravings and relapse prevention.

Case 2: substance use disorder with several substances

Mr ZA is a 43-year-old man, living in a nursing home. He has paraplegia, chronic sacral decubitus, multiple hospitalizations for osteomyelitis, chronic pain, and malnutrition. He has a long history of addiction to methamphetamine and currently uses marijuana and smokes cigarettes. He reports "severe pain" even after being on high-dose opioids (oxycodone ER, 20 mg, twice daily, oxycodone, 10 mg, every 4 hours) and wants more opioids. He also reports "severe anxiety" and wants more alprazolam (he is on 1 mg 3 times daily). Because of the high complexity of the case, the PCP referred the patient to the consultant psychiatrist. The consultant psychiatrist after assessment provided education to the patient that cannabis use along with opioids, BZD, puts him at high risk for delirium, falls, overdose death, and worsening of his anxiety disorder. The consultant psychiatrist recommended switching oxycodone to buprenorphine (Mr ZA declined), very slow taper over months and eventual discontinuation of alprazolam (Mr ZA declined even a small dose reduction), to quit smoking and start a nicotine patch (Mr ZA agreed), to quit using cannabis (Mr ZA reluctantly agreed), addiction treatment including individual counseling, group therapy, support groups (Mr ZA declined all of them), duloxetine for chronic pain and chronic anxiety (Mr ZA agreed to it), individual counseling (Mr ZA agreed), and naloxone for emergency use to treat opioid-induced respiratory depression or central nervous system (CNS) depression. The consultant psychiatrist provided staff education on the importance of naloxone and importance of not giving more opioids or BZD and that addiction is a disease of the brain and body and not a personal failure or a moral defect.

Teaching points: polysubstance use disorder is not uncommon in PALTC settings, especially in younger population with preexisting SUD. Its management is complex and best done in collaboration with a consultant psychiatrist.

Addressing Co-occurring Physical Health Conditions

Stress from poorly managed medical comorbidity (especially acute and chronic pain, frailty, sarcopenia) may trigger SUD relapse.[3,20] Optimal control of pain, ideally without opioids, is important in individuals with SUD, as undertreated pain is a risk factor for

SUD exacerbation or relapse.[6] Compared with other substances, alcohol has the most drug-drug interactions. It takes less alcohol to cause impairment in older adults and PALTC population due to high rates of multiple medical and psychiatric conditions and polypharmacy in this population.[5] For PALTC populations, there may be no level of safe alcohol use. Although vaping nicotine is less harmful than smoking tobacco, there are growing concerns that vaping nicotine may damage lungs, and hence its use in PALTC populations should be discouraged.[21] For patients in PALTC settings who insist on using cannabis, edible forms of cannabis (where legally available) should replace smoking and vaping cannabis to reduce the risk of respiratory system complications.[21] Close monitoring is recommended in such situations, as some edible forms of cannabis may contain higher than expected concentrations of tetrahydrocannabinol that may pose significant risks.

Deprescribing Benzodiazepine Receptor Agonists

BZD and Z-drug use is prevalent in older adults and PALTC populations.[24,31] In the PALTC settings, it is not uncommon for patients to be admitted who have been on long-term BZD treatment for years or even decades for management of anxiety disorder and or insomnia. The authors recommend the BZD deprescribing protocol as a guide that needs to be tailored to the unique individual needs of patient in PALTC population. Inappropriate or unnecessary BZD use needs to be identified and a tapering plan developed together with the patient and their support system. The pace of BZD taper should be individually tailored and generally done over weeks to months. In general, reduction is 5% to 25% of the daily dose every 2 weeks initially.[32] The amount of dose being tapered and the pace of taper needs to be gradually lowered as the taper progresses. In complex cases, a lower dose may need to be maintained for several months before resuming taper and completing discontinuation. Patients with BZD use disorder are expected to have more difficulty tapering BZD due to craving and may report intolerable withdrawal symptoms and that they cannot function without BZD. In such cases, it is important to clarify if the increases in anxiety symptoms are related to preexisting anxiety or trauma-related disorders and if so, these need to be treated. Involving a consultant psychiatrist and or referral to local addiction centers for comprehensive treatment is recommended in such cases. Long-term use of Z-drugs is also not recommended in older adults and PALTC populations because the risks (eg, falls and injury) are higher than potential benefits.[33] Deprescribing Z-drugs needs to follow the same principles as BZD deprescribing— the longer the patient has been on Z-drug, the slower the taper.

Opioid Crises in Postacute and Long-Term Care Population and Deprescribing Opioids

Older adults and PALTC population are ignored in our national opioid crisis reporting.[6,34] Use of LTOT (long-term opioid therapy—use of opioids on most days for more than 3 months) for chronic noncancer pain is prevalent in older adults and PALTC populations and so is use of opioid doses higher than the manufactured recommended maximum dose.[6,34] Guidelines for pain management in PALTC settings strongly discourage use of opioids for management of chronic noncancer pain (except during palliative and end-of-life care) because of minimal benefits and serious risks associated with LTOT in this population.[27] It is important to note that many individuals in PALTC settings on opioids have become dependent (meaning they will experience withdrawal symptoms if opioids are tapered or discontinued) on opioids but dependence is not addiction. It would not be right to tell these individuals that they have become addicted to opioids or diagnose them with OUD. Having strict prescribing limits for opioids in PALTC population is recommended even at the cost of some patients not being happy and choosing to leave and find care elsewhere.

PCPs should be diligent in avoiding the co-prescription of opioids and BZD and minimizing co-prescription of opioids and gabapentinoids.[6] Deprescribing of CNS depressants used concomitantly with opioids (eg, BZD, gabapentin, pregabalin, muscle relaxants, sedating antipsychotics [eg, quetiapine, olanzapine]) should be considered routinely in PALTC residents. Appropriate dose reduction or discontinuation of LTOT should follow the guidelines published in October 2019 by the United States department of Health and Human Services.[35]

Case 3: opioid use disorder and benzodiazepine misuse
Mr CM is a 66-year-old nursing home resident with history of chronic noncancer pain, OUD, and BZD misuse. He has a history of suicidal ideation and has been demanding an increase in his diazepam (currently he is on 5 mg twice daily as needed). He is also on scheduled opioids and has also been asking for more opioids. Mr CM was homeless, developed pneumonia, and after stabilization in the hospital, was discharged to the nursing home for rehabilitation. The PCP in collaboration with the consultant psychiatrist gradually tapered and discontinued diazepam and started pregabalin for neuropathic pain and informed Mr CM that pregabalin may also help with his anxiety. Mr CM was also connected to Narcotics Anonymous and accepted individual addiction counseling via telemedicine. Staff were educated about SUD and to see Mr CM's "behavioral challenges" as manifestations of SUD.

Teaching points: opioid misuse, OUD, and BZD misuse often co-occur, and risk of overdose death is very high when opioids and BZD are used concurrently.

Medical Cannabis/Medical Marijuana for Patients with Substance Use Disorder Living in Postacute and Long-Term Care Settings

Medical cannabis (medical marijuana) refers to use of the unprocessed marijuana plant or its basic extracts (eg, cannabidiol, tetrahydrocannabinol) to treat symptoms of illness or other conditions.[36] The FDA has not recognized or approved the marijuana plant as medicine. Medical cannabis may have potential benefits for some PALTC patients (eg, management of chronic severe pain) but its use should be in compliance with state and federal laws. The PALTC staff need to be educated about risks of cannabis and what signs and symptoms to monitor to identify adverse effects early. Educating residents and families about potential benefits and serious risks of cannabis (including risk of developing CUD) is also important. Patients with SUD should not be deprived of appropriate treatment with medical cannabis, but closer monitoring is recommended to ensure that medical cannabis is being used appropriately.

Addressing Co-occurring Mental Health Conditions

Based on preliminary research in PALTC settings, extrapolation from studies in older adults, and the authors' clinical experience, the 4 most common co-occurring conditions in residents with SUD are anxiety, depression, insomnia, and executive neurocognitive impairment.[2–6,15–17] Appropriate pharmacologic and nonpharmacological treatments for these conditions need to happen simultaneously with treatment of SUD. Presence of suicidal ideas should be assessed and taken seriously, as suicide rates are elevated in older adults with SUD.[2,3] Suicide risk is especially elevated in older adults with both AUD and depression.[5] Delirium and dementia are prevalent in PALTC population and in the authors' experience, patients with SUD living in PALTC settings have a higher risk of both delirium and dementia due to direct effects of substances (eg, alcohol) as well as indirect effects (eg, neglect of cardiovascular conditions such as hypertension due to preoccupation with activities to obtain and consume substance; traumatic brain injury caused by falls that were caused by use of alcohol).[2,3,14] Even moderate alcohol intake has been shown to worsen depression, anxiety, insomnia, and cognitive impairment in older adults.[5] Individuals with history of SUD may experience exacerbation or relapse of their underlying SUD, MM as well as mental health disorder after experiencing a significant stressor (eg, death of a family member or a close friend, family conflict, new illness or disability). Helping the patient address these stressors should include inquiring about craving and monitoring for signs and symptoms of relapse. Alcohol use policies in PALTC settings should take into account the legal right of individuals to consume alcohol, the risk of AUD, the possibility of liability in negligence and the use of substitute decision-makers for individuals with impaired decision-making capacity.[37]

Case 4: opioid misuse and major depression
Mr SD is a 38-year-old nursing home resident with chronic noncancer pain, spina bifida, diabetes, and end-stage kidney disease requiring dialysis. He has a history of misusing opioids before coming to the nursing home, and in the nursing home, he has asked for his as-needed oxycodone even when he seems to not be in any pain. The PCP explained to Mr SD the risk of overdose and other adverse effects and need to taper and discontinue oxycodone. The PCP also found that Mr SD had treatment-resistant major depression. His venlafaxine ER, 150 mg, daily along with individual counseling had helped him only partially. The PCP added aripiprazole for treatment-resistant major depression, and over subsequent weeks, Mr SD's depression gradually improved, his pain also improved, and his seeking opioids for "pain" became rare.

Teaching points: comorbid depression is prevalent in patients with chronic noncancer pain, especially in younger PALTC populations and needs to be treated vigorously.

SUMMARY

Managing SUDs in PALTC populations should be a routine part of clinical care. Managing SUDs successfully takes a team due to multiple comorbidities, polypharmacy, and time pressure on PCPs. PCPs need to be vigilant in recognizing signs and symptoms as well as taking preventative efforts. Ongoing advocacy is needed to support the reimbursement not only of medications but of supportive and telemedicine services. Expanded telemedicine services need to be maintained in order to support PALTC residents especially in medically underserved communities. By addressing SUD with evidence-based treatments, we can improve lives of individuals living in PALTC settings.

CLINICS CARE POINTS

- PCPs play a key role in promoting hope to patients with SUDs.
- Collaborative psychiatric care (via telemedicine if necessary) can greatly improve outcomes in complex cases.
- Co-morbid psychiatric disorders are common causes of treatment resistance and need to be identified early and optimally treated.

DISCLOSURE

The author receives book royalties from Cambridge University Press for his book titled *Psychiatric consultation in long-term care: A guide for healthcare professionals*, 2nd edition. 2017. The book has been mentioned as one of the references.

REFERENCES

1. American Psychiatric Association. Diagnostic and statistical manual of mental disorders. 5th edition. Arlington, VA: American Psychiatric Publishing; 2013.
2. Yarnell S, Li L, MacGrory B, et al. Substance use disorders in later life: a review and synthesis of the literature of an emerging public health concern. Am J Geriatr Psychiatry 2020;28(2):226–36.
3. Sorrell JM, Sorrell JM. Substance use disorders in long-term care settings: a crisis of care for older adults. J Psychosoc Nurs Ment Health Serv 2017; 55(1):24–7.
4. Bulut EA, Isik AT. Abuse/misuse of prescription medications in older adults. Clin Geriatr Med 2022;38(1):85–98.
5. Maldonado GF, Brown D, Hoffman H, et al. Alcohol use disorder in older adults. Clin Geriatr Med 2022;38(1):1–22.
6. Duggirala R, Khushalani S, Palmer T, et al. Screening for and management of opioid use disorder in older adults in primary care. Clin Geriatr Med 2022; 38(1):23–38.
7. Ghantous Z, Ahmad V, Khoury R. Illicit drug use in older adults: an invisible epidemic? Clin Geriatr Med 2022;38(1):39–54.
8. Redden WM, Paracha S, Sheheryar Q. Hallucinogen use and misuse in older adults. Clin Geriatr Med 2022;38(1):55–66.
9. Khoury R, Maliha P, Ibrahim R. Cannabis use and misuse in older adults. Clin Geriatr Med 2022;38(1):67–84.
10. Bassil NK, Ohanian LK, Saba TGB. Nicotine use disorder in older adults. Clin Geriatr Med 2022;38(1):119–32.
11. Kim E, Robinson NM, Newman BM. A brewed awakening: neuropsychiatric effects of caffeine in older adults. Clin Geriatr Med 2022;38(1):133–44.
12. Werner RM, Templeton Z, Apathy N, et al. Trends in post-acute care in US nursing homes: 2001-2017. JAMDA 2021;22:2491–5.
13. Shieu BM, Almusajin JA, Dictus C, et al. Younger nursing home residents: a scoping review of their lived experiences, needs, and quality of life. JAMDA 2021;22:2296–312.
14. Desai AK, Grossberg GT. Psychiatric consultation in long-term care: a guide for healthcare professionals. 2nd edition. New York, NY: Cambridge University Press; 2017.
15. Lemke S, Schaefer JA. VA nursing home residents with substance use disorders: mental health comorbidities, functioning, and problem behaviors. Aging Ment Health 2010;14(5):593–602.
16. Johannessen A, Tevik K, Engedal K, et al. Health professional's experience of nursing home residents' consumption of alcohol and use of psychotropic drugs. Nordic Stud Alcohol Drugs 2021;38(2):161–74.
17. Jutkowitz E, Halladay C, McGeary J, et al. Homeless veterans in nursing homes: care for complex medical, substance use and social needs. J Am Geriatr Soc 2019;67(8):1707–12.
18. Han BH, Moore AA. Prevention and screening of unhealthy substance use by older adults. Clin Geriatr Med 2018;34(1):117–29.
19. Hayek SE, Geagea L, Bourj HE, et al. Prevention strategies of alcohol and substance use disorders in older adults. Clin Geriatr Med 2022;38(1):169–79.
20. Substance Abuse and Mental Health Services Administration. Treating substance use disorder in older adults. treatment improvement protocol (TIP) series No. 26,

SAMHSA publication No. EPE20-02-01-011. Rockville, MD: Substance Abuse and Mental Health Services Administration; 2020.

21. Bertram JR, Porath A, Seitz D, et al. Canadian guidelines on cannabis use disorder among older adults. Can Geriatr J 2020;23(1):135–42.

22. Satre DD, Hirschtritt ME, Silverberg MJ, et al. Addressing problems with alcohol and other substances among older adults during the COVID-19 pandemic. Am J Geriatr Psychiatry 2020;28(7):780–3.

23. Butt PR, White-Campbell M, Canham S, et al. Canadian guidelines for alcohol use disorder in older adults. Can Geriatr J 2020;23(1):143–8.

24. Conn DK, Hogan DB, Amdam L, et al. Canadian guidelines on benzodiazepine receptor agonist use disorder among older adults. Can Geriatr J 2020;23(1): 116–22.

25. American Geriatrics Society 2019 updated AGS beers criteria for potentially inappropriate medication use in older adults. J Am Geriatr Soc 2019;67(4):674–94.

26. O'Mahony D. STOPP/START criteria for potentially inappropriate medications/potential prescribing omissions in older people: origin and progress. Expert Rev Clin Pharmacol 2020;13(1):15–22.

27. Levenson S, Resnick B, Cryst S, et al. Pain management in the post-acute and long-term care setting: a clinical practice guideline from the society of post-acute and long-term care medicine. J Am Med Dir Assoc 2021;22:2407.

28. Smith PC, Schmidt SM, Allendsworth-Davies D, et al. A single-question screening test for drug use in primary care. Arch Intern Med 2010;170(13):1155–60.

29. Aalto M, Alho H, Halme JT, et al. The alcohol use disorders identification test (AUDIT) and its derivatives in screening for heavy drinking among the elderly. Int J Geriatr Psychiatry 2011;26(9):881–5.

30. Webster LR, Webster RM. Predicting aberrant behaviors in opioid-treated patients: preliminary validation of the Opioid Risk Tool. Pain Med 2005;6(6):432–42.

31. Evrard P, Henrard S, Foulon V, et al. Benzodiazepine use and deprescribing in Belgian nursing homes: Results from the COME-ON study. J Am Geriatr Soc 2020;68(12):2768–77.

32. Ogbonna CI, Lembke A. Tapering patients off of benzodiazepines. Am Fam Physician 2017;96(9):606–8.

33. Pottie K, Thompson W, Davies S, et al. Deprescribing benzodiazepine receptor agonists. Evidence-based clinical practice guideline. Can Fam Physician 2018; 64:339–51.

34. Pruskowski J, Hanlon JT. Is there an opioid crisis in nursing homes? J Am Dir Assoc 2019;20(3):273–4.

35. Health and Human Services. HHS guide for clinicians on appropriate dosage reduction or discontinuation of long-term opioid analgesics. Available at: https://www.hhs.gov/opioids/sites/default/files/2019-10/Dosage_Reduction_Discontinuation.pdf last. accessed January 10, 2022.

36. Palace ZJ, Reingold DA. Medical cannabis in the skilled nursing facility: a novel approach to improving symptom management and quality of life. J Am Med Dir Assoc 2019;20(1):94–8.

37. Grossi A, Holmes A, Ibrahim JE. Use of alcohol in long-term care settings: a comparative analysis of personal choice, public health advice and the law. J Am Med Dir Assoc 2021;22(1):9–14.

Update on Gambling Disorder

Elina A. Stefanovics, PhD[a,b], Marc N. Potenza, MD, PhD[a,c,d,e,f,g,h],*

KEYWORDS

- Gambling disorder • Addictive behaviors • Substance-related disorders
- Epidemiology • Treatment • Regulation

KEY POINTS

- Gambling is prevalent and a sizable minority experiences gambling disorder (GD).
- Sociodemographic, environmental, and genetic factors contribute to GD.
- Populations vulnerable to GD (e.g., adolescents) warrant particular attention.
- Promoting engagement in effective GD treatments is needed.

INTRODUCTION

Gambling disorder (GD; formally termed pathologic gambling) is characterized by persistent and recurrent maladaptive pattern of gambling (betting or wagering) that persists despite negative consequences in major areas of life functioning.[1] The estimated lifetime prevalence of GD among U.S. adults ranges from 0.2% to 2.0%,[1] whereas problem gambling (i.e., subthreshold GD) is estimated to fall between 1% and 4%.[2]

Gambling involves risking something of value (often money) on events of uncertain outcomes with intents of winning something of greater value.[3] Gambling includes considerations (amounts of bet), risks (chance elements), and prizes (outcomes). Numerous

[a] Department of Psychiatry, Yale University School of Medicine, New Haven, CT, USA; [b] U.S. Department of Veterans Affairs New England Mental Illness Research and Education Clinical Center (MIRECC), West Haven, CT, USA; [c] Yale Child Study Center, Yale University, New Haven, CT, USA; [d] Connecticut Mental Health Center, New Haven, CT, USA; [e] Connecticut Council on Problem Gambling, Wethersfield, CT, USA; [f] Department of Neuroscience, Yale University, New Haven, CT, USA; [g] Wu Tsai Institute, Yale University, New Haven, CT, USA; [h] Division on Addictions Research at Yale, Yale Impulsivity Research Program, Yale Center of Excellence in Gambling Research, Women and Addictions Core of Women's Health Research at Yale, Neuroscience and Child Study, Yale University School of Medicine, 1 Church Street, Room 726, New Haven, CT 06510, USA
* Corresponding author. Division on Addictions Research at Yale, Yale Impulsivity Research Program, Yale Center of Excellence in Gambling Research, Women and Addictions Core of Women's Health Research at Yale, Neuroscience and Child Study, Yale University School of Medicine, 1 Church Street, Room 726, New Haven, CT 06510.
E-mail address: marc.potenza@yale.edu

Psychiatr Clin N Am 45 (2022) 483–502
https://doi.org/10.1016/j.psc.2022.04.004
0193-953X/22/© 2022 Elsevier Inc. All rights reserved.
psych.theclinics.com

gambling types exist, both legal and illegal including casino table gambling (eg, poker, blackjack), electronic gambling machines [EGMs] (EGMs like "slots"), bingo, lotteries, and sports betting, among others. Various gambling opportunities exist on the Internet, and games that have features similar to gambling also exist. For example, social casino games are online games that may have features like EGMs that are available through stand-alone Web sites, social networking platforms, and mobile device applications.[4]

Gambling is prevalent among adults.[5] Most adults gamble without developing problems.[6] However, gambling may escalate to problematic levels characterized by persistent maladaptive risk-taking leading to negative consequences in multiple domains (e.g., occupational, financial, social, health). Gambling typically takes years to progress to GD, although more rapid progression has been noted in women with rapid forms of gambling like EGMs.[7]

Multiple terms have been used to describe levels of problem gambling severity. Recreational and low-risk gambling have described wagering patterns without adverse consequences. At-risk gambling has described individuals with some but few features of GD. Problem gambling has referred to a broader spectrum of difficulties defined by harms from gambling,[8] sometimes inclusive of GD.[9] GD is a psychiatric disorder characterized by continued gambling despite significant adverse consequences.[10] GD is currently classified as an addictive disorder as it shares clinical features with substance-use disorders (SUDs).[11] In the 11th revision of the International Classification of Diseases (ICD-11), GD includes predominantly off-line and predominantly online types.[12]

Also included in the ICD-11, hazardous gambling is mutually exclusive of GD and is characterized by gambling that substantially increases the risk of harmful physical or mental health consequences. The criteria for hazardous gambling may aid in public health efforts aimed at reducing gambling-related harms.

POTENTIAL RISK FACTORS FOR GAMBLING DISORDER
Sociodemographic Factors

Frequently documented sociodemographic factors include younger age and male gender. Traditionally, males have been more likely than females to experience GD, with a 2:1 ratio. This holds true for adolescents, young adults, college students, veterans, and Indigenous groups, although gender-related differences may be gradually narrowing and, in some populations, female gender may be a risk factor.[13] For example, women in the military may be more vulnerable to GD than men.[14] Being female may also be a risk factor for GD in adults aged 50 years and older.[15] Men and women often differ with respect to gambling motivations and preferences.[16] Women tend to prefer luck or chance-based games[17] that may provide relaxation, a way of managing emotions, or escape from problems.[18] Men are often more oriented toward excitement or competitive skill-based forms of gambling.[19] Among women, low levels of family support may be risk factors.[20]

Sociodemographic factors linked to GD across many groups include low incomes or living in poverty,[21] unemployment,[22] and low educational attainment.[23] Poverty and financial hardships may influence decision-making in manners that may exacerbate poverty.[24] Poverty may have particular psychological consequences, which, in turn, may perpetuate the cycle of poverty.[25]

Co-occurring Disorders

Other potential risk factors found across many groups are psychiatric comorbidity and physical health problems. Like in the general population, most treatment-seeking patients with GD experienced other psychiatric disorders including anxiety, mood, and personality disorders.[26] Gambling may be used as a maladaptive coping mechanism, helping to escape from stress, anxiety, and depression in the short term.[27] GD has been strongly associated with Substance Use Disorders, with odds ratios ranging from 3.9 for nicotine dependence to 5.8 for alcohol or drug dependence in a nationally representative adult U.S. sample.[28] An independent nationally representative U.S. survey found that 73% of adults with GD have co-occurring alcohol-use disorders, 38% co-occurring drug-use disorders, and 60.4% nicotine dependence.[29] Alcohol-use problems and conduct disorder statistically predicted GD in a representative sample of U.S. adolescents, with odds ratios of 3.9 and 2.9, respectively.[30] In most cases, co-occurring disorders precede GD.[28] Prevalence estimates for GD of 4.3% have been reported in individuals receiving treatment of SUDs and 6.9% in psychiatric inpatients[31] and 3.4% to 7% in patients with neurologic conditions, including Parkinson disease.[32] One study found that 45% of treatment-seeking individuals with GD had at least one co-occurring behavioral addiction relating to work, exercise, food bingeing, sex, or shopping.[33] Problem gambling severity and gambling-related cognitions have been linked to poor emotion regulation and coping strategies.[34] GD and substance use appear interrelated but with incomplete overlap in associated factors.[35]

Environmental Factors

Among environmental factors, availability of gambling should be considered. Data suggest that with the introduction of some new forms of gambling (eg, integrated resort casinos) rates of GD may remain stable over time.[1] However, continued research is needed, especially with newer forms of gambling. For example, online accessibility in a seemingly anonymous environment may be a potential risk factor for some individuals.

Isolation and social connectedness may constitute seemingly contradictory risk factors for GD. Isolation resulting from loneliness, low family connectedness, and unmarried status has been linked to GD in younger individuals. In contrast, gambling for entertainment purposes and social engagement was most common among older adults who gamble, suggesting age-related differences in possible risk factors for GD. Such considerations may also apply to specific Indigenous groups, where being marginalized socially[36] and connected socially[37] may constitute risk factors for GD.

Trauma and traumatic experiences have been linked to GD across demographic groups, although trauma may manifest differently in specific groups. For example, Indigenous groups have historically been vulnerable to trauma such as displacement and have been more likely to experience discrimination.[38] Veterans who have been in active duty and combat-exposed may be particularly likely to have Posttraumatic Stress Disorder (PTSD).[39] Sexual abuse may be a strong risk factor, including among younger individuals[40] and loss of a partner a factor for older adults.[41] Gambling as a coping mechanism has been reported by women to manage domestic violence and abusive relationships.[42]

Genetics

Population-based studies implicate both environmental and genetic factors. A recent meta-analysis of 18 twin studies[43] estimates genetic and non-shared environmental contributors to GD. Gambling factors, age, and sex may moderate how factors influence the development of GD. The contribution of genetic factors was greater for GD diagnosed via symptom-oriented assessment (53%) than for general gambling diagnosed via behavior-oriented assessment (41%). Heritability was found to be lower in adolescents (42%) than in adults (53%) and increased with age. Environmental factors (eg, peer pressure) appeared to contribute more in adolescents compared with adults. Higher heritability in adults may reflect genetic predispositions for prolonged problematic engagement in gambling. Higher heritability was found in men (47%) compared with women (28%). Shared environmental factors were implicated in females but not in males, suggesting that targeting environmental factors may be particularly for girls and women. However, another earlier study found that a contribution of genetic, shared, and non-shared environmental factors to GD were comparable in men and women.[44] In addition, personality features and life experiences are important to consider with respect to the genetics of GD.[45]

VULNERABLE POPULATIONS

Specific populations may be particularly vulnerable to gambling-related problems. These include adolescents/young adults,[46] military and veteran populations, older adults, members of ethnic and racial minority groups, individuals with mental/physical health concerns, and prison and homeless populations.[47] Information on potentially vulnerable groups is tabulated (**Table 1**).

SCREENING INSTRUMENTS

Although the Diagnostic and Statistical Manual of Mental Disorders-5 (DSM-5) criteria represent the current gold standard for diagnosing GD, multiple screening instruments have been developed and used in clinical practice and research settings. They vary in length and psychometric properties, including sensitivity and specificity (**Table 2**).

INTERVENTION AND TREATMENT

A small minority of people (less than 10%) with GD seek treatment.[1] Motivation for treatment may vary, and motivating factors may include financial, legal, or relational problems. Sometimes family members enquire about treatment options on behalf of a family member. Multiple factors should be considered in GD treatment including co-occurring psychiatric conditions. Treatments may include behavioral (**Box 1**) and pharmacologic (**Box 2**) therapies, although no medication has a formal indication for GD.

Behavioral Interventions

Self-help interventions include gambling anonymous, and empirically supported psychotherapies include cognitive-behavioral therapy (CBT), motivational interviewing (MI), imaginal desensitization, and contingency management.[1]

Pharmacotherapies

Several medications, including serotonergic antidepressants, lithium, glutamatergic agents, catechol-O-methyl transferase (COMT) inhibitors, neuroleptics, dopamine-1 receptor and dopamine-2 receptor antagonists, and opioid receptor antagonists, have been investigated based on available neurochemical, neurocognitive, or neuroimaging data. Results from double-blind, placebo-controlled trials have often demonstrated mixed findings, providing limited support for the use of specific pharmacologic agents.[95] However, pharmacotherapies based on co-occurring disorders and approved indications suggest treatment algorithms[1]

RESPONSIBLE GAMBLING INITIATIVES

Responsible gambling (RG) initiatives have been developed in response to community concerns about negative social and personal consequences associated with GD,[118]

Table 1
Prevalence of, and potential risk factors for, gambling disorder in possibly vulnerable populations

Possibly Vulnerable Population	Prevalence	Potential Risk Factors
Adolescents	0.2%–12.3%	Male gender, substance use, cognitive biases and cognitive distortions, delinquent behaviors, smoking, exposure to gambling through family and community, having friends who gamble, impulsiveness and excitement-seeking, local availability/accessibility and geographic proximity of gambling venues, low family connectedness, low peer support, and deprivation, having a personal relationship with someone who gambles, low self-esteem and low self-control, poor parental attachment, being an only child, medication related to nervousness, loneliness, negative life events, depression and anxiety, sexual abuse and maltreatment, childhood hyperactivity and Attention-deficit/hyperactivity disorder (ADHD), emotion dysregulation, and maladaptive coping strategies, learning disorders, conduct problems, antisocial behaviors (fighting, illegal car racing, committing crimes, sexual promiscuity, carrying a weapon), consuming alcohol with energy drinks, involvement in competitive sports, exposure to advertisements, poor school performance, presence of cyberbullying
College students (individuals aged 18–25 y)	6.13%–11.26%	Male gender, non-White individuals, the proximity of a college or university to a casino; alcohol and drug use and other impulsive and compulsive behaviors, and ADHD
Older Adults (50+ years)	0.01%–10.6%	Male gender, accessibility, age of onset, medical and psychiatric comorbidity, spending more on gambling in a single session, quantities of gambling activities, alcohol or substance use problems, loneliness, social isolation and boredom, family and friend acceptance of gambling and participation in more types of gambling types, childhood maltreatment, physical and mental health problems, role limitations due to physical health, cognitive distortions, emotional escape, and overspending
Military personnel	0.03% of active-duty service members	Male gender, age over 24 years, Asian/Black/Hispanic race, not-married, military-specific factors include enlisted rank, service in Air Force, Marine, or Navy, prior substance use or mental health conditions, feelings of isolation, proximity to gambling venues and availability of EGM on bases, and post-deployment difficulties

(continued on next page)

Table 1
(continued)

Possibly Vulnerable Population	Prevalence	Potential Risk Factors
Veterans	0.2%–9.0% (including at-risk/problem gambling)	Younger age, male gender, minority status, trauma exposure, trauma-related conditions, impulsivity and adverse childhood experiences, psychiatric disorders, homelessness, substance use, anxiety and depressive disorders, posttraumatic stress disorder (PTSD), lower social support post-deployment, and traumatic brain injury, having friends and family members engaged in gambling
Indigenous people	2.3% 10%–20% (Australian Indigenous), 2.0% (Indigenous Canadians (2.0%)	In North America with Canadian Aboriginal peoples: childhood sexual abuse, type (EGM, instant lotteries and bingo) and intensity of gambling, gambling availability and familiarity, traumatic life events, social trauma (racism and colonization), unemployment, anxiety, depression and drug/alcohol abuse. In American Indian/Alaska natives: current and lifetime psychiatric disorders. For Native Americans: male gender, younger age, lifetime tobacco use disorder, neighborhood disadvantage, lower socioeconomic status, mental and substance use disorders, and nonmedical use of drugs
Prisoners	5.3%–42.0%	Younger age, low educational attainment, drug/alcohol addiction and other psychiatric conditions, lower levels of perceived health, poor social functioning, impulsiveness and poor decision-making in risky situation with reduced sense of regret, needing money to pay debts, and boredom
Homeless individuals	11%–12%, combined lifetime problem and pathologic gambling ranging from 29.8% to 58.2%	Easy access to gambling, availability of specific forms of gambling (EGM, lotteries), substance use, and reward without work consideration
Women	0.06%–10%, and 15.3% (Indigenous women) 3.6% (female veterans)	Older age, low income, unemployment, history of trauma or abuse, living in an abusive home environment with a violent partner, or having a violent partner, substance use problems, low self-esteem, having never been married, poor coping skills, higher levels of baseline aggression in female adolescents, lack of family support, emotional distress, financial problems, loss chasing, online gambling, availability and access

| *Black individuals* | 2.2%–4.4% | Alcohol and tobacco use disorders, low socioeconomic status, and unemployment |
| *Hispanic individuals* | 0.8%–1.4% | Alcohol and tobacco use disorders, major depression disorder, PTSD, substance use, low socioeconomic status, and unemployment |

Table 2
Screening tools for GD

Screening Instrument	Description
The South Oaks Gambling Screen (SOGS)	The SOGS is a widely used 20-item screening tool.[48] It has been shown to accurately identify people with gambling problems. It was developed using DSM-III criteria, so it does not reflect the DSM-5 criteria.[49] The SOGS has also been revised and validated for use in adolescents.[50]
The Early Intervention Gambling Health Test (EIGHT)	The EIGHT was developed as a screening instrument for GD to be used in general medical settings.[51,52]
Problem Gambling Severity Index (PGSI)	The PGSI is a 9-item screening tool can be self-administered or administered by a clinician.[53] It is a briefer version of the 31-item Canadian Problem Gambling Index.[54] It uses to describe gambling behavior over the previous 12 months.[55] An online version of this instrument, called the Gambling Quiz, is available in English and in French.
The Massachusetts Gambling Screen (MAGS-DSM-IV)	The MAGS-DSM-IV is a brief screening instrument that can produce an index of non-pathologic and pathologic gambling during a 5–10 min survey or interview. It reflects the first translation of the DSM-IV criteria for pathologic gambling into a survey or clinical interview questionnaire.[56]
The Brief Biosocial Gambling Screen (BBGS);	The BBGS is a 3-item screen derived from the Alcohol Use Disorder and Associated Disabilities Interview Schedule-IV.[57]
The Case-finding and Help Assessment Tool (CHAT)	A 2-item screen to detect gambling problems is contained in the CHAT, a multipurpose screening tool for addictive behaviors for use in primary care settings.[58]
Brief Problem Gambling Screen (BPGS)	The BPGS is a 5-item screening tool that combines items from other widely used tools to capture different levels of gambling behavior.[59] Although the BPGS has not been fully validated, it is the only tool to accurately identify all levels of problem gambling in individuals seeking mental health treatment.[60]
The Self-Administered National Opinion Research Center (NORC) Diagnostic Screen for Gambling Problem (NODS-SA)	The NORC Diagnostic Screen for Gambling Problem-Self Administered (NODS-SA) is a self-administered 10-item version of the NODS, a validated instrument for assessing DSM-IV pathologic gambling[61]
The Lie-Bet Questionnaire	The Lie-Bet Questionnaire is a 2-item brief screening instrument.[62,63]
NORC DSM-IV Screen for Gambling Problems (NODS-CLiP)	This 3-item screening tool is a subset of the 17-item NODS.[64] The "CLiP" refers to the three questions in the tool, which focus on diminished control, lying, and preoccupation with gambling. The NORC DSM-IV Screen for Gambling Problems (NODS-CLiP) may be used to identify people with moderate to severe gambling problems.[65]

Box 1
Behavioral interventions

Gamblers Anonymous
Gamblers anonymous (GA), a recovery fellowship program resembling Alcoholics Anonymous, is the most common intervention for GD. GA consists of a 12-step program, requires regular attendance of group meetings, and involves obtaining a sponsor. In addition, some groups provide peer assistance with managing financial problems related to gambling. The underlying theory of GA is that GD is a disease requiring abstinence. Relatively little is known about the effectiveness of GA, partly because anonymity is a central feature. However, a few randomized controlled trials assessing the effectiveness of GA have reported mixed findings, with one study showing that GA was not as effective as imaginal desensitization and MI.[66] Given high levels of psychiatric comorbidity with GD, it is also possible that GA as a single form of therapy may not be as effective as in conjunction with other therapies.

Cognitive Behavioral Therapy
Cognitive behavioral therapy (CBT) is a widely used treatment of GD. The focus of CBT is on cognitive components of gambling, such as cognitive distortions, cravings, or urges and is accompanied by modifying behaviors. CBT is efficacious in shorter and medium terms,[67] and it may be more effective if combined with motivational interviewing (MI). Few studies have examined the long-term efficacy of CBT.[68,69] CBT may be successfully combined with money management and target other factors related to gambling.

Motivational Interviewing
MI is designed to enhance engagement in treatment and seeks to meet people at their motivational stage, understand barriers, and promote behavioral change. Elements include the assessment of a person's readiness for change, assuming a nonjudgmental, nonconfrontational, and non-adversarial position and using interventions that involve open-ended questions, affirmations, reflective listening, and brief summarizations.[70] Although a literature review found that the effect of MI may declines over time, it may be helpful in the shorter term,[71] particularly if used with other therapies like self-help workbooks or self-directed online programs.[72] One randomized control trial examining MI versus CBT found no difference at any point in time. Instead, both MI and CBT produced significant within-group improvements on most outcome measures up to the 12-month follow-up. Both forms of intervention were superior to the nontreatment control group.[73] Culturally sensitive treatment options such as MI and CBT have been identified as effective treatments for GD in culturally diverse populations.[74]

Mindfulness-Based Interventions
Mindfulness-based interventions are currently being examined in GD. These involve internalized processes including nonjudgmental awareness and attention to the present moment.[75] Mindfulness-based interventions may target experiential avoidance (EA) that may occur when people try to suppress unwanted internal experiences and aims steps to reduce them.[76] EA functions as a core mechanism in the progressive course of some psychological conditions including gambling.[77] Treatment components addressing EA may focus on maladaptive responding (i.e, escape and/or avoidance) rather than the form of the response to increase an adaptive response to an aversive stimulus.

Self-Directed Interventions
Several self-directed interventions for GD have been investigated, including a self-help workbook for GD based on cognitive-behavioral principles and several guided and unguided Internet intervention options that may not be particularly helpful, possibly due to insufficient contact with therapists.[78] Differential improvement has been reported when online treatments have been accompanied by brief telephone calls[79] or personalized e-mails[80] providing instructions and support. Finally, recent randomized controlled trials suggest that supplementing online self-directed treatment programs with a single digitally delivered MI session may be beneficial.[72] Other emerging therapies include ecological momentary interventions (EMIs). EMIs are smartphone-based, individual-directed, real-time-delivered interventions aimed to provide intervention in individuals' natural environments at specifically identified moments of everyday life.[81] To identify when an EMI is needed, apps

administer real-time ecological momentary assessments (EMAs) of relevant situations at random or prespecified times. Based on EMA results, apps apply decision rules to determine the time, type, and intensity of the EMI delivered.[82] Although EMIs are increasingly used in the mental health and addiction field, there are only two known smartphone app-delivered EMIs for gambling.[83,84] The first app, Jeu-contrôle, aims to help people adhere to their gambling time and money limits by delivering personalized feedback about current gambling behavior compared with preset limits recorded during EMAs.[83] GamblingLess: Curb Your Urge targets gambling urges and is tailored by responses to prompted EMAs.[84] The results of one of the recent study[85] support the acceptability and preliminary efficacy of this app-delivered intervention for preventing gambling episodes through craving management.

Neuromodulation

Noninvasive brain stimulation techniques that induce neuromodulation are being examined in GD treatment.[86] Two main types include rapid transcranial magnetic stimulation (rTMS) and transcranial direct current stimulation (tDCS). To date, six studies have investigated neuromodulation effects on gambling urges, craving, cognitive flexibility, decision-making, and gambling behavior.[87–93] Specifically, findings suggest neuromodulation involving rTMS may reduce craving[87–89] and tDCS may improve decision-making.[93]

Cognitive remediation

Cognitive remediation (CR), an approach with efficacy in treating SUDs,[94] is being studied in GD treatment. The goal of CR is to induce neuroplastic changes by using cognitive training either by using hard copy or computer exercises to generate cognitive/behavioral changes. In contrast to CBT, CR aims to improve cognitive processing. Three types of CR include compensatory/strategy-based, restorative, and social-cognitive approaches. Consensus has not been reached on optimal CR parameters (e.g, duration, intensity, frequency, group vs. individual, pencil-and-paper vs. computerized delivery). CR interventions may represent a promising adjunct treatment of GD, although they have not been systematically examined. CR could supplement existing interventions, such as CBT and MI, with prospects of making therapies more effective and longer lasting

as responsible drinking initiatives have been for alcohol.[119] RG involves the use of programs and policies that aim to provide fair and safe gambling environments and experiences to prevent or minimize gambling-related harms.[120]

RG initiatives involve multiple stakeholders (governments, regulators, industry operators, and consumers), all of whom may share degrees of accountability in individuals gamble within affordable social and personal limits.[121] For example, governments establish laws permitting or restricting gambling, and regulators need to follow government standards. Industry operators must comply with regulatory requirements, and communities influence policy and public health initiatives. Ultimately, individuals make personal decisions regarding gambling.

The Reno Model[118] first proposed and described principles underlying RG strategies. These strategies suggest that governments through legislation and regulation have responsibilities for protecting consumers. Concurrently, the gambling industry has responsibility for implementing RG strategies to minimize harm and provide sufficient and necessary information for consumers to make informed choices.[122]

There are several types of RG programs. One is customer-oriented and designed to reduce the prevalence and incidence of gambling-related problems.[123] This program exists for behavioral tracking of gambling, and a precommitment gambling tool enables people to preset monetary and time limits with both approaches based on analyzing behavioral tendencies. Another program involves loss and deposit limit

---

Box 2
Pharmacotherapies

Opioid receptor antagonists
  Opioid receptor antagonists, such as naltrexone or nalmefene, have been investigated in the treatment of GD,[96] in part based on data from SUDs and proposed mechanisms of action, including reductions of cravings and urges.[97] Opioid receptor antagonists may indirectly influence dopaminergic neurons, although their precise mechanism of action in GD is currently speculative.[98] Four randomized controlled trials have supported the efficacy of opioid receptor antagonists to varying degrees.[99–102] Analysis of 284 participants from two studies demonstrated that a positive response to either nalmefene or naltrexone was associated with a positive family history of AUD and stronger gambling urges at treatment onset.[101] However, a trial of as-needed naltrexone failed to identify differences from placebo.[103]

Monoaminergic drugs
  Early models proposed a role for serotonin in GD, particularly with respect to impulse control.[104] Five placebo-controlled studies of serotonin reuptake inhibitors for GD have demonstrated mixed findings. Although initial studies of fluvoxamine and paroxetine reported some benefits over placebo, the subsequent studies of fluvoxamine, paroxetine, and sertraline have not.[105,106]
  Given early proposed roles for dopaminergic and serotoninergic systems in GD,[107] olanzapine, a dopamine receptor and serotonin receptor antagonist, was examined in GD treatment, and two studies did not demonstrate superiority of olanzapine over placebo.[108,109] These findings resonate with those from studies of the dopamine receptor antagonist haloperidol, which was found to increase gambling urges in GD.[110] Prefrontal dopamine could represent a potential target in GD treatment.[64] Dopamine reuptake transporters and catechol-O-methyl transferase (COMT) are in part responsible regulating synaptic dopamine in the frontal cortex.[111] In an open-label study, tolcapone (a COMT inhibitor) was associated with GD improvement that was linked to planning-related frontoparietal brain activity and a common *COMT* polymorphism.[112] Although the findings resonate with precision medicine initiatives, placebo-controlled trials are needed.

Glutamatergic drugs
  Preclinical data suggest a role for glutamate in reward, reinforcement, and relapse,[113] and glutamate systems have been targeted in medication development for addictions.[114] Preliminary data suggest glutamate dysfunction in GD.[115] N-acetylcysteine, a glutamate-modulating agent with promise in treating SUDs, has shown promise in studies of individuals with GD[116] and co-occurring GD and tobacco-use disorder.[117]

---

settings and player precommitment to deposits, based on voluntary limit settings and choices, with budgeting software intended to help people gamble within their limits.[124] Other approaches focus on tracking losses, wins, or time gambling, use warning messages and provide education and information.[119]

Other types of RG programs are employee-oriented, focusing on training casino staff on regulations and codes of practice. These programs often review regulatory requirements, legal obligations, and problem gambling. Such programs aim to promote safe gambling and intervene when problematic gambling is suspected.[125]

The last type of RG programs, onsite RG programs, serves both customers and employees concurrently. Onsite RG programs involve areas within gambling venues where people can find information about gambling and gambling-related consequences and resources for help managing their gambling.[126]

Although RG programs have shown potential in reducing gambling-related harms, long-term effects are understudied.

FUTURE CONSIDERATIONS
Internet Gambling

Digital technologies are changing many behaviors, including gambling. Internet gambling has been becoming increasingly common perhaps in part given its availability and accessibility.[127] Despite increased research of online gambling, most studies rely on self-reports and use convenience or self-selected samples.

Sociodemographic data suggest that GD involving the Internet may not constitute a distinctly different entity than non-Internet-based GD, although the ICD-11 includes specifiers for online versus off-line gambling. Potential risk factors for Internet-based GD include being younger, male, unmarried/separated/divorced, and from a culturally diverse background.[128] Men and women differ in online gambling, with women gambling for shorter durations and experiencing more feelings of guilt and shame.[129] Men typically prefer online sports betting, horse/dog race betting, and skill-based gambling, whereas women typically prefer online bingo.[130] Internet gambling, as compared with off-line gambling, has been associated with higher educational attainment.[131]

The online gambling environment may pose risk to vulnerable individuals like adolescents. Between 0.77% and 57.5% of adolescents present with some degree of online GD.[132] Prevalence estimates of GD were five times higher among youth who gamble online versus off-line.[133] Online gambling often occurs in the absence of age verification and parental control. New technologies not only have been associated with online gambling,[134] but also cyberbullying[135] or problematic use of the Internet, with social environments contributing[136]

SUMMARY

GD is a relatively rare diagnosis compared with prevalence of gambling. Nonetheless, impacts can be severe, and many people with GD do not currently receive treatment. The Internet has altered many behaviors, including gambling. In this setting, regulations and RG initiatives warrant evaluation and modification. Improving prevention and treatment strategies should involve considering at-risk populations and advances in understanding factors underlying GD so that they may be effectively targeted.

CLINICS CARE POINTS

- Individuals with gambling disorder (GD) may not disclose their gambling problems due to shame, ambivalence, or other factors. These factors likely contribute to low rates of treatment-seeking observed among people with GD.

- Active screening is important to help identify people with GD, and this may be particularly relevant for high-risk groups (e.g, people with other psychiatric conditions).

- Behavioral therapies, including cognitive-behavioral therapy and motivational interviewing, have empirical support in the treatment of GD.

- Although no medications have formal indications for treating people with GD, co-occurring psychiatric disorders may inform decision-making regarding psychopharmacological treatments, and this situation is clinically relevant given the frequent co-occurrence of GD with other psychiatric disorders.

DISCLOSURE

The authors declare no conflicts of interest with respect to the content of this article. Dr M.N. Potenza has: consulted for and advised Game Day Data, the Addiction Policy Forum, AXA, BariaTek, Idorsia, and Opiant/Lakelight Therapeutics; received research support from the Veteran's Administration, Mohegan Sun Casino, and the National Center for Responsible Gaming (no the International Center for Responsible Gambling); has been involved in a patent application with Yale University and Novartis; participated in surveys, mailings, or telephone consultations related to drug addiction, impulse-control disorders or other health topics; consulted for law offices and the federal public defender's office in issues related to impulse-control and addictive disorders; provided clinical care in the Connecticut Department of Mental Health and Addiction Services Problem Gambling Services Program; performed grant reviews for the National Institutes of Health and other agencies; edited journals and journal sections; given academic lectures in grand rounds, CME events and other clinical/scientific venues; and generated books or chapters for publishers of mental health texts.

REFERENCES

1. Potenza MN, Balodis IM, Derevensky J, et al. Gambling disorder. Nat Rev Dis Primers 2019;5(1). 51-21.
2. Kessler R, Berglund PA, Chiu W, et al. The National Comorbidity Survey Replication (NCS-R): cornerstone in improving mental health and Mental Health Care in the United States. The WHO world mental health surveys: global perspectives on the epidemiology of mental disorders, 2008: p. 165–210.
3. Whelan JP, Meyers AW, Steenbergh TA. Problem and pathological gambling, vol. 8. Cambridge MA: Hogrefe & Huber; 2007.
4. Gainsbury SM. A taxonomy of gambling and casino games via social media and online technologies. Int Gambling Stud 2014;14(2):196–213.
5. Binde P. Gambling across cultures: Mapping worldwide occurrence and learning from ethnographic comparison. Int Gambling Stud 2005;5(1):1–27.
6. Potenza MN, Kosten TR, Rounsaville BJ. Pathological gambling. Jama 2001; 286(2):141–4.
7. Allami Y, Hodgins DC, Young M, et al. A meta-analysis of problem gambling risk factors in the general adult population. Addiction, 2021.116(11):2968-77.
8. Delfabbro P. Problem and pathological gambling: a conceptual review. J Gambling Business Econ 2013;7(3):35–53.
9. Lorains FK, Cowlishaw S, Thomas SA. Prevalence of comorbid disorders in problem and pathological gambling: Systematic review and meta-analysis of population surveys. Addiction 2011;106(3):490–8.
10. American Psychiatric Association DS, Association AP. Diagnostic and statistical manual of mental disorders: DSM-5. Washington, DC: American psychiatric association; 2013.
11. Grant JE, Potenza MN, Weinstein A, et al. Introduction to behavioral addictions. Am J Drug Alcohol Abuse 2010;36(5):233–41.
12. WHO, ICD-11: International classification of diseases 11th revision. WHO. 2018. Available at: https://icd.who.int/en. Accessed January 12, 2022.
13. Merkouris SS, Thomas AC, Shandley KA, et al. An update on gender differences in the characteristics associated with problem gambling: A systematic review. Curr Addict Rep 2016;3(3):254–67.

14. Westermeyer J, Canive J, Thuras P, et al. Pathological and problem gambling among veterans in clinical care: Prevalence, demography, and clinical correlates. Am J Addict 2013;22(3):218–25.

15. Marks KR, Clark CD. The telescoping phenomenon: Origins in gender bias and implications for contemporary scientific inquiry. Subst Use Misuse 2018;53(6): 901–9.

16. Nordmyr J, Forsman AK, Wahlbeck K, et al. Associations between problem gambling, socio-demographics, mental health factors and gambling type: Sex differences among Finnish gamblers. Int Gambling Stud 2014;14(1):39–52.

17. Svensson J, Romild U. Problem gambling features and gendered gambling domains amongst regular gamblers in a Swedish population-based study. Sex Roles 2014;70(5–6):240–54.

18. Pattinson J, Parke A. The experience of high-frequency gambling behavior of older adult females in the United Kingdom: an interpretative phenomenological analysis. J Women Aging 2017;29(3):243–53.

19. Grant JE, Chamberlain SR, Schreiber LR, et al. Gender-related clinical and neurocognitive differences in individuals seeking treatment for pathological gambling. J Psychiatr Res 2012;46(9):1206–11.

20. González-Ortega I, Echeburúa E, Corral P, et al. Predictors of pathological gambling severity taking gender differences into account. Eur Addict Res 2013;19(3):146–54.

21. Hahmann T, Hamilton-Wright S, Ziegler C, et al. Problem gambling within the context of poverty: a scoping review. Int Gambling Stud 2020;1–37.

22. Spångberg J, Svensson J. Associations Between Youth Unemployment and Underage Gambling in Europe. J Gambling Issues 2020;45.

23. Hing N, Russell A, Tolchard B, et al. Risk factors for gambling problems: An analysis by gender. J Gambling Stud 2016;32(2):511–34.

24. Mani A, Mullainathan S, Shafir E, et al. Poverty impedes cognitive function. science 2013;341(6149):976–80.

25. Haushofer J, Fehr E. On the psychology of poverty. science 2014;344(6186): 862–7.

26. Dowling NA, Cowlishaw S, Jackson AC, et al. Prevalence of psychiatric comorbidity in treatment-seeking problem gamblers: A systematic review and meta-analysis. Aust N Z J Psychiatry 2015;49(6):519–39.

27. Jauregui P, Onaindia J, Estévez A. Adaptive and maladaptive coping strategies in adult pathological gamblers and their mediating role with anxious-depressive symptomatology. J Gambling Stud 2017;33(4):1081–97.

28. Kessler RC, Hwang I, LaBrie R, et al. DSM-IV pathological gambling in the National Comorbidity Survey Replication. Psychol Med 2008;38(9):1351–60.

29. Petry NM, Stinson FS, Grant BF. Comorbidity of DSM-IV pathological gambling and other psychiatric disorders: results from the National Epidemiologic Survey on Alcohol and Related Conditions. J Clin Psychiatry 2005;66(5):564–74.

30. Barnes GM, Welte JW, Hoffman JH, et al. The co-occurrence of gambling with substance use and conduct disorder among youth in the United States. Am J Addict 2011;20(2):166–73.

31. Cowlishaw S, Hakes JK. Pathological and problem gambling in substance use treatment: Results from the National Epidemiologic Survey on Alcohol and Related Conditions (NESARC). Am J Addict 2015;24(5):467–74.

32. Weintraub D, Koester J, Potenza MN, et al. Impulse control disorders in Parkinson disease: a cross-sectional study of 3090 patients. Arch Neurol 2010;67(5): 589–95.

33. Tang KT, Kim HS, Hodgins DC, et al. Gambling disorder and comorbid behavioral addictions: Demographic, clinical, and personality correlates. Psychiatry Res 2020;284:112763.
34. Estevez A, Jáuregui P, Lopez-Gonzalez H, et al. The severity of gambling and gambling related cognitions as predictors of emotional regulation and coping strategies in adolescents. J Gambling Stud 2021;37(2):483–95.
35. Caldeira KM, Arria AM, O'Grady KE, et al. Risk factors for gambling and substance use among recent college students. Drug and alcohol dependence 2017;179:280–90.
36. Abbott M. The changing epidemiology of gambling disorder and gambling-related harm: public health implications. Public health 2020;184:41–5.
37. Stevens M, Young M. Independent correlates of reported gambling problems amongst Indigenous Australians. Social Indicators Res 2010;98(1):147–66.
38. Gill KJ, Heath LM, Derevensky J, et al. The social and psychological impacts of gambling in the Cree communities of Northern Quebec. J gambling Stud 2016; 32(2):441–57.
39. Fulton JJ, Calhoun PS, Wagner HR, et al. The prevalence of posttraumatic stress disorder in Operation Enduring Freedom/Operation Iraqi Freedom (OEF/OIF) veterans: A meta-analysis. J anxiety Disord 2015;31:98–107.
40. Hayatbakhsh MR, Clavarino AM, Clavarino GM, et al. Early life course predictors of young adults' gambling. Int Gambling Stud 2013;13(1):19–36.
41. Botterill E, Gill PR, McLaren S, et al. Marital status and problem gambling among Australian older adults: The mediating role of loneliness. J gambling Stud 2016;32(3):1027–38.
42. Hing N, O'Mullan C, Nuske E, et al. The relationship between gambling and intimate partner violence against women. [Research Report]: Australia's National Research Organisation for Women's Safety Limited (ANROWS); 2020.
43. Xuan Y-H, Li S, Tao R, et al. Genetic and environmental influences on gambling: A meta-analysis of twin studies. Front Psychol 2017;8:2121.
44. Slutske WS, Zhu G, Meier MH, et al. Genetic and environmental influences on disordered gambling in men and women. Arch Gen Psychiatry 2010;67(6): 624–30.
45. Savage JE, Slutske WS, Martin NG. Personality and gambling involvement: a person-centered approach. Psychol Addict Behav 2014;28(4):1198.
46. Calado F, Alexandre J, Griffiths MD. Prevalence of adolescent problem gambling: A systematic review of recent research. J gambling Stud 2017; 33(2):397–424.
47. Sharman S. Gambling and Homelessness: Prevalence and Pathways. Curr Addict Rep 2019;6(2):57–64.
48. Lesieur HR, Blume SB. The South Oaks Gambling Screen (SOGS): A new instrument for the identification of pathological gamblers. Am J Psychiatry 1987; 144(9):I.
49. Toneatto T, Millar G. Assessing and treating problem gambling: Empirical status and promising trends. Can J Psychiatry 2004;49(8):517–25.
50. Edgren R, Castrén S, Mäkelä M, et al. Reliability of instruments measuring at-risk and problem gambling among young individuals: A systematic review covering years 2009–2015. J Adolesc Health 2016;58(6):600–15.
51. Sullivan S. GPs take a punt with a brief gambling screen: development of the early intervention gambling health test (Eight Screen). in Culture and the gambling phenomenon: Proceedings of the 12th annual conference of the

National Association for Gambling Studies. Sydney, Australia: National Association for Gambling Studies; 1999.

52. Sullivan S. Don't let an opportunity go by: Validation of the EIGHT gambling screen. Int J Ment Health Addict 2007;5(4):381–9.

53. Jackson AC, Wynne H, Dowling NA, et al. Using the CPGI to determine problem gambling prevalence in Australia: Measurement issues. Int J Ment Health Addict 2010;8(4):570–82.

54. Abbott MW, Volberg RA. The measurement of adult problem and pathological gambling. Int Gambling Stud 2006;6(2):175–200.

55. Callan MJ, Shead NW, Olson JM. The relation between personal relative deprivation and the urge to gamble among gamblers is moderated by problem gambling severity: A meta-analysis. Addict behaviors 2015;45:146–9.

56. Shaffer HJ, LaBrie R, Scanlan KM, et al. Pathological gambling among adolescents: Massachusetts gambling screen (MAGS). J Gambling Stud 1994;10(4): 339–62.

57. Gebauer L, LaBrie R, Shaffer HJ. Optimizing DSM-IV-TR classification accuracy: A brief biosocial screen for detecting current gambling disorders among gamblers in the general household population. Can J Psychiatry 2010;55(2):82–90.

58. Goodyear-Smith F, Arroll B, Coupe N. Asking for help is helpful: validation of a brief lifestyle and mood assessment tool in primary health care. Ann Fam Med 2009;7(3):239–44.

59. Volberg RA, Williams RJ. Developing a brief problem gambling screen using clinically validated samples of at-risk, problem and pathological gamblers. Boston, MA: Health Sciences; Report to the Alberta Gambling Research Institute; 2011.

60. Dowling NA, Merkouris SS, Manning V, et al. Screening for problem gambling within mental health services: a comparison of the classification accuracy of brief instruments. Addiction 2018;113(6):1088–104.

61. Fager M. How does one measure gambling problems. Int J Test 2007;6:25–39.

62. Johnson EE, Hamer R, Nora RM, et al. The Lie/Bet Questionnaire for screening pathological gamblers. Psychol Rep 1997;80(1):83–8.

63. Johnson EE, Hamer RM, Nora RM. The Lie/Bet Questionnaire for screening pathological gamblers: a follow-up study. Psychol Rep 1998;83(3_suppl): 1219–24.

64. Hodgins DC, Stea JN, Grant JE. Gambling disorders. Lancet 2011;378(9806): 1874–84.

65. Cowlishaw S, McCambridge J, Kessler D. Identification of gambling problems in primary care: properties of the NODS-CLiP screening tool. J Addict Med 2018; 12(6):442–6.

66. Grant JE, Donahue CB, Odlaug BL, et al. Imaginal desensitisation plus motivational interviewing for pathological gambling: randomised controlled trial. Br J Psychiatry 2009;195(3):266–7.

67. Petry NM, Ginley MK, Rash CJ. A systematic review of treatments for problem gambling. Psychol Addict Behav 2017;31(8):951.

68. Cowlishaw S, Merkouris S, Dowling N, et al. Psychological therapies for pathological and problem gambling. Cochrane Database Syst Rev 2012;(11):CD008937.

69. Oei TP, Raylu N, Casey LM. Effectiveness of group and individual formats of a combined motivational interviewing and cognitive behavioral treatment program for problem gambling: A randomized controlled trial. Behav Cogn psychotherapy 2010;38(2):233–8.

70. Miller WR, Rollnick S. Motivational interviewing: helping people change. New York, NY: Guilford press; 2012.
71. Yakovenko I, Quigley L, Hemmelgarn BR, et al. The efficacy of motivational interviewing for disordered gambling: systematic review and meta-analysis. Addict Behaviors 2015;43:72–82.
72. Brazeau BW, Hodgins DC, Cunningham JA, et al. Augmenting an online self-directed intervention for gambling disorder with a single motivational interview: Study protocol for a randomised controlled trial 2021;22(1):1–10.
73. Carlbring P, Jonsson J, Josephson H, et al. Motivational interviewing versus cognitive behavioral group therapy in the treatment of problem and pathological gambling: A randomized controlled trial. Cogn Behav Ther 2010;39(2):92–103.
74. Richard K, Baghurst T, Faragher JM, et al. Practical treatments considering the role of sociocultural factors on problem gambling. J gambling Stud 2017;33(1): 265–81.
75. Maynard BR, Wilson AN, Labuzienski E, et al. Mindfulness-based approaches in the treatment of disordered gambling: A systematic review and meta-analysis. Res Social Work Pract 2018;28(3):348–62.
76. Riley B. Experiential avoidance mediates the association between thought suppression and mindfulness with problem gambling. J Gambling Stud 2014;30(1): 163–71.
77. Dixon MR. Acceptance and commitment therapy. Carbondale (IL): Shawnee Scientific Press; 2014.
78. Cunningham JA, Hodgins DC, Mackenzie CS, et al. Randomized controlled trial of an Internet intervention for problem gambling provided with or without access to an Internet intervention for co-occurring mental health distress. Internet Interv 2019;17:100239.
79. LaBrie RA, Peller AJ, LaPlante DA, et al. A brief self-help toolkit intervention for gambling problems: A randomized multisite trial. Am J Orthop 2012;82(2):278.
80. Luquiens A, Tanguy ML, Lagadec M, et al. The efficacy of three modalities of Internet-based psychotherapy for non–treatment-seeking online problem gamblers: a randomized controlled trial. J Med Internet Res 2016;18(2):e4752.
81. Loo Gee B, Griffiths KM, Gulliver A. Effectiveness of mobile technologies delivering Ecological Momentary Interventions for stress and anxiety: a systematic review. J Am Med Inform Assoc 2016;23(1):221–9.
82. Heron KE, Smyth JM. Ecological momentary interventions: incorporating mobile technology into psychosocial and health behaviour treatments. Br J Health Psychol 2010;15(1):1–39.
83. Khazaal Y, Monney G, Richter F, et al. «Jeu-contrôle», rationnel d'une application de soutien aux limites de jeux. J de thérapie comportementale Cogn 2017;27(3): 129–37.
84. Merkouris SS, Hawker CO, Rodda SN, et al. GamblingLess: Curb Your Urge: Development and usability testing of a smartphone-delivered ecological momentary intervention for problem gambling. Int Gambling Stud 2020;20(3): 515–38.
85. Hawker CO, Merkouris SS, Youssef GJ, et al. A smartphone-delivered ecological momentary intervention for problem gambling (GamblingLess: Curb Your Urge): Single-arm acceptability and feasibility trial. J Med Internet Res 2021; 23(3):e25786.
86. Goudriaan AE, Schluter RS. Non-invasive Neuromodulation in Problem Gambling: What Are the Odds? Curr Addict Rep 2019;6(3):165–74.

87. Gay A, Boutet C, Sigaud T, et al. A single session of repetitive transcranial magnetic stimulation of the prefrontal cortex reduces cue-induced craving in patients with gambling disorder. Eur Psychiatry 2017;41(1):68–74.

88. Sauvaget A, Bulteau S, Guilleux A, et al. Both active and sham low-frequency rTMS single sessions over the right DLPFC decrease cue-induced cravings among pathological gamblers seeking treatment: A randomized, double-blind, sham-controlled crossover trial. J Behav Addict 2018;7(1):126–36.

89. Zack M, Cho SS, Parlee J, et al. Effects of high frequency repeated transcranial magnetic stimulation and continuous theta burst stimulation on gambling reinforcement, delay discounting, and stroop interference in men with pathological gambling. Brain Stimulation 2016;9(6):867–75.

90. Daneshparvar H, Sadat-Shirazi MS, Fekri M, et al. NMDA receptor subunits change in the prefrontal cortex of pure-opioid and multi-drug abusers: a postmortem study. Eur Arch Psychiatry Clin Neurosci 2019;269(3):309–15.

91. Dickler M, Lenglos C, Renauld E, et al. Online effects of transcranial direct current stimulation on prefrontal metabolites in gambling disorder. Neuropharmacology 2018;131:51–7.

92. Rosenberg O, Klein LD, Dannon PN. Deep transcranial magnetic stimulation for the treatment of pathological gambling. Psychiatry Res 2013;206(1):111–3.

93. Soyata AZ, Aksu S, Woods AJ, et al. Effect of transcranial direct current stimulation on decision making and cognitive flexibility in gambling disorder. Eur Arch Psychiatry Clin Neurosci 2019;269(3):275–84.

94. Challet-Bouju G, Bruneau M, Victorri-Vigneau C, et al. Cognitive remediation interventions for gambling disorder: A systematic review. Front Psychol 2017;8:1961.

95. Bartley CA, Bloch MH. Meta-analysis: pharmacological treatment of pathological gambling. Expert Rev neurotherapeutics 2013;13(8):887–94.

96. Kraus SW, Etuk R, Potenza MN. Current pharmacotherapy for gambling disorder: a systematic review. Expert Opin Pharmacother 2020;21(3):287–96.

97. Bosco D, Plastino M, Colica C, et al. Opioid antagonist naltrexone for the treatment of pathological gambling in Parkinson disease. Clin neuropharmacology 2012;35(3):118–20.

98. Theile JW, Morikawa H, Gonzales RA, et al. Ethanol enhances GABAergic transmission onto dopamine neurons in the ventral tegmental area of the rat. Alcohol Clin Exp Res 2008;32(6):1040–8.

99. Kim SW, Grant JE, Adson DE, et al. Double-blind naltrexone and placebo comparison study in the treatment of pathological gambling. Biol Psychiatry 2001;49(11):914–21.

100. Grant JE, Kim SW, Hartman BK. A double-blind, placebo-controlled study of the opiate antagonist naltrexone in the treatment of pathological gambling urges. J Clin Psychiatry 2008;69(5):4784.

101. Grant JE, Kim SW, Hollander E, et al. Predicting response to opiate antagonists and placebo in the treatment of pathological gambling. Psychopharmacology 2008;200(4):521–7.

102. Grant JE, Odlaug BL, Potenza MH, et al. Nalmefene in the treatment of pathological gambling: multicentre, double-blind, placebo-controlled study. Br J Psychiatry 2010;197(4):330–1.

103. Kovanen L, Basnet S, Castrén S, et al. A randomised, double-blind, placebo-controlled trial of as-needed naltrexone in the treatment of pathological gambling. Eur Addict Res 2016;22(2):70–9.

104. Potenza MN. Neurobiology of gambling behaviors. Curr Opin Neurobiol 2013; 23(4):660–7.

105. A Bullock S, Potenza MN. Pathological gambling: neuropsychopharmacology and treatment. Curr Psychopharmacol 2012;1(1):67–85.

106. Grant JE, Schreiber LR, Odlaug BL. Phenomenology and treatment of behavioural addictions. Can J Psychiatry 2013;58(5):252–9.

107. Goudriaan AE, Oosterlaan J, de Beurs E, et al. Pathological gambling: a comprehensive review of biobehavioral findings. Neurosci Biobehavioral Rev 2004;28(2):123–41.

108. Fong T, Kalechstein A, Bernhard B, et al. A double-blind, placebo-controlled trial of olanzapine for the treatment of video poker pathological gamblers. Pharmacol Biochem Behav 2008;89(3):298–303.

109. McElroy SL, Nelson EB, Welge JA, et al. Olanzapine in the, Treatment of Pathological Gambling: A Negative Randomized Placebo-Controlled Trial. J Clin Psychiatry 2008;69(3):433–40.

110. Zack M, Poulos CX. A D2 antagonist enhances the rewarding and priming effects of a gambling episode in pathological gamblers. Neuropsychopharmacology 2007;32(8):1678–86.

111. Tunbridge E, Bannerman DM, Sharp T, et al. Catechol-o-methyltransferase inhibition improves set-shifting performance and elevates stimulated dopamine release in the rat prefrontal cortex. J Neurosci 2004;24(23):5331–5.

112. Grant JE, Odlaug BL, Chamberlain SR, et al. A proof of concept study of tolcapone for pathological gambling: relationships with COMT genotype and brain activation. Eur Neuropsychopharmacol 2013;23(11):1587–96.

113. Kalivas P, Volkow N, Seamans J. Unmanageable motivation in addiction: a pathology in prefrontal-accumbens glutamate transmission. Neuron 2005;45(5): 647–50.

114. Kalivas P, Volkow N. New medications for drug addiction hiding in glutamatergic neuroplasticity. Mol Psychiatry 2011;16(10):974–86.

115. Nordin C, Gupta RC, Sjödin I. Cerebrospinal fluid amino acids in pathological gamblers and healthy controls. Neuropsychobiology 2007;56(2–3):152–8.

116. Grant JE, Kim SW, Odlaug BL. N-acetyl cysteine, a glutamate-modulating agent, in the treatment of pathological gambling: a pilot study. Biol Psychiatry 2007; 62(6):652–7.

117. Grant JE, Odlaug BL, Chamberlain SR, et al. A randomized, placebo-controlled trial of N-acetylcysteine plus imaginal desensitization for nicotine-dependent pathological gamblers. J Clin Psychiatry 2013;74(1).

118. Blaszczynski A, Ladouceur R, Shaffer HJ. A science-based framework for responsible gambling: The Reno model. J Gambling Stud 2004;20(3):301–17.

119. Blaszczynski A, Collins P, Fong D, et al. Responsible gambling: General principles and minimal requirements. J gambling Stud 2011;27(4):565–73.

120. Harris A, Parke A. The interaction of gambling outcome and gambling harm-minimisation strategies for electronic gambling: The efficacy of computer generated self-appraisal messaging. Int J Ment Health Addict 2016;14(4):597–617.

121. Blaszczynski A, Shaffer HJ, Ladouceur R, et al. Clarifying responsible gambling and its concept of responsibility. Int J Ment Health Addict 2021;1–7.

122. Shaffer HJ, Blaszczynski A, Ladouceur R. Truth, alternative facts, narrative, and science: What is happening to responsible gambling and gambling disorder? Int J Ment Health Addict 2017;15(6):1197–202.

123. Percy C, França M, Dragičević S, et al. Predicting online gambling self-exclusion: an analysis of the performance of supervised machine learning models. Int Gambling Stud 2016;16(2):193–210.

124. Ivanova E, Magnusson K, Carlbring P. Deposit limit prompt in online gambling for reducing gambling intensity: a randomized controlled trial. Front Psychol 2019;10:639.

125. Quilty LC, Robinson J, Blaszczynski A. Responsible gambling training in Ontario casinos: employee attitudes and experience. Int Gambling Stud 2015;15(3): 361–76.

126. Gray HM, Juliver J, LaPlante DA. Gambling industry employees' experiences with an onsite responsible gambling program. J Gambling Stud 2021;37(2): 369–86.

127. Gainsbury S. Online gambling addiction: the relationship between internet gambling and disordered gambling. Curr Addict Rep 2015;2(2):185–93.

128. Hing N, Russell AMT, Gainsbury SM, et al. Characteristics and help-seeking behaviors of Internet gamblers based on most problematic mode of gambling. J Med Internet Res 2015;17(1):e3781.

129. McCormack A, Shorter GW, Griffiths MD. An empirical study of gender differences in online gambling. J Gambling Stud 2014;30(1):71–88.

130. Håkansson A, Widinghoff C. Gender differences in problem gamblers in an online gambling setting. Psychol Res Behav Management 2020;13:681.

131. Hayer T, Meyer G. Internet self-exclusion: Characteristics of self-excluded gamblers and preliminary evidence for its effectiveness. Int J Ment Health Addict 2011;9(3):296–307.

132. Montiel I, Ortega-Barón J, Basterra-González A, et al. Problematic online gambling among adolescents: A systematic review about prevalence and related measurement issues. J Behav Addict 2021;10(3):566–86.

133. Shi J, Colder Carras M, Potenza MN, et al. A Perspective on Age Restrictions and Other Harm Reduction Approaches Targeting Youth Online Gambling, Considering Convergences of Gambling and Videogaming. Front Psychiatry 2021;11:1650.

134. Calado F, Griffiths MD. Problem gambling worldwide: An update and systematic review of empirical research (2000–2015). J Behav Addict 2016;5(4):592–613.

135. Makri-Botsari E, Karagianni G. Cyberbullying in Greek adolescents: The role of parents. Procedia-Social Behav Sci 2014;116:3241–53.

136. Faltýnková A, Blinka L, Ševčíková A, et al. The associations between family-related factors and excessive internet use in adolescents. Int J Environ Res Public Health 2020;17(5):1754.

Attention-Deficit Hyperactivity Disorder and Therapeutic Cannabis Use Motives

Mariely Hernandez, PhD[a],*, Frances R. Levin, MD[b]

KEYWORDS

- Attention-deficit hyperactivity disorder • Cannabis • Marijuana

KEY POINTS

- Attention-deficit hyperactivity disorder (ADHD) is a risk factor for cannabis use problems.
- Widespread decriminalization of cannabis in the United States (US) has led to increased use in young adults and lower perceptions of harm, augmenting the risk for developing cannabis use problems.
- Cannabis users with ADHD report the therapeutic use of cannabis to treat sleep problems and physical pain.
- Clinicians should inquire about motivations for cannabis use.

INTRODUCTION

Attention-deficit hyperactivity disorder (ADHD) is a neurodevelopmental disorder characterized by impairing symptoms of age-inappropriate inattention and impulsivity across multiple settings.[1] It is primarily a disorder of executive dysfunction that manifests as poor regulation of attentional, behavioral, and emotional processes. The estimated prevalence of a lifetime ADHD diagnosis in the United States (US) pediatric population (ages 2–17 years) is 8.4%, with a global prevalence estimated at 5%.[2–4] While it is believed that most youth exhibit remittance from ADHD symptoms over time, recent findings from the Multimodal Treatment Study of ADHD (MTA) demonstrated fluctuating patterns of ADHD symptomology and impairment for 90% of the sample over the course of 16 years, with only 9.1% of participants evincing sustained remission from ADHD symptoms into young adulthood.[5] The prevalence of ADHD in adults is estimated to be between 2.5% and 4.4% in the US and 3.4% globally.[6,7]

Childhood ADHD is a widely identified risk factor for substance use and its associated problems.[8–10] Longitudinal studies on ADHD trajectories have shown that

[a] Columbia University Medical Center, New York State Psychiatric Institute, 1051 Riverside Drive, Unit 43, New York, NY 10032, USA; [b] Columbia University Vagelos College of Physicians and Surgeons, New York State Psychiatric Institute, 1051 Riverside Drive, Unit 66, New York, NY 10032, USA
* Corresponding author.
E-mail address: mariely.hernandez@nyspi.columbia.edu

Psychiatr Clin N Am 45 (2022) 503–514
https://doi.org/10.1016/j.psc.2022.05.010
0193-953X/22/© 2022 Elsevier Inc. All rights reserved.

adolescents with ADHD are more likely to initiate substance use earlier, and escalate to regular use more quickly than their neurotypical peers, placing them at risk of developing a substance use disorder (SUD).[11,12] Additionally, ADHD is over-represented in substance use treatment settings and is often associated with more severe pathology.[13,14] While alcohol and nicotine (both legal and widely available) are the most commonly used psychoactive substances, cannabis use has been increasing as more states decriminalize marijuana for personal use, particularly in young adults aged 18 to 25 years.[15] Genetic and longitudinal study findings strongly suggest ADHD is a risk factor for cannabis use and developing a cannabis use disorder (CUD). A recent study found a causal relation between ADHD and lifetime cannabis use, with a staggering odds ratio of 7.9 for cannabis use in those with ADHD compared with non-ADHD peers (95% CI: 3.72, 15.51, $P = 5.88$ x10^{-5}).[16] Another study of 483 adolescents referred for SUD treatment reported that 32% and 47% of participants met DSM-IV criteria for cannabis abuse and dependence, respectively.[17] Furthermore, those with CUDs were twice as likely to be diagnosed with ADHD compared with their peers without a CUD.[17] Given the growing accessibility and decreasing perceptions of harm, individuals with ADHD may be at an increased risk for cannabis use problems, particularly due to shared deficits in self-regulation found in externalizing disorders such as ADHD and SUDs.[15,18]

Adolescents and young adults with ADHD are at great risk for substance use problems due to neurodevelopmental processes underlying the impulsivity and emotional lability characteristic of these developmental stages. This risk is conceptualized here as multi-pronged: first, symptoms of impulsivity and inattention may predispose individuals with ADHD to experience negative consequences following use, such as using more than intended and subsequently being unable to fulfill social, academic, or occupational responsibilities. Second, individuals with ADHD may self-medicate with cannabis to treat symptoms of psychological distress (eg,: insomnia, anxiety) that may cooccur with or exist independently of ADHD.[19] Others diagnosed with ADHD may prefer to use cannabis instead of pharmacologic interventions or alongside them to temper unwanted side effects of ADHD medication.[20]

While experimentation with psychoactive substances is relatively normative for adolescents and young adults, those with ADHD are more likely to experience negative consequences of use compared with neurotypical peers and despite comparable rates of use.[21,22] A closer look at the worsening risk of cannabis use problems in ADHD populations is warranted, starting with cannabis use trends, effects on cognition, and motivators for use. As the availability of cannabis grows alongside the increasing diversity of formulations and routes of administration (ROA), clinicians are tasked with consolidating concerns of neurodevelopmental effects of substance use in adolescents with the reductions in perceived harm and decriminalization of cannabis. The following questions arise:

- What are the trends in cannabis use across age groups?
- What are the effects of cannabis use on cognition in teenagers and emerging adults? Are these effects related to recreational or chronic use?
- What are the perceived benefits of cannabis use, particularly for those with ADHD? What are the harms? Is there a dose-dependent threshold for therapeutic vs harmful?

Cannabis Use Trends

Cannabis, also known as marijuana, is a psychoactive drug originating from the cannabis plant. Numerous derivatives and isolates are being assessed for therapeutic benefit across mental and physical problems; for the purposes of this summary, we will focus on the uses of tetrahydrocannabinol (THC) and cannabidiol (CBD), the 2 most common phytocannabinoids of the cannabis plant, and the most frequently found in cannabis products.[23,24] THC is the most potent and well-known psychoactive element of the cannabis plant, associated with a "high." CBD does not share those psychoactive properties but has gained widespread popularity for alleviating pain, anxiety, and facilitating sleep.[23]

In the US, whereby an increasing number of states have adapted medical marijuana laws and are decriminalizing cannabis for personal use, the 2020 National Survey on Drug Use and Health (NSDUH) reports show steadily increasing rates of individuals using cannabis. Trends in NSDUH 2020 reports shows an overall increase in past-year cannabis use initiation for individuals 12 and older, with 2.8 million people reporting first time use in the past year. Nearly 25% of these new users were $\geq$ 26 years of age.[15] Findings reveal past-year cannabis use was greatest in the 18 to 25 age group (34.5%), followed by 16.3% in adults 26 years and older, and 10.1% in adolescents 12 to 17 years of age.[15] In 2020, 4% of respondents reported daily or almost daily cannabis use in the past month, compared with 1.3% in 2002.[15] Finally, the 2020 NSDUH Highlights noted only 27.4% of respondents aged 12 and older reported they perceived great risk of harm from smoking cannabis 1-2x/week while emerging adults aged 18 to 25 were less likely than their counterparts to regard weekly cannabis use as harmful.[15] Although the NSDUH data do not show increased cannabis use in adolescents, longitudinal and cohort studies suggest growing trends of cannabis use in this age group. A recent systematic review and meta-analysis of adolescent vaping of cannabis in the US and Canada shows dramatic increases in lifetime (6.1% to 13.6%), past year (7.2% to 13.2%), and past month (1.6% to 8.4%) prevalence from 2013 to 2020.[25] The authors raised concerns that preference for cannabis products may be shifting from dried herb to cannabis oil, which is more potent due to higher concentrations of THC.[25] These data may support the high percentage of adolescents with cannabis use problems found in substance use treatment settings.[17] Roehler and colleagues (2022) recently published data showing a steady average 12.1% increase in cannabis use-related ER visits from 2006 to 2014,[26] highlighting a rising public health burden likely associated with increasing use.

Thus, with the growing decriminalization of cannabis, reported rates of initiation, use, and frequency of use have increased over the past 2 decades, especially among those 18 and older. Cannabis use initiation may be due to several factors, such as decriminalization making it more socially acceptable to use or disclose cannabis use, greater availability of products, as well as possible therapeutic use. With no consensus on dosing and reduced perceptions of harm, individuals using cannabis recreationally may be particularly vulnerable to using more than intended, with potentially serious consequences.

Cannabis and Cognition

As with any psychoactive substance, clinicians and researchers alike have concerns about the effects of repeated cannabis use on the brain. For individuals with ADHD, a disorder associated with both neuroanatomical and functional differences in comparison to neurotypical peers,[27] it is important to investigate whether cannabis use has any effect on preexisting neurocognitive vulnerabilities in ADHD. Cannabinoid receptors are typically concentrated in the temporal and midbrain regions of the brain, structures associated with memory, emotion regulation, and reward processing. Cannabis use affects not only cortical and subcortical structures but also functional connectivity between regions. How harmful is occasional recreational use compared with chronic, problem use? Can cannabis instigate structural changes in the brain? These are difficult questions researchers have been trying to answer, with imaging studies reporting conflicting findings. A recent review found no net differences, between cannabis users and nonusers, in volumetric changes in the whole brain, the amygdala, striatum, cerebellum, prefrontal cortex, or anterior cingulate cortex.[28] The most consistent findings on morphologic changes in regular cannabis users (compared with nonusers) are volumetric reductions in the hippocampus and orbitofrontal cortex,[29] as well as atypical structural connectivity and diffusivity.[28] Other studies have published findings on both increased and decreased cerebellar and striatal volumes in cannabis users compared with nonusers, highlighting the need for further research to better characterize these effects.

Cognitive effects of both occasional and chronic cannabis use include impaired verbal learning, memory, and attention, with psychomotor reduction in acute intoxication.[30] Importantly, several studies found that acute THC administration impaired decision making by increasing risk taking in both recreational and regular cannabis users compared with nonusers.[31] For individuals with ADHD, who are already predisposed to riskier choices, lowering this threshold elevates the likelihood of adverse consequences. Some studies show that cannabis effects on brain volume and cognition can persist following periods of abstinence in non-ADHD users, but more research is needed.[30,31]

Findings from studies comparing substance use in individuals with and without ADHD (also ADHD users and nonusers) in terms of brain structure and function suggest that ADHD neurocognitive effects are significantly more pronounced than the perhaps more subtle influence of recreational substance use.[32,33] Prospective longitudinal studies (beyond adolescence and young adulthood) of ADHD and cannabis use trajectories are needed to better understand the neural underpinnings of regular cannabis use in the ADHD brain.

A potential explanation for the inconsistent outcomes is the possibility that cannabinoids may have both neurotoxic and neuroprotective attributes, particularly CBD.[28,34] Baseline and posttreatment structural imaging of 18 adult regular cannabis users participating in a 10-week trial of daily 200 mg of cannabidiol showed significantly *increased* volume in hippocampal subregions, especially for the heavy users.[35]

Taken together, these results present compelling evidence of structural and functional differences in the brains of chronic cannabis users compared with nonusers. Adolescents are at greatest risk due to the critical neurodevelopmental period and the potentially long-lasting neurotoxic effects of psychoactive substances, which may persist even after prolonged periods of abstinence.[31,36] In terms of cannabis use and ADHD, findings have been inconsistent across studies, possibly due to variability in substance use histories, and differences in cannabis use quantity, frequency, formulation, and ROA. Chronic cannabis users with ADHD may worsen preexisting deficits in working memory and executive function in ways that may not become apparent until later in life, with long-lasting, persistent effects despite discontinuing use.[31] More studies of cannabis users with comparable use histories and co-occurring ADHD are needed to better elucidate the effects of cannabis on cognition in this population, *especially* considering general beliefs about the therapeutic benefits of cannabis-derived products.

Cannabis Use Motives

The expanding decriminalization of cannabis in the US and concurrent reductions in perceptions of harm have impacted reported initiation and escalation in the use of cannabis, particularly for young adults.[15] With greater availability and destigmatization of cannabis products, as well as a diverse array of options for ingesting (tinctures, concentrates, edibles, and so forth), users are now able to tailor their use to their needs, potentially leading to increases in new users due to more discreet methods of delivery (eg, edibles). For those with ADHD, a disorder characterized by deficits in self-regulation and impulsivity, greater access to cannabis products may accelerate trajectories to a CUD.

Recent studies have shown that individuals with ADHD and concurrent cannabis use may do so to treat other ailments.[19,20,37] To date, the FDA has only approved the prescription use of 3 cannabis-derived products: one CBD medication (Epidiolex) for severe epilepsy, nabilone (Cesamet) and dronabinol (Marinol, Syndros) for nausea related to chemotherapy.[38] Despite the short list of FDA approved indications, there is a widespread use of cannabis-derived products for treating nausea and somatic pain, with some research support.[39,40] Unfortunately, there is still a dearth of consistent evidence in favor of the therapeutic use of cannabis for psychiatric illness. Studies examining ADHD and cannabis use have noted an association between greater hyperactive/impulsive symptoms and likelihood of heavy cannabis use.[41,42] While this finding is consistent with reported therapeutic use motivations to treat sleep problems and anxiety, individuals with more severe ADHD presentations may be chronically undertreated and use drugs to manage mood and ADHD symptoms.

Mitchell and colleagues completed a qualitative analysis of online discussion forums related to cannabis use and ADHD, finding that 25% reported therapeutic benefits of cannabis for ADHD symptoms, compared with 8% of posts stating cannabis was harmful to ADHD, 5% who believed it was both, and 2% who believe it had no effect.[19] Importantly, the spread in these findings did not extend to mood symptoms and other psychiatric disorders. For example, while 14% stated that cannabis is therapeutic for their mood, 13% stated it was harmful and 3% of posts indicated that it was both harmful and therapeutic.

Sleep. One of the most frequently reported motives for cannabis use is to treat sleep problems.[20,37] Individuals with ADHD may be especially drawn to using cannabis therapeutically to address sleep issues, due to the increased likelihood of experiencing sleep problems if one has ADHD,[43] and the soporific effects of cannabis. A Dutch national survey study found individuals with ADHD were significantly more likely than their non-ADHD peers to report insomnia and alterations in sleep duration.[43]

A prospective study examined multiple motivational pathways from baseline ADHD symptomology to 12-month cannabis use problems in 361 veterans with a lifetime history of cannabis use.[37] Findings revealed sleep motives at 6 months to be a strong mediator for frequency of use, while coping with negative affect emerged as a proximal predictor of cannabis use problems. Cannabis use problems were defined as interpersonal conflict, job loss, financial problems, and so forth, resulting from cannabis use. Thus, a CUD is measured more by the negative consequences related to how one accommodates the drug use into their lifestyle, at the expense of relationships, responsibilities, physical health, and safety. As individuals with ADHD build tolerance to substances, even if it is cannabis for sleep, they may be susceptible to cannabis use problems that can affect all aspects of their daily lives, especially in the absence of other behavioral coping strategies.

Importantly, there is insufficient data to support the therapeutic use of cannabis for sleep. A recent review of cannabinoids and sleep disorders noted that with short-term use, THC can increase sleep duration, reduce sleep onset latency (SOL), and reduce wakefulness after sleep onset (WASO), while long-term use of THC for sleep was associated with longer SOL and reduced overall sleep duration.[44] The authors posited that tolerance to THC from chronic use may underlie these changes and further noted that withdrawal from cannabis was associated with sleep disturbances. Although CBD can have alerting effects, it has been associated with improved sleep. CBD and THC formulations to treat insomnia are currently being studied, and authors note improvement in sleep with the therapeutic use of cannabis for insomnia secondary to chronic pain conditions, though it is unclear whether cannabis effects on sleep are direct or indirect, via pain relief.[44]

Pain relief

Individuals may also use cannabis therapeutically for its analgesic properties, as there is a significant overlap in the distribution of endogenous opioid and cannabinoid receptors in the brain.[45] There is a nascent literature suggesting an association between ADHD and chronic pain disorders. One national survey study of community-dwelling adults in England reported a significant association between elevated ADHD symptoms and extreme pain, an effect which was sustained even after controlling for common comorbid mental disorders (depression, anxiety) also associated with somatic pain.[46] In the US, an interim analysis of 37 adult patients using cannabis therapeutically via a medical marijuana certification for chronic pain showed reductions in pain after 6 months of treatment, which was associated with improved sleep, mood, anxiety, and overall quality of life.[39] These findings suggest an indirect pathway whereby at least short-term therapeutic use of cannabis to alleviate chronic pain conditions can also lead to improvements in sleep, mood, and cognition.

One potentially overlooked motive for cannabis use in women is to treat somatic pain, particularly pelvic pain associated with relatively common medical conditions, such as endometriosis.[47] Dorani and colleagues (2021) investigated hormone-related mood problems in 209 women with ADHD, finding that participants had high rates of co-occurring premenstrual dysphoric disorder, postpartum depression, and more severe climacteric (peri-menopausal, menopausal) symptoms than the general population.[48] These studies suggest that cannabis products are potent analgesics in women with severe pelvic pain. Additional research is needed on the long-term use of cannabis to treat somatic pain, as tolerance to the effects of THC may result in more frequent use, increasing the risk of CUD. There is research suggesting that cannabis is a "gateway drug" to opioid use,[49] particularly for youth. However, there is also evidence that supports cannabis as an analgesic alternative to opioids and its utility in treating opioid use disorders (OUD).[45] More research is needed on the therapeutic use of cannabis and progression to other psychoactive substances.

Other studies have reported high rates of childhood ADHD in chronic pain treatment settings. One study of 106 women with Fibromyalgia Syndrome (FMS) found nearly 25% of the sample had ADHD, which was associated with higher ratings of FMS symptom severity and diminished functioning, especially in the occupational/academic domain; 38.5% of patients with FMS and co-occurring ADHD also had a SUD (primarily opioid use), compared with only 3.8% of patients with FMS alone.[50] The greater use of opioids in the ADHD + FMS participants in addition to reports of more severe pain in this group, suggests that even with opioid treatment, the pain is not being well-managed. Kerekes and colleagues (2021) hypothesized that neuroinflammation underlies pain perception and sensitization in ADHD, proposing a mechanism whereby inflammation in the brain can affect dopamine levels and subsequent pro or antiinflammatory cellular processes that can lead to ADHD and sensitization to pain.[51]

Future research studies should investigate whether interventions that reduce neuroinflammation are a potential therapeutic target to treat ADHD and chronic pain.

In summary, there is burgeoning evidence that individuals with ADHD are more likely to report somatic pain and experience more severe symptoms of chronic pain disorders. Alleviating this pain is a potential pathway for developing substance use problems with cannabis and/or opioid products.

Attention-deficit hyperactivity disorder symptoms and side effects of attention-deficit hyperactivity disorder treatment

Another motive for cannabis use may be to treat ADHD symptoms, and, although it is believed that treating ADHD can reduce the risk of substance use problems, individuals with ADHD may use cannabis therapeutically to treat symptoms missed by ADHD medication and/or unpleasant side effects of medication. A recent study analyzed online survey data of cannabis effects on ADHD symptoms, ADHD medication side effects, and ADHD-related executive function from predominantly female college students with ADHD who reported using cannabis to manage ADHD symptoms.[20] Participants reported that acute cannabis use improved ADHD symptoms of restlessness (88.17%), hyperactivity (80.47%), and mental frustration (75.74%) while it worsened memory (66.86%) and inattention (43.20% compared with 39.64% reporting it improved inattention). Nearly 92% of respondents reported acute cannabis use improved ADHD symptoms overall. Participant-reported effects of chronic cannabis use on ADHD symptoms were more modest, with about 35% reporting overall improvement with chronic use, 14.20% reporting an overall worsening of ADHD symptoms, and nearly 37% reporting no effect.[20] The limited appraisals of how cannabis use impacts ADHD symptoms in chronic users may reflect an increased tolerance for the psychoactive effects of cannabis. Notably, few participants reported an overall worsening of ADHD symptoms. The stark contrast in perceived benefit between acute and chronic use begs the question of what motives underlie continued cannabis use when there is low perception of the improvement of ADHD symptoms, suggesting other motives for chronic use and/or physical dependence. For the subset of participants with ADHD who reported using cannabis to treat adverse side effects of ADHD medication (n = 72), cannabis improved many of the negative side effects.[20] Nearly 82% reported that cannabis improved loss of appetite and about 67% reported that cannabis improved sleep problems.

Executive dysfunction, a core component of ADHD, may pose as both a motive and by-product of cannabis use. Analyses of cannabis use frequency, ADHD symptoms, and executive dysfunction showed cannabis use frequency was a significant moderator of the association between executive dysfunction and ADHD symptom total scores, with a trending decrease in the strength of the association between ADHD total score and executive dysfunction as the frequency of cannabis use increased.[20] The authors unexpectedly found that for the top 0.08% of cannabis users, there was no significant relation between impulsivity or hyperactivity symptom severity and executive dysfunction. These findings underscore the challenge of determining whether for chronic cannabis users who report improvement in ADHD symptomology, the subjective impression is consistent with their actual functioning. It may be that the mood-altering effects of cannabis may desensitize users to the negative effect/distress associated with ADHD symptoms and/or that users modify their required tasks to accommodate frequent use.

To date, there is one known randomized placebo-controlled trial of cannabis to treat ADHD. A 6-week placebo-controlled RCT compared cognitive performance in 30 adults with ADHD 1-h after the administration of Sativex , an oral mucosal spray with low dose of THC, or placebo.[52] Participants exhibited comparable cognitive performance with placebo vs active treatment, with trends toward improved performance in the active treatment arm. The authors noted the absence of any worsening of performance on the cognitive task in active treatment participants compared with placebo.[52] The strength and generalizability of the findings were limited by a small sample size, emphasizing the need for more studies with larger samples.

DISCUSSION

ADHD is a complex, highly heritable neurodevelopmental disorder with significant heterogeneity in presentations over time. The moniker "ADHD" may be misleading, since, for many, ADHD is experienced as difficulty in *regulating* attention. This can manifest as hypersensitivity to both internal and external distractors, making it difficult to prioritize attentional targets, as well as perseverative hyper-focus on a rewarding activity or hobby, even at the expense of food and sleep. These seemingly opposite presentations of an attentional problem can be confusing and frustrating for parents of children and adolescents with ADHD, as well as partners and friends of adults with persistent ADHD. The same attentional dysregulation can predispose those with ADHD to use psychoactive substances, such as cannabis. For those with ADHD seeking relief from boredom, cannabis (and other drugs) may be appealing due to known psychoactive effects of lowering the threshold for amusement. Individuals with ADHD may also turn to substances to cope with negative affect related to interpersonal conflict, and address some of the undesirable sequelae of the attentional dysregulation, such as anxiety and disruptive sleep patterns.

In co-occurring CUD and ADHD, it is important to consider the perceived benefits of cannabis, particularly its effects on relieving pain and anxiety, as well as facilitating sleep. The use of illicit substances to address these symptoms likely reflects inadequately treated conditions necessitating adjunctive behavioral interventions, dose adjustments, or changes in medication regimen. While a harm reduction approach respects the individual's decision to use illicit substances and attempts to mitigate risks related to use, there is evidence that cannabis use by those with ADHD can be motivated by untreated or inadequately treated symptoms of ADHD, pain, anxiety, and sleep disturbances.

In the US, the privatized health care system and financial barriers to quality psychiatric care may compel individuals with undiagnosed ADHD to use substances to treat symptoms, as they are more readily accessible than a diagnostic evaluation and pharmacologic treatment under the care of a qualified practitioner. Further, as cannabis is increasingly legalized in the US, prevailing public discourse about the therapeutic benefits of cannabis and diminishing perceptions of harm can overshadow scientific findings on the negative impact that chronic cannabis use has on neuroanatomy,[37] cognition,[36] and risk for cardiovascular and pulmonary diseases associated with smoking cannabis.[53] While increasing access to psychiatric treatment of underserved populations is paramount in addressing therapeutic use of illicit drugs, exploring motivations for use in existing patients gives clinicians the opportunity to discuss alternative treatment options that are potentially more effective and less risky for those with ADHD.

One of the shared traits in ADHD and SUD is impulsivity and deficits in inhibitory control. Psychoactive substances can lower the threshold for impulsivity and risk-taking in many individuals, but it can lead to more serious consequences for those with ADHD, who may accidently overuse cannabis while waiting to feel the psychoactive effects of edible formulations. Therefore, one of the clinical concerns about the increasing availability of cannabis and perceptions of benefit is that individuals with ADHD are vulnerable to excessive, impulsive use that can result in adverse physical outcomes.

Potential impediments to attentional focus and overall functioning in individuals with and without ADHD are sleep disturbances, pain, and physical restlessness. For those with hyperactive symptoms, the sedating effects of cannabis can sufficiently reduce physical restlessness for an individual to attend to a task. Similarly, for individuals with ADHD and chronic pain, the severity of the pain may be disabling in the absence of therapeutic intervention, and thus impair functioning more than any cognitive effects of acute cannabis use. So, as clinicians deliberate cannabis's potential for harm against the potential for therapeutic benefit, patients with ADHD, chronic pain, and co-occurring cannabis use may be weighing the immediate and persistent pain symptoms against a potent and effective analgesic, despite the unclear long-term effects. More research on both recreational and therapeutic cannabis use effects in ADHD populations are needed.

CLINICS CARE POINTS

- There is evidence that cannabis use by those with ADHD can be motivated by untreated or inadequately treated symptoms of ADHD, pain, anxiety, and sleep disturbances.
- Practitioners should inquire about motivations for cannabis use, such as to help with sleep, anxiety, or physical pain. These symptoms may be more effectively treated by pharmacologic or behavioral interventions, which can be part of a treatment plan alongside reducing cannabis use. Changes in conventional medication regimens may be warranted.

ACKNOWLEDGEMENT

The content is solely the responsibility of the authors and does not necessarily represent the official views of the National Institute of Drug Abuse. This research was supported by a grant from the National Institute on Drug Abuse (5R25DA035161, Multiple PIs: Ruglass and Hien).

DISCLOSURE

The authors have no conflicts of interest to disclose.

REFERENCES

1. American Psychiatric Association. Diagnostic and Statistical Manual of Mental Disorders. 5th edition. Washington, DC: American Psychiatric Publishing; 2013.
2. Danielson ML, Bitsko RH, Ghandour RM, et al. Prevalence of Parent-Reported ADHD Diagnosis and Associated Treatment Among U.S. Children and Adolescents, 2016. J Clin Child Adolesc Psychol 2018;47(2):199–212.
3. Sayal K, Prasad V, Daley D, et al. ADHD in children and young people:prevalence, care pathways, and service provision. Lancet Psychiatry 2018;5(2): 175–86.
4. Polanczyk G, de Lima MS, Horta BL, et al. The worldwide prevalence of ADHD: a systematic review and metaregression analysis. Am J Psychiatry 2007;164(6): 942–8.
5. Sibley MH, Arnold LE, Swanson JM, et al. Variable Patterns of Remission From ADHD in the Multimodal Treatment Study of ADHD. Am J Psychiatry 2022; 179(2):142–51.

6. Kessler RC, Adler L, Barkley R, et al. The prevalence and correlates of adult ADHD in the United States: results from the National Comorbidity Survey Replication. Am J Psychiatry 2006;163(4):716–23.

7. Fayyad J, De Graaf R, Kessler R, et al. Cross-national prevalence and correlates of adult attention-deficit hyperactivity disorder. Br J Psychiatry 2007;190:402–9.

8. Lee SS, Humphreys KL, Flory K, et al. Prospective association of childhood attention-deficit/hyperactivity disorder (ADHD) and substance use and abuse/dependence: a meta-analytic review. Clin Psychol Rev 2011;31(3):328–41.

9. Charach A, Yeung E, Climans T, et al. Childhood attention-deficit/hyperactivity disorder and future substance use disorders: comparative meta-analyses. J Am Acad Child Adolesc Psychiatry 2011;50(1):9–21.

10. Molina BS, Pelham WE Jr. Attention-deficit/hyperactivity disorder and risk of substance use disorder: developmental considerations, potential pathways, and opportunities for research. Annu Rev Clin Psychol 2014;10:607–39.

11. Elkins IJ, Saunders GRB, Malone SM, et al. Associations between childhood ADHD, gender, and adolescent alcohol and marijuana involvement: A causally informative design. Drug Alcohol Depend 2018;184:33–41.

12. Hechtman L, Swanson JM, Sibley MH, et al. Functional Adult Outcomes 16 Years After Childhood Diagnosis of Attention-Deficit/Hyperactivity Disorder: MTA Results. J Am Acad Child Adolesc Psychiatry 2016;55(11):945–52.e2 [published correction appears in J Am Acad Child Adolesc Psychiatry. 2018 Mar;57(3):225].

13. van Emmerik-van Oortmerssen K, van de Glind G, Koeter MW, et al. Psychiatric comorbidity in treatment-seeking substance use disorder patients with and without attention deficit hyperactivity disorder: results of the IASP study. Addiction 2014;109(2):262–72.

14. Notzon DP, Pavlicova M, Glass A, et al. ADHD Is Highly Prevalent in Patients Seeking Treatment for Cannabis Use Disorders. J Atten Disord 2020;24(11):1487–92.

15. Substance Abuse and Mental Health Services Administration. Key substance use and mental health indicators in the United States: Results from the 2020 National Survey on Drug Use and Health. Rockville, MD: Center for Behavioral Health Statistics and Quality; 2021. Retrieved from. https://www.samhsa.gov/data/. Substance Abuse and Mental Health Services Administration.

16. Soler Artigas M, Sánchez-Mora C, Rovira P, et al. Attention-deficit/hyperactivity disorder and lifetime cannabis use: genetic overlap and causality. Mol Psychiatry 2020;25(10):2493–503, published correction appears in Mol Psychiatry. 2021 Jul;26(7):3663.

17. Zaman T, Malowney M, Knight J, et al. Co-Occurrence of Substance-Related and Other Mental Health Disorders Among Adolescent Cannabis Users. J Addict Med 2015;9(4):317–21.

18. Karlsson Linnér R, Mallard TT, Barr PB, et al. Multivariate analysis of 1.5 million people identifies genetic associations with traits related to self-regulation and addiction. Nat Neurosci 2021;24(10):1367–76.

19. Mitchell JT, Sweitzer MM, Tunno AM, et al. "I Use Weed for My ADHD": A Qualitative Analysis of Online Forum Discussions on Cannabis Use and ADHD. PLoS One 2016;11(5):e0156614.

20. Stueber A, Cuttler C. Self-Reported Effects of Cannabis on ADHD Symptoms, ADHD Medication Side Effects, and ADHD-Related Executive Dysfunction. J Atten Disord 2022;26(6):942–55.

21. Goldstein AL, Shifrin A, Katz JL, et al. Exploring the Relationship Between ADHD Symptoms and Daily Cannabis Consequences in Emerging Adulthood: The Role of Cannabis Motives. J Stud Alcohol Drugs 2021;82(2):228–36.

22. Rooney M, Chronis-Tuscano A, Yoon Y. Substance use in college students with ADHD. J Atten Disord 2012;16(3):221–34.

23. Navarrete F, García-Gutiérrez MS, Gasparyan A, et al. Role of Cannabidiol in the Therapeutic Intervention for Substance Use Disorders. Front Pharmacol 2021;12: 626010.

24. Atakan Z. Cannabis, a complex plant: different compounds and different effects on individuals. Ther Adv Psychopharmacol 2012;2(6):241–54.

25. Lim CCW, Sun T, Leung J, et al. Prevalence of Adolescent Cannabis Vaping: A Systematic Review and Meta- analysis of US and Canadian Studies. JAMA Pediatr 2022;176(1):42–51.

26. Roehler DR, Hoots BE, Holland KM, et al. Trends and characteristics of cannabis-associated emergency department visits in the United States, 2006-2018. Drug Alcohol Depend 2022;232:109288.

27. Adisetiyo V, Gray KM. Neuroimaging the neural correlates of increased risk for substance use disorders in attention-deficit/hyperactivity disorder-A systematic review. Am J Addict 2017;26(2):99–111.

28. Chye Y, Kirkham R, Lorenzetti V, et al. Cannabis, Cannabinoids, and Brain Morphology: A Review of the Evidence. Biol Psychiatry Cogn Neurosci Neuroimaging 2021;6(6):627–35.

29. Lorenzetti V, Chye Y, Silva P, et al. Does regular cannabis use affect neuroanatomy? An updated systematic review and meta-analysis of structural neuroimaging studies. Eur Arch Psychiatry Clin Neurosci 2019;269:59–71.

30. Broyd SJ, van Hell HH, Beale C, et al. Acute and Chronic Effects of Cannabinoids on Human Cognition-A Systematic Review. Biol Psychiatry 2016;79(7):557–67.

31. Burggren AC, Shirazi A, Ginder N, et al. Cannabis effects on brain structure, function, and cognition: considerations for medical uses of cannabis and its derivatives. Am J Drug Alcohol Abuse 2019;45(6):563–79.

32. Paraskevopoulou M, van Rooij D, Batalla A, et al. Effects of substance misuse on reward- processing in patients with attention-deficit/hyperactivity disorder. Neuropsychopharmacology 2021;46(3):622–31.

33. Rasmussen J, Casey BJ, van Erp TGM, et al. ADHD and cannabis use in young adults examined using fMRI of a Go/NoGo task. Brain Imaging Behav 2016;10: 761–71.

34. Solowij N, Broyd S, Greenwood LM, et al. A randomised controlled trial of vaporised Δ9- tetrahydrocannabinol and cannabidiol alone and in combination in frequent and infrequent cannabis users: acute intoxication effects. Eur Arch Psychiatry Clin Neurosci 2019;269(1):17–35.

35. Beale C, Broyd SJ, Chye Y, et al. Prolonged Cannabidiol Treatment Effects on Hippocampal Subfield Volumes in Current Cannabis Users. Cannabis Cannabinoid Res 2018;3(1):94–107.

36. Ashtari M, Avants B, Cyckowski L, et al. Medial temporal structures and memory functions in adolescents with heavy cannabis use. J Psychiatr Res 2011;45: 1055–66.

37. Stevens AK, Gunn RL, Jackson KM, et al. Examining motivational pathways from adult attention-deficit/hyperactivity disorder symptoms to cannabis use: Results from a prospective study of veterans. Psychol Addict Behav 2021;35(1):16–28.

38. gov FDA. FDA Regulation of Cannabis and Cannabis-Derived Products, Including Cannabidiol (CBD). Content current as of January. 2022. Available at:

https://www.fda.gov/news-events/public-health-focus/fda-regulation-cannabis-and-cannabis-derived-products-including-cannabidiol-cbd#approved.   Accessed March 23, 2022.

39. Gruber SA, Smith RT, Dahlgren MK, et al. No pain, all gain? Interim analyses from a longitudinal, observational study examining the impact of medical cannabis treatment on chronic pain and related symptoms. Exp Clin Psychopharmacol 2021;29(2):147–56.

40. Sarris J, Sinclair J, Karamacoska D, et al. Medicinal cannabis for psychiatric disorders: a clinically-focused systematic review. BMC Psychiatry 2020;20(1):24.

41. MacDonald B, Sadek J. Naturalistic exploratory study of the associations of substance use on ADHD outcomes and function. BMC Psychiatry 2021;21(1):251.

42. Brandt A, Rehm J, Lev-Ran S. Clinical correlates of cannabis use among individuals with attention deficit hyperactivity disorder. J Nerv Ment Dis 2018;206(9): 726–32.

43. Wynchank D, Ten Have M, Bijlenga D, et al. The Association Between Insomnia and Sleep Duration in Adults With Attention-Deficit Hyperactivity Disorder: Results From a General Population Study. J Clin Sleep Med 2018;14(3):349–57.

44. Kaul M, Zee PC, Sahni AS. Effects of Cannabinoids on Sleep and their Therapeutic Potential for Sleep Disorders. Neurotherapeutics 2021;18(1):217–27.

45. Wiese B, Wilson-Poe AR. Emerging Evidence for Cannabis' Role in Opioid Use Disorder. Cannabis Cannabinoid Res 2018;3(1):179–89.

46. Stickley A, Koyanagi A, Takahashi H, et al. ADHD symptoms and pain among adults in England. Psychiatry Res 2016;246:326–31.

47. Carrubba AR, Ebbert JO, Spaulding AC, et al. Use of Cannabis for Self-Management of Chronic Pelvic Pain. J Womens Health (Larchmt) 2021;30(9): 1344–51.

48. Dorani F, Bijlenga D, Beekman ATF, et al. Prevalence of hormone- related mood disorder symptoms in women with ADHD. J Psychiatr Res 2021;133:10–5.

49. Williams AR. Cannabis as a Gateway Drug for Opioid Use Disorder. J Law Med Ethics 2020;48(2):268–74.

50. Pallanti S, Porta F, Salerno L. Adult attention deficit hyperactivity disorder in patients with fibromyalgia syndrome: Assessment and disabilities. J Psychiatr Res 2021;136:537–42.

51. Kerekes N, Sanchéz-Pérez AM, Landry M. Neuroinflammation as a possible link between attention-deficit/hyperactivity disorder (ADHD) and pain. Med Hypotheses 2021;157:110717.

52. Cooper RE, Williams E, Seegobin S, et al. Cannabinoids in attention- deficit/hyperactivity disorder: A randomised-controlled trial. Eur Neuropsychopharmacol 2017;27(8):795–808.

53. Hall W, Degenhardt L. Adverse health effects of non-medical cannabis use. Lancet 2009;374(9698):1383–91.

Practical Technology for Expanding and Improving Substance Use Disorder Treatment

Telehealth, Remote Monitoring, and Digital Health Interventions

Mary M. Sweeney, PhD[a], August F. Holtyn, PhD[a],
Maxine L. Stitzer, PhD[a,b], David R. Gastfriend, MD[c,*]

KEYWORDS

- Technology • Telehealth • Digital health • Digital therapeutics • Mobile health
- Substance use disorder • Alcohol use disorder • Smoking

KEY POINTS

- The US opioid and stimulant epidemics create expanding need for substance use disorder (SUD) treatment.
- COVID-19 has imposed new demand for telehealth, remote monitoring, and digital health interventions for SUD to enhance clinical practice.
- Technology offers potential to mitigate health-related disparities in SUD care by addressing the needs of diverse patient groups and increasing access to care.
- A strong evidence base supports the feasibility and potential effectiveness of technology-based interventions.
- Patient satisfaction suggests that technology can be accepted and even preferred to conventional approaches to interventions.

INTRODUCTION

This review describes 3 major uses of technology to support treatment of substance use disorder (SUD): telehealth, remote biometric monitoring, and digital health interventions. *Telehealth* uses telecommunication technology such as 2-way interactive video to provide services to patients with SUD from a distance.[1] The coronavirus

[a] Department of Psychiatry and Behavioral Sciences, Behavioral Pharmacology Research Unit, Johns Hopkins University School of Medicine, 5510 Nathan Shock Drive, Baltimore, MD 21224, USA; [b] Friends Research Institute, 1040 Park Avenue, Suite 103, Baltimore, MD 21201, USA; [c] DynamiCare Health, 6 Liberty Square, Suite 2102, Boston, MA 02109, USA
* Corresponding author.
E-mail address: drgastfriend@dynamicarehealth.com

Psychiatr Clin N Am 45 (2022) 515–528
https://doi.org/10.1016/j.psc.2022.05.006
0193-953X/22/© 2022 Elsevier Inc. All rights reserved.
psych.theclinics.com

disease 2019 (COVID-19) global pandemic necessitated the expansion of SUD tele-health, and although current evidence supports telehealth as an effective method of SUD treatment delivery,[2,3] greater utilization is needed.[4,5] *Remote monitoring* can now be accomplished via state-of-the-art devices for breath alcohol concentration (BrAC) and biological fluid drug testing. This approach allows frequent biometric assessment of patient substance use without need for in-person contact. *Digital health interventions* including smartphone applications (apps) have adapted behavioral interventions with a strong evidence base such as contingency management and cognitive behavioral therapy (CBT) for digitally streamlined implementation.

With the opioid and stimulant epidemics[6] there is an enormous gap between treatment need and treatment reach. Of 40 million Americans with an SUD in the United States in 2020, only 6.5% received any SUD treatment.[7] Technology-based treatments both complement in-person treatments and may access an untapped population of patients who are unreachable or uninterested in traditional treatment. This practical, rather than systematic,[3,8–14] review provides a condensed discussion of technology-based SUD interventions with strong empirical support.

TELEHEALTH
Provider Visits

Patients use telehealth to connect to clinicians, peer recovery coaches, nurses, pharmacists, and prescribers for opioid use disorder (OUD).[1] Strategies for real-time, synchronous communications can include telephone (audio-only) and 2-way video. Telehealth software can be stand-alone or integrated with an electronic health record. Many telehealth-ready software platforms comply with the Health Insurance Portability and Accountability Act (HIPAA), including free and subscription services (eg, Doxy.Me, Mend, AMC Health). Other telehealth products can be used without incurring HIPAA penalties, such as Apple FaceTime, Google Hangouts video, or Zoom. These platforms use end-to-end encryption that allows only the specified parties to communicate and is thus sufficient for a good faith effort to protect a patient's health information during telehealth visits under current regulations. Public-facing applications do not offer the expectation of privacy (eg, Facebook Live, Tik-Tok) and are not appropriate for telehealth. Telehealth reimbursement varies by insurer and state, and current regulations should be consulted but are trending toward flexibility.[4,15]

A systematic review of SUD telehealth effectiveness evaluated 13 studies including 7 randomized controlled trials (RCTs) across a range of substances and settings.[3] Telehealth was used with individual psychotherapy counseling and opioid pharmacotherapy visits. No study observed a significant difference in substance use outcomes between in-person care and SUD telehealth. Two studies found superior treatment retention with telehealth versus in-person treatments, although one study observed substantial dropout before receiving telehealth treatment. When reported, treatment satisfaction and therapeutic alliance were generally comparable between telehealth and in-person treatments.

A review of buprenorphine OUD telehealth pharmacotherapy examined 69 empirical papers and commentaries published both before and during COVID-19.[16] It concluded that telehealth for OUD can increase buprenorphine access and utilization and patient satisfaction, decrease health care costs, and achieve comparable retention relative to in-person treatment. Analysis of a large sample ($n = 28,791$) of veterans with OUD receiving buprenorphine treatment before the pandemic found that telehealth was associated with a reduced risk of treatment attrition relative to in-person services.[17] Despite the unplanned transition to telehealth necessitated by COVID-19, providers have reported improvements in treatment attendance and telehealth patient volumes meeting or exceeding prepandemic (in-person) patient volumes following a brief initial disruption.[18,19]

Group Therapy

Group therapy, the most commonly used therapy format for SUD treatment, has also been implemented virtually.[3,19,20] Several commercially available software options are HIPAA-compliant platforms for delivering group therapy alongside e-prescribing, patient scheduling, online patient portals, and other electronic record-keeping (eg, Mend, Kareo, and inSync Healthcare Solutions).

Across different software and patient populations, current evidence suggests virtual group therapy can be an effective treatment approach for SUD,[3,19,20] although there is a clear need for further randomized trials. A systematic review of telehealth strategies for SUD included 3 studies using group therapy among patients with tobacco, alcohol, and opioid use.[3] One of the included studies was a small (n = 37) randomized trial using virtual group therapy delivered as part of methadone treatment. There was no difference in substance use, treatment adherence, or satisfaction among patients randomized to receive group therapy via videoconferencing versus participants receiving in-person therapy. During COVID-19, a retrospective analysis from an emergency response treatment program for SUD including peer-led group recovery meetings observed an initial disruption with subsequent increased group meeting attendance when transitioning to virtual group meetings.[19] Taken together, existing evidence supports the acceptability and efficacy of virtual group therapy for SUD.

Best Practices for Substance Use Disorder Telehealth

SUD telehealth visits should include (1) sufficient technology/bandwidth speed to support video conferencing, (2) sufficient privacy for the patient at both sides of the patient-provider contact, (3) appropriate visual environment including eye-level contact and an uncluttered workspace, and (4) careful attention to a supportive interaction including a positive attitude and gesticulation that suggests engagement.[12] Standards of in-person treatments should be applied to telehealth visits wherever possible, including detailed assessments, patient histories, and use of standardized measures. Strategies have been developed to determine patient level of risk using traditional and computerized assessments, as well as for safe at-home initiation of OUD buprenorphine treatment.[12] With appropriate structure and safeguards in place, telehealth holds tremendous promise for improving convenience and expanding treatment access.

REMOTE MONITORING

On-site testing is an obstacle in telehealth and for patients with mobility, transportation, work, or childcare challenges—disproportionately affecting underserved populations and further exacerbating health disparities. Testing is critical in one of the most effective SUD interventions, contingency management, which provides monetary incentives contingent on verified substance abstinence.[21] Frequent random substance tests are generally recognized as more effective than predictable testing,[22] but feasibility can be a challenge. Wearable devices or patient-provided self-videos (selfies) may overcome barriers to frequent testing.

Alcohol

Wearable alcohol biosensors

Alcohol biosensor devices can be passively worn by individuals in their daily lives while providing a continuous measure of alcohol use. The Secure Continuous Remote Alcohol Monitor (SCRAM) ankle bracelet is the only commercially available wearable alcohol biosensor. The bracelet is tamper-evident, that is, it cannot be removed by the wearer without cutting the strap or breaking the closure clip, and it detects device removal and tampering through skin temperature and reflectivity changes. It provides a continuous estimate of blood alcohol concentration by sampling alcohol vapor just above the skin. Results are provided on a secure Web site provided by Alcohol Monitoring Systems, Inc. SCRAM has demonstrated feasibility, reliably detecting consumption at a level of 2 or more standard drinks and treatment-related changes in drinking.[23–25]

Broad use of SCRAM in clinical settings has been limited due to its large size and weight (about 6 oz and about the size of a deck of cards), high cost ($1500 per device plus a daily service fee of approximately $5), and social stigma due to its use with criminal justice–involved populations.

Remote breathalyzers

Alcohol use can also be objectively measured using remote breathalyzers.[26] Soberlink uses a wireless handheld breathalyzer and facial recognition to verify the patient's identity. When patients perform a BrAC test, a photo is automatically taken and facial recognition software verifies that the uploaded picture matches their reference picture. BrAC results can be sent in real time to treatment providers and an approved list of patient support contacts. Two controlled trials demonstrated acceptability, feasibility, and efficacy when combined with contingency management.[26,27]

Another remote breathalyzer is the BACtrack Mobile Pro. This police-grade device has good sensitivity at low BrAC levels (ie, 95% of measurements underestimate venous blood alcohol concentrations by no more than 0.02%).[28] Results are transmitted via Bluetooth to a smartphone. Unlike the larger and heavier (5.3–8.4 ounces) Soberlink, the BACtrack is palm- or purse-sized (1.7 ounces). For a witnessed remote test, the user performs a video selfie, which is reviewed for validation.[29]

Tobacco

Smokerlyzer

Smoking status can be objectively measured via breath carbon monoxide (CO).[30,31] Because breath CO is cleared rapidly from the body, handheld, smartphone-compatible monitors offer frequent testing to detect smoking lapses. The iCO Smokerlyzer is small and portable, plugging directly into a smartphone and providing reliable and valid CO measurement comparable to professional-grade CO monitors.[31] The Smokerlyzer has a range of 0 to 100 parts per million (ppm) and a suggested smoking abstinence cutoff of 6 ppm. The software facilitates self-monitoring and sharing of results with designated contacts.[31] Studies have shown its effectiveness for detecting smoking reductions and abstinence.[30–32]

Other Drugs

Oral fluid panels

Oral fluid drug testing can verify patients' substance use with video-selfie testing administered on a random schedule.[30] Premier Biotech, Inc.'s OralTox rapid saliva test kits have a 510(k) clearance from the Food and Drug Administration (FDA) for in vitro diagnostic use for amphetamine, cocaine, methamphetamine, cannabis, methadone, opiates, oxycodone, and phencyclidine. Oral fluid testing offers a shorter window of detection (12–48 hours for most substances) relative to urine; however, it is unobtrusive, requires no toilet facilities, and thus far seems less susceptible to sample tampering.[33]

Oral fluid testing is necessary with electronic cigarette use (vaping), because breath CO will not detect noncombustible tobacco use.[34] For example, the Alere iScreen OFD Oral Fluid Cotinine Test, measuring the primary metabolite of nicotine in saliva, can be performed at the office or remotely via selfie video and will yield a positive result for 1 to 2 days after nicotine use (whether via e-cigarettes, ie, vaping, or nicotine replacement therapy medication).

Medication Adherence

Remote monitoring of methadone and buprenorphine adherence has used electronic pill dispensers. Electronic pill dispensers contain individual dosing compartments that open only during preprogrammed times. The dispensers can provide notices when medication is available and alerts for missed doses. Effective remote monitoring has been achieved with methadone take-home doses using the MedMinder ("Jon")[35] and with buprenorphine, using the Med-O-Wheel.[36]

Video directly observed therapy (Video DOT) has been used as an alternative to electronic pill dispensers.[37–39] For example, a commercially available Video DOT platform offered by emocha Mobile Health allows patients to use a smartphone app to securely submit videos of themselves taking medication, which providers then review to confirm adherence. Pilot studies have shown that Video DOT for buprenorphine is feasible and acceptable and results in similar rates of illicit opioid use and treatment engagement compared with treatment-as-usual.[37–39]

DIGITAL HEALTH INTERVENTIONS

Many health and wellness Web sites and smartphone apps are marketed to treat SUD.[8] Unfortunately, most are of poor quality and lack research validation,[13] whereas researchers have developed many digital tools with outcome data but not availability or support.[14] There are, however, several technology-based SUD interventions that are evidence based and freely or commercially available.[21]

Computer- and Web-Based Interventions

Programs that aim to develop cognitive and behavioral skills to reduce substance use or promote abstinence can be accessed via web-browser from laptop or desktop computers through a health care provider or direct patient access.[8] Computer-based training for CBT (CBT4CBT; https://cbt4cbt.com/) is a self-guided, web-based training that uses games, cartoons, interactive video exercises, and quizzes to promote understanding of substance use patterns, skills for coping with craving, and improvements in decision-making about substance use.[40] RCTs favor CBT4CBT as an improvement over treatment-as-usual for persons who use alcohol, cannabis, cocaine, and opioids.[40] CBT4CBT is currently available in conjunction with office-based treatments for SUD at a low cost (approximately $100) and has also demonstrated potential efficacy as a standalone treatment.[41]

Other computer- and web-based trainings include CheckUp & Choices (https://checkupandchoices.com/) and Vorvida (https://us.vorvida.com/) for alcohol use disorder and Breaking Free Online (https://www.breakingfreeonline.com/) for opioid, cannabis, alcohol and other SUDs.[42] The DEAL project (https://dealproject.org.au/) and the SHADE program (https://shadetreatment.com/) address co-occurring depressive symptoms and alcohol use.[43]

Several effective computerized/web-based trainings serve as the backbone of smartphone app interventions for SUDs. Therapeutic Education System (TES) is a web-based computerized intervention that can use incentives to support drug abstinence and the community reinforcement approach to enhance nondrug sources of reinforcement for long-term recovery.[44] TES is supported by several RCTs and served as the basis for the reSET and reSET-O apps. For tobacco use, the web-based contingency management program Motiv8, which incentivizes smoking abstinence, was supported by several randomized trials and served as the basis for the novel mMotiv8 mobile app.[32]

Smartphone Applications for Tobacco Cessation

Several research-supported smoking cessation apps are available for consumers at the Apple App Store and Google Play. The most robust treatment effect sizes for smoking cessation smartphone apps incorporate abstinence incentives contingent on providing negative breath CO.[21]

QuitGuide and quitSTART

The QuitGuide (for adults) and quitSTART (for adolescents and young adults) apps are free digital smoking cessation tools through the US Centers for Disease Control (CDC) created by the National Cancer Institute (NCI). Both applications provide tools for addressing craving, tracking progress and milestones, providing helpful notifications and location alert triggers when a person is at a prespecified high-risk location, as well as tools to incorporate sharing goals with a support network (eg, text messaging your quit date to friends, sharing progress on social media). In addition, quitSTART has brief games to "distract" from cravings.

iCanQuit

iCanQuit is a mobile app for smoking cessation that incorporates strategies from Acceptance and Commitment Therapy[45] that includes (1) allowing urges to smoke pass rather than actively avoiding smoking urges and (2) motivating smokers to quit based on alignment with personal values. Efficacy of iCanQuit for long-term smoking cessation was supported in a randomized trial such that past-30-days abstinence at the 12-month follow-up was greater with iCanQuit (28%) relative to the CDC/NCI Quit-Guide app (21%).[45]

Pivot

Pivot is a smoking cessation tool using CO monitoring and smoking cessation coaches that tailors its strategy according to each person's readiness to quit.[46] The intervention guides users to use pharmacotherapies, log cigarettes, and monitor CO values using the app in collaboration with their coach. Cohort studies have provided encouraging data for Pivot with respect to increasing likelihood of making a quit attempt, increasing confidence to quit, and reducing cigarettes per day.[46]

Quit Genius

Quit Genius was developed in the United Kingdom based on CBT for smoking cessation. It includes self-monitoring (with or without breath CO), goal-setting, feedback on progress, pharmacotherapy encouragement, video/audio lessons and quizzes, and access to a smoking cessation coach via phone contact and in-app chat. A randomized trial found that participants assigned to Quit Genius reported a significantly higher rate of smoking abstinence (past-14-days) at 4 weeks after quit day (34%) relative to those who received only brief advice (23%).[47]

DynamiCare Health

The DynamiCare Health app incentivizes treatment attendance, completion of in-app CBT, and nicotine cessation. The app monitors remote videos of breath CO for smoking[30] and salivary cotinine for e-cigarettes.[34] The company's staff provide feedback and reinforcement for abstinence. In a cohort study, pregnant smokers who were assigned to DynamiCare plus a best-practice quit line referral (vs quit line alone) had quit rates of 37% versus 13% during late pregnancy with 40% versus 10% abstinence at 4 weeks postdelivery.[30] The app has received FDA Breakthrough Device designation for pregnant smokers.

Smartphone Applications for Alcohol and Substance Use Disorder

Smartphone apps have been developed for alcohol and other SUDs by standardizing and automating effective aspects of in-person substance use treatment, including CBT, substance testing, pharmacotherapy, and abstinence incentives. Some interventions are specifically targeted for alcohol, but others such as reSET and DynamiCare Health can target multiple substances simultaneously. Many apps are designed to be combined with in-person SUD treatment, but some may have independent treatment utility. Apps that are currently available and with some level of research support are reviewed in the following section.

VetChange

VetChange is a free mobile app created by the VA's National Center for Posttraumatic Stress Disorder (PTSD) for veterans and other service members to address problem drinking, smoking, and PTSD symptoms. VetChange is a fully automated self-guided program incorporating CBT including personalized feedback on alcohol use and PTSD symptoms, alcohol tracking, goal-setting, coping tips, and building a support system.[48] VetChange is supported by research evidence from an RCT and convenience samples from nationwide implementation of the web-based version of the VetChange intervention.[48,49] VetChange resulted in significantly greater reductions in drinking and PTSD symptoms over an 8-week intervention period relative to a wait-list control.[49] VetChange has demonstrated larger treatment effect size relative to other brief interventions to address alcohol use among veterans, including telephone-, web-, and in-person treatments.[50]

Connections: from Comprehensive Health Enhancement Support System Health

Connections is a recovery support and relapse prevention tool that has been developed from Addiction-Comprehensive Health Enhancement Support System (A-CHESS).[51] Designed for persons leaving residential treatment, it offers educational information about recovery, communications with designated providers and support groups/discussions, breathing and refusal exercises, and alert messages triggered by prespecified high-risk locations. In an RCT, patients who were assigned to use the A-CHESS app during treatment-as-usual had significantly fewer risky drinking days and greater odds of reporting abstinence at 8- and 12-month follow-up relative to patients assigned to treatment-as-usual only.[51] A-CHESS has also been adapted for OUD treatment[52] and patients who speak Spanish.[53]

reSET and reSET-O

reSET and reSET-O deliver 2 evidence-based interventions: CBT lessons based on TES (see earlier discussion on Computer and Web-Based Interventions) and contingency management.[54] CBT topics relevant to abstinence and recovery incorporate fluency training, with comprehension tests. Patients earn small amounts of money on a probability schedule (eg, 50% of rewards result in money; the remainder acknowledge "good job") for completing lessons and providing evidence of recent abstinence via drug-negative urinalysis (when results are entered by the clinician). reSET is designed for treatment of alcohol, stimulants, or cannabis use disorder, whereas reSET-O is designed for patients receiving buprenorphine for OUD. Both apps allow patients to track recent drug use, cravings, and triggers. reSET-O also includes self-reports of medication adherence and can provide medication dosing notifications. reSET products are designated Breakthrough Devices and are FDA authorized for prescription by a licensed clinician. The clinician submits an enrollment form to the manufacturer, whose staff then guides patients in using the app. A 12-week course may be reimbursable by insurance.

DynamiCare Health

The DynamiCare Health app delivers remote contingency management incentives to treat alcohol,[29] opioid,[55] and stimulant use.[56] Abstinence is monitored remotely via selfie video of randomly scheduled breathalyzer and/or saliva tests. It incentivizes attendance (validated via GPS), medication adherence, self-assessment, and self-directed CBT lessons. Recovery coaches transition participants from monetary incentives to community reinforcers (eg, employment, savings, independent housing, and healthy relationships) over 4 to 8 months.[57] Monetary rewards of $100 to $200 per month are delivered via a smart debit card that blocks use at bars, liquor stores, casinos, and other high-risk situations. The app has been determined not to violate Federal anti-kickback and inducement regulations.[58] Costs may be covered by insurance, Medicaid, employers, or the patient or family. Prospective cohort studies and RCTs demonstrate significant findings for alcohol, opioid, stimulant, tobacco, and nicotine cessation.[29,30,34,55,56]

DISCUSSION
Strengths of Technology-Based Approaches

Technology offers many advantages for providers and patients. Patients have greater access to tools and services, avoiding objective obstacles, including transportation limitations, work schedule conflicts, and childcare disruptions. Technology-based treatments can be delivered even to patients who lack smartphones, because Medicaid covers phones and data plans under the Affordable Care Act.[59] Convenience for providers is enhanced as well, with work-from-home and flex-time scheduling. Telehealth may also yield useful insights into patients' home life.[60,61] Technology-based treatments can be preprogrammed, which means increased fidelity and improved scalability. Automation reduces the burdens of specialized SUD training and complex infrastructure. More frequent patient contact becomes feasible, with opportunities for real-time alerts and interventions. Technology supports personalization based on use status and readiness to change. Finally, as most of the individuals with SUD do not seek treatment in brick-and-mortar programs, digital interventions may prove to be a more feasible and attractive option.

Limitations of Technology-Based Approaches

Few randomized trials have compared in-person versus technology-based treatments for SUD. Prospectively designed noninferiority trials are needed.[3,14] Practically, establishing new patients via telehealth may be challenging for patients with housing instability or limited access to technology. Treatment hotlines where mobile or landline phones can be used to initiate longer-term telehealth treatments may help with onboarding new patients.[62] Clinicians speculate that in-person visits provide structure, accountability, rapport, and evidence of substance use or withdrawal that is not achieved with telehealth.[61] However, technology-based treatments do not preclude some in-person interaction (eg, a hybrid model of care),[5] supplementation of telehealth with additional remote monitoring,[4] or providing access to structured digital health interventions.[4] Care must be taken that technology-based treatments do not exacerbate treatment access gaps among persons with limited technology access or literacy. Even so, data collected among low-income populations or those without smartphones suggest that technology-based SUD treatments are feasible, acceptable, and effective among these patients.[51,56,63] Although privacy and software security must be continually monitored and strengthened,[64] many digital interventions have extensive privacy-protection features including end-to-end encryption, host and cloud firewalls, virtual private networks, physically hardened servers, and antivirus and anti-malware software.

Evolving Policies

During the pandemic, Federal regulations were loosened to permit remote initiation of buprenorphine and methadone OUD treatment.[65] The Centers for Medicare & Medicaid Services intends to extend expanded regulations for SUD treatment via telehealth (eg, audio-only reimbursement, removal of geographic licensure restrictions) through 2023, and appeals are being made to permanently increase telehealth reimbursement for SUDs.[4,15,65] The Biden administration has noted barriers to use of certain evidence-based treatments and has formally called on the Office of National Drug Control Policy to "identify and address policy barriers related to contingency management interventions," and to "explore reimbursement for motivational incentives and digital treatment for addiction."[66] These initiatives will help to rectify the underutilization of effective evidence-based treatments and are well aligned with the emergence of digital health interventions.

SUMMARY

Most people with SUDs do not seek treatment. The pandemic has created other obstacles due to social distancing and other stressors that amplify the incidence of SUD. Patients with SUDs need improved access and acceptability of effective SUD treatment. Telehealth, remote biometric monitoring, and digital health interventions are transforming the delivery of SUD treatment. Technology has the potential to greatly expand access to both usual care and complementary evidence-based interventions. Future research will evaluate generalizability and the implementation models needed to realize the potential of these new treatment delivery tools.

CLINICS CARE POINTS

- Technology-assisted SUD care is available, feasible, and effective in the era of the opioid and stimulant epidemics, COVID-19, and beyond.
- Providers have multiple technology options to support telehealth and adjunctive digital health interventions for SUD including evidence-based smartphone apps.
- Patients may accept, like, and even prefer services and tools that are technology based.
- The effectiveness, quality, and security of technology-based services and tools should continue to accumulate supporting evidence via valid scientific research.

DISCLOSURE

This work was funded by the NIH/NIAAA Small Business Innovative Research and Small Business Technology Transfer Grants R43AA026234, R44AA026234, and R44DA055396. The funding source was not involved in the study design, research, or the preparation of the article. Dr M.M. Sweeney is now employed by the National Institutes of Health, National Institute of Mental Health. This article was prepared while Dr M.M. Sweeney was employed at Johns Hopkins University. The opinions expressed in this article are the authors' own and do not reflect the view of the National Institutes of Health, the Department of Health and Human Services, or the United States government. Dr M.M. Sweeney has received support from DynamiCare Health through her faculty position at Johns Hopkins University School of Medicine. Dr A.F. Holtyn has received support from DynamiCare Health and Pear Therapeutics through her faculty position at Johns Hopkins University School of Medicine. Dr M.L. Stitzer has served as consultant to DynamiCare Health. Dr D.R. Gastfriend is co-founder and Chief Medical Officer of DynamiCare Health.

REFERENCES

1. Substance Abuse and Mental Health Services Administration (SAMHSA). Telehealth for the treatment of serious mental illness and substance use disorders. Rockville, MD: National Mental Health and Substance use Policy Laboratory, SAMHSA; 2021.
2. Chan B, Bougatsos C, Priest KC, et al. Opioid treatment programs, telemedicine and COVID-19: A scoping review. Subst Abuse 2021;1–8. https://doi.org/10.1080/08897077.2021.1967836.
3. Lin L, Casteel D, Shigekawa E, et al. Telemedicine-delivered treatment interventions for substance use disorders: A systematic review. J Subst Abuse Treat 2019;101:38–49.
4. McDonnell A, MacNeill C, Chapman B, et al. Leveraging digital tools to support recovery from substance use disorder during the COVID-19 pandemic response. J Subst Abuse Treat 2021;124:108226.
5. Melamed OC, deRuiter WK, Buckley L, et al. COVID-19 and the impact on substance use disorder treatments. Psychiatr Clin North Am 2021. https://doi.org/10.1016/j.psc.2021.11.006. S0193953X21000848.
6. Strickland JC, Havens JR, Stoops WW. A nationally representative analysis of "twin epidemics": Rising rates of methamphetamine use among persons who use opioids. Drug Alcohol Depend 2019;204:107592.
7. Substance Abuse and Mental Health Services Administration (SAMHSA). Key substance use and mental health indicators in the United States: results from the 2020 national survey on drug use and health. Rockville, MD: Center for Behavioral Health Statistics and Quality, SAMHSA; 2021. Available at: https://samhsa.gov/data.
8. Lemley SM, Marsch LA. Towards addiction treatment: technological advances & applying technology. In: el-Guebaly N, Carrà G, Galanter M, et al, editors. Textbook of addiction treatment. Cham, Switzerland: Springer International Publishing; 2021. p. 505–18.
9. Chu KH, Matheny SJ, Escobar-Viera CG, et al. Smartphone health apps for tobacco Cessation: A systematic review. Addict Behav 2021;112:106616.
10. Staiger PK, O'Donnell R, Liknaitzky P, et al. Mobile Apps to Reduce Tobacco, Alcohol, and Illicit Drug Use: Systematic Review of the First Decade. J Med Internet Res 2020;22(11):e17156.

11. Steinkamp JM, Goldblatt N, Borodovsky JT, et al. Technological Interventions for Medication Adherence in Adult Mental Health and Substance Use Disorders: A Systematic Review. JMIR Ment Health 2019;6(3):e12493.
12. Oesterle TS, Kolla B, Risma CJ, et al. Substance Use Disorders and Telehealth in the COVID-19 Pandemic Era. Mayo Clin Proc 2020;95(12):2709–18.
13. Tofighi B, Chemi C, Ruiz-Valcarcel J, et al. Smartphone Apps Targeting Alcohol and Illicit Substance Use: Systematic Search in in Commercial App Stores and Critical Content Analysis. JMIR MHealth UHealth 2019;7(4):e11831.
14. Carreiro S, Newcomb M, Leach R, et al. Current reporting of usability and impact of mhealth interventions for substance use disorder: A systematic review. Drug Alcohol Depend 2020;215:108201.
15. Stringer KL, Langdon KJ, McKenzie M, et al. Leveraging COVID-19 to sustain regulatory flexibility in the treatment of opioid use disorder. J Subst Abuse Treat 2021;123:108263.
16. Guillen AG, Reddy M, Saadat S, et al. Utilization of Telehealth Solutions for Patients with Opioid Use Disorder Using Buprenorphine: A Scoping Review. Telemed E-health 2021. https://doi.org/10.1089/tmj.2021.0308. tmj.2021.0308.
17. Vakkalanka JP, Lund BC, Ward MM, et al. Telehealth Utilization Is Associated with Lower Risk of Discontinuation of Buprenorphine: a Retrospective Cohort Study of US Veterans. J Gen Intern Med 2021. https://doi.org/10.1007/s11606-021-06969-1.
18. Fiacco L, Pearson BL, Jordan R. Telemedicine works for treating substance use disorder: The STAR clinic experience during COVID-19. J Subst Abuse Treat 2021;125:108312.
19. Langabeer JR, Yatsco A, Champagne-Langabeer T. Telehealth sustains patient engagement in OUD treatment during COVID-19. J Subst Abuse Treat 2021; 122:108215.
20. Gentry MT, Lapid MI, Clark MM, et al. Evidence for telehealth group-based treatment: A systematic review. J Telemed Telecare 2019;25(6):327–42.
21. Getty CA, Morande A, Lynskey M, et al. Mobile telephone-delivered contingency management interventions promoting behaviour change in individuals with substance use disorders: a meta-analysis. Addict Abingdon Engl 2019;114(11): 1915–25.
22. Jarvis M, Williams J, Hurford M, et al. Appropriate Use of Drug Testing in Clinical Addiction Medicine. J Addict Med 2017;11(3):163–73.
23. Dougherty DM, Lake SL, Hill-Kapturczak N, et al. Using contingency management procedures to reduce at-risk drinking in heavy drinkers. Alcohol Clin Exp Res 2015;39(4):743–51.
24. Alessi SM, Barnett NP, Petry NM. Objective continuous monitoring of alcohol consumption for three months among alcohol use disorder treatment outpatients. Alcohol Fayettev N 2019;81:131–8.
25. Barnett NP, Celio MA, Tidey JW, et al. A preliminary randomized controlled trial of contingency management for alcohol use reduction using a transdermal alcohol sensor. Addict Abingdon Engl 2017;112(6):1025–35.
26. Koffarnus MN, Bickel WK, Kablinger AS. Remote Alcohol Monitoring to Facilitate Incentive-Based Treatment for Alcohol Use Disorder: A Randomized Trial. Alcohol Clin Exp Res 2018;42(12):2423–31.
27. Koffarnus MN, Kablinger AS, Kaplan BA, et al. Remotely administered incentive-based treatment for alcohol use disorder with participant-funded incentives is effective but less accessible to low-income participants. Exp Clin Psychopharmacol 2021;29(5):555–65.

28. Delgado MK, Shofer F, Wetherill R, et al. Accuracy of Consumer-marketed smartphone-paired alcohol breath testing devices: A laboratory validation study. Alcohol Clin Exp Res 2021;45(5):1091–9.

29. Hammond AS, Sweeney MM, Chikosi TU, et al. Digital delivery of a contingency management intervention for substance use disorder: A feasibility study with DynamiCare Health. J Subst Abuse Treat 2021;126:108425.

30. Kurti AN, Tang K, Bolivar HA, et al. Smartphone-based financial incentives to promote smoking cessation during pregnancy: A pilot study. Prev Med 2020;140: 106201.

31. Wong HY, Subramaniyan M, Bullen C, et al. The mobile-phone-based iCOTM Smokerlyzer®: Comparison with the piCO+ Smokerlyzer® among smokers undergoing methadone-maintained therapy. Tob Induc Dis 2019;17:65.

32. Dallery J, Stinson L, Bolívar H, et al. mMotiv8: A smartphone-based contingency management intervention to promote smoking cessation. J Appl Behav Anal 2021;54(1):38–53.

33. Bosker WM, Huestis MA. Oral Fluid Testing for Drugs of Abuse. Clin Chem 2009; 55(11):1910–31.

34. Palmer AM, Tomko RL, Squeglia LM, et al. A pilot feasibility study of a behavioral intervention for nicotine vaping cessation among young adults delivered via telehealth. Drug Alcohol Depend 2022;109311. https://doi.org/10.1016/j.drugalcdep. 2022.109311.

35. Dunn KE, Brooner RK, Stoller KB. Technology-assisted methadone take-home dosing for dispensing methadone to persons with opioid use disorder during the Covid-19 pandemic. J Subst Abuse Treat 2021;121:108197.

36. Sigmon SC, Ochalek TA, Meyer AC, et al. Interim Buprenorphine vs. Waiting List for Opioid Dependence. N Engl J Med 2016;375(25):2504–5.

37. Godersky ME, Klein JW, Merrill JO, et al. Acceptability and Feasibility of a Mobile Health Application for Video Directly Observed Therapy of Buprenorphine for Opioid Use Disorders in an Office-based Setting. J Addict Med 2020;14(4): 319–25.

38. Tsui JI, Leroux BG, Radick AC, et al. Video directly observed therapy for patients receiving office-based buprenorphine – A pilot randomized controlled trial. Drug Alcohol Depend 2021;227:108917.

39. Holtyn AF, Toegel F, Novak MD, et al. Remotely delivered incentives to promote buprenorphine treatment engagement in out-of-treatment adults with opioid use disorder. Drug Alcohol Depend 2021;225:108786.

40. Carroll KM, Kiluk BD, Nich C, et al. Computer-Assisted Delivery of Cognitive-Behavioral Therapy: Efficacy and Durability of CBT4CBT Among Cocaine-Dependent Individuals Maintained on Methadone. Am J Psychiatry 2014; 171(4):436–44.

41. Kiluk BD, Devore KA, Buck MB, et al. Randomized Trial of Computerized Cognitive Behavioral Therapy for Alcohol Use Disorders: Efficacy as a Virtual Stand-Alone and Treatment Add-On Compared with Standard Outpatient Treatment. Alcohol Clin Exp Res 2016;40(9):1991–2000.

42. Elison S, Davies G, Ward J. An Outcomes Evaluation of Computerized Treatment for Problem Drinking using Breaking Free Online. Alcohol Treat Q 2015;33(2): 185–96.

43. Deady M, Mills KL, Teesson M, et al. An Online Intervention for Co-Occurring Depression and Problematic Alcohol Use in Young People: Primary Outcomes From a Randomized Controlled Trial. J Med Internet Res 2016;18(3):e71.

44. Campbell ANC, Nunes EV, Matthews AG, et al. Internet-Delivered Treatment for Substance Abuse: A Multisite Randomized Controlled Trial. Am J Psychiatry 2014;171(6):683–90.

45. Bricker JB, Watson NL, Mull KE, et al. Efficacy of Smartphone Applications for Smoking Cessation: A Randomized Clinical Trial. JAMA Intern Med 2020; 180(11):1472.

46. Marler JD, Fujii CA, Galanko JA, et al. Durability of Abstinence After Completing a Comprehensive Digital Smoking Cessation Program Incorporating a Mobile App, Breath Sensor, and Coaching: Cohort Study. J Med Internet Res 2021;23(2): e25578.

47. Webb J, Peerbux S, Smittenaar P, et al. Preliminary Outcomes of a Digital Therapeutic Intervention for Smoking Cessation in Adult Smokers: Randomized Controlled Trial. JMIR Ment Health 2020;7(10):e22833.

48. Enggasser JL, Livingston NA, Ameral V, et al. Public implementation of a web-based program for veterans with risky alcohol use and PTSD: A RE-AIM evaluation of VetChange. J Subst Abuse Treat 2021;122:108242.

49. Brief DJ, Rubin A, Keane TM, et al. Web intervention for OEF/OIF veterans with problem drinking and PTSD symptoms: a randomized clinical trial. J Consult Clin Psychol 2013;81(5):890–900.

50. Doherty AM, Mason C, Fear NT, et al. Are brief alcohol interventions targeting alcohol use efficacious in military and veteran populations? A meta-analysis. Drug Alcohol Depend 2017;178:571–8.

51. Gustafson DH, McTavish FM, Chih MY, et al. A smartphone application to support recovery from alcoholism: a randomized clinical trial. JAMA Psychiatry 2014; 71(5):566–72.

52. Hochstatter KR, Gustafson DH, Landucci G, et al. Effect of an mHealth Intervention on Hepatitis C Testing Uptake Among People With Opioid Use Disorder: Randomized Controlled Trial. JMIR MHealth UHealth 2021;9(2):e23080.

53. Muroff J, Robinson W, Chassler D, et al. An Outcome Study of the CASA-CHESS Smartphone Relapse Prevention Tool for Latinx Spanish-Speakers with Substance Use Disorders. Subst Use Misuse 2019;54(9):1438–49.

54. Maricich YA, Gerwien R, Kuo A, et al. Real-world use and clinical outcomes after 24 weeks of treatment with a prescription digital therapeutic for opioid use disorder. Hosp Pract 2021;49(5):348–55.

55. DeFulio A, Rzeszutek MJ, Furgeson J, et al. A smartphone-smartcard platform for contingency management in an inner-city substance use disorder outpatient program. J Subst Abuse Treat 2021;120:108188.

56. DeFulio A, Furgeson J, Brown HD, et al. A Smartphone-Smartcard Platform for Implementing Contingency Management in Buprenorphine Maintenance Patients With Concurrent Stimulant Use Disorder. Front Psychiatry 2021;12:778992.

57. Meyers RJ, Miller WR, Hill DE, et al. Community reinforcement and family training (CRAFT): engaging unmotivated drug users in treatment. J Subst Abuse 1998; 10(3):291–308.

58. U.S. Department of Health and Human Services, Office of the Inspector General. Advisory Opinion 22-04. Issued March 2, 2022. Available at: https://oig.hhs.gov/compliance/advisory-opinions/22-04/. Accessed March 3, 2022.

59. Federal Communications Commission. Lifeline Support for Affordable Communications. Last updated October, 2021. Available at: https://www.fcc.gov/lifeline-consumers. Accessed March 3, 2022.

60. Hunter SB, Dopp AR, Ober AJ, et al. Clinician perspectives on methadone service delivery and the use of telemedicine during the COVID-19 pandemic: A qualitative study. J Subst Abuse Treat 2021;124:108288.

61. Uscher-Pines L, Sousa J, Raja P, et al. Treatment of opioid use disorder during COVID-19: Experiences of clinicians transitioning to telemedicine. J Subst Abuse Treat 2020;118:108124.

62. Clark SA, Davis C, Wightman RS, et al. Using telehealth to improve buprenorphine access during and after COVID-19: A rapid response initiative in Rhode Island. J Subst Abuse Treat 2021;124:108283.

63. Johnston DC, Mathews WD, Maus A, et al. Using Smartphones to Improve Treatment Retention Among Impoverished Substance-Using Appalachian Women: A Naturalistic Study. Subst Abuse Res Treat 2019;13. 117822181986137.

64. Shachar C, Engel J, Elwyn G. Implications for Telehealth in a Postpandemic Future: Regulatory and Privacy Issues. JAMA 2020;323(23):2375.

65. Wang L, Weiss J, Ryan EB, et al. Telemedicine increases access to buprenorphine initiation during the COVID-19 pandemic. J Subst Abuse Treat 2021;124: 108272.

66. Executive Office of the President, Office of National Drug Control Policy. The Biden-Harris Administration's Statement of Drug Policy Priorities for Year One. Published April 2021. Available at: https://www.whitehouse.gov/wp-content/uploads/2021/03/BidenHarris-Statement-of-Drug-Policy-Priorities-April-1.pdf. Accessed March 3, 2022.

Harm Reduction
Not Dirty Words Any More

Avinash Ramprashad, MD[a],
Gregory Malik Burnett, MD, MBA, MPH[b,c,]*, Christopher Welsh, MD[c]

KEYWORDS

• Harm reduction • Harm minimization • Risk reduction

KEY POINTS

• Harm reduction refers to a collection of principles, practices, and policies that aim to minimize the negative health, social, and legal impacts associated with drug use.
• Harm reduction practices have been shown to significantly reduce negative consequences of substance use such as infectious diseases and overdoses.
• Harm reduction principles and practices should be integrated with all traditional medical, psychiatric, and addiction treatment programs.

DEFINITIONS/PRINCIPLES

Harm reduction is a conceptual framework that has increased reach and application at the individual, public health, and public policy settings in the twenty-first century. With a history rooted in reducing harms associated with substance use and contemporary applications around reducing pandemic contagion,[1] the framework is principally centered around reducing risk to the health of individuals without eliminating the risk entirely. The globally recognized leading civil society organization in the field, Harm Reduction International, defines harm reduction as "policies, programs, and practices that aim to minimize the negative health, social, and legal impacts associated with drug use, drug policies, and drug laws."[2] In North America, harm reduction has historically been viewed with significant controversy, with opponents stating that these strategies enable drug use despite overwhelming evidence to the contrary. The US-based Harm Reduction Coalition similarly defines harm reduction as a set of principles that reduce the negative consequences associated with drug use but broaden

a Division of Addiction Research and Treatment, Department of Psychiatry, University of Maryland School of Medicine, 701 W Pratt St, 2nd Floor Suite 289, Baltimore, MD 21201, USA; b Center for Addiction Medicine, University of Maryland Midtown Campus, 827 Linden Avenue 4th Floor, Suite 405, Baltimore MD 21201 USA; c Division of Addiction Research and Treatment, Department of Psychiatry, University of Maryland School of Medicine, 22 S. Greene Street S-1-D-04, Baltimore, MD 21201, USA
* Corresponding author.
E-mail address: gregory.burnett@umm.edu

Psychiatr Clin N Am 45 (2022) 529–546
https://doi.org/10.1016/j.psc.2022.04.005
0193-953X/22/© 2022 Elsevier Inc. All rights reserved.
psych.theclinics.com

the concept to include the movement for social justice and respect for the rights of individuals who use drugs.[3] Despite the lack of a universal definition, there is agreement around a universal set of principles which support the conceptual framework and allow for its broad application across settings. Scholars have attempted to contextualize these principles for general application across health care settings to include humanism, pragmatism, autonomy, incrementalism, individualism, and accountability without termination[4] (**Box 1**).

Overall, the conceptual framework of harm reduction allows individuals, providers, and policy makers to develop strategies to objectively address issues in the real world as they exist today. The framework removes the dichotomy of good and bad as it pertains to people and their decisions, allowing a more nuanced approach to the behaviors that accompany substance use disorders. What follows is a review of the history of harm reduction and the practical applications of the concept across the spectrum of substance use and public health management.

Infectious Disease Prevention

There is evidence of efforts to reduce harms related to substance use for thousands of years. Various cultures have used rituals and taboos to protect community and individual health from known harms from opium (Asia) and hallucinogens and coca (Central & South America). The conceptual framework of more "modern" harm reduction efforts is inextricably linked to the goal of infectious disease prevention, largely due to the inherent risks associated with injection drug use from communicable diseases such as hepatitis and human immunodeficincy virus (HIV) to the seeding of various parts of the body with bacteria which lead to skin, soft tissue, vascular, and valvular infections. Epidemiological estimates of the disease burden associated with injection drug use are notoriously difficult to capture, however, the burden is significant.[5] There are high levels of regional variation in skin and soft tissue infections (SSTIs) burden, largely attributable to the variation in the type of illicit substances available in the drug supply, with greater burdens in areas where black tar heroin is more prevalent.

Box 1 Harm reduction principles[4]	
Humanism	Providers treat patients with care and respect and take time to understand why patients make the decisions they make, taking into account that patients may derive benefit from otherwise harmful behaviors
Pragmatism	Providers understand that perfect health decisions are not achievable and the capacity for patients to make change is highly influenced by social determinants
Autonomy	Providers allow for patient-centered decision-making
Incrementalism	Providers understand that change happens over time and any positive change should be acknowledged
Individualism	Providers recognize that every person has their own needs, strengths, receptivity, to change along the continuum of harmful behaviors and requires unique strategies to facilitate change
Accountability without termination	Providers let patients know they are responsible for their own health choices and providers should not withhold care from patients for not achieving health goals but should instead help patients understand and take ownership of the consequences of their decisions

International efforts to reduce the incidence of drug-related infectious disease originally centered around reducing syringe sharing. Needle exchange began in the Netherlands in the early 1980s[6] and has evolved over time to meet the growing needs of the population, becoming the prevailing harm reduction practice.

In North America, given the stigma associated with injection drug use and the criminalization of drug paraphernalia, access to clean needles was, historically, significantly constrained. During the mid-1980s and early 1990s, in the context of the emerging HIV/acquired immunodeficiency syndrome (AIDS) epidemic, harm reduction efforts centered around cleaning available needles with bleach and other crude antimicrobial agents. However, given the unrelenting spread of HIV, harm reduction activists realized that this effort was insufficient and began to distribute needles in violation of the law. Activists like Johnny Parker and civil society organizations such as ACT UP and ADAPT significantly advanced the cause of needle exchange programs, ultimately winning a court ruling overturning New York state's ban on syringe sharing[6] which paved the way for organizations like the North American Syringe Exchange Network to finance the development of syringe service programs (SSPs) across the country.[7] As more SSPs emerged, these programs quickly adapted to include a wide range of health services beyond access to clean needles, including condom and drug paraphernalia distribution, referrals to substance abuse treatment, infectious disease counseling and testing, and naloxone distribution for the prevention of overdose.

The efficacy of SSPs in reducing infectious disease burden was demonstrated in dramatic fashion in 2014 in Scott County, Indiana, where the establishment of an SSP program facilitated the end of an outbreak of HIV in the community.[8] The success of this effort had a significant impact on Congress's decision in 2016 to partially repeal the ban on the use of federal funding to support SSPs.[9] Currently, SSPs continue to proliferate around the country and are also beginning to incorporate strategies like co-locating wound care and substance use disorder service programs to connect the traditionally difficult to reach populations serviced by these programs to advanced medical care.[10]

As syringe service programs became a more established part of public health strategy, people who inject drugs (PWID) and their supporters began to advocate for the establishment of safe spaces to inject drugs. Through the work of advocates like Ann Livingston and the Vancouver Area Drug User Network, leveraging evidence from countries in Europe (where the first such program opened in Switzerland in 1986) the first North American supervised consumption site (SCS) (also referred to as supervised injection facilities or overdose prevention sites) was established in 2003.[11] Although the primary goal of SCSs is to reduce overdose mortality, SCSs play a significant role in reducing infectious disease burden by providing a hygienic space for injection, clean injection equipment, a prohibition on equipment sharing, and education on safe injection practices. Data from around the world support the efficacy of SCSs in reducing infectious disease burden, with 75% of SCS users adopting safer injection practices outside of SCSs and 80% of SCS users reporting a decrease in rushed injections, where users fail to use safe injection practices due to fear of prosecution and needle sharing. The overall incidence of SSTI was found to be lower in PWID who use SCSs (6%–10%) than in the broader PWID population (10%–30%).[12] Despite this positive evidence, SCSs are not without significant controversy and have been effectively banned in the United States until November 2021 when New York City opened the first two sanctioned SCSs in the country.[13]

Outside of the aforementioned traditional harm reduction interventions, additional efforts at reducing infectious disease burden among PWID have been attempted which would appropriately be categorized as harm reduction albeit at a smaller scale. For PWID requiring long-term intravenous antibiotics, the use of peripherally inserted central catheters (PICC) is controversial with some physicians viewing the strategy as increasing the risk of intravenous use through the PICC itself, whereas other physicians view the use of PICC lines as a potential harm reduction strategy for individuals who otherwise cannot obtain vascular access themselves and resort to intramuscular use and subdermal injection or "skin popping."[14] Additional novel antibiotics, like the lipoglycopeptide dalbavancin, have promise as an effective antimicrobial for PWID who require long-term intravenous antibiotics and are at risk for leaving the hospital against medical advice.[15]

Opioids

The opioid epidemic and its resultant increase in nonfatal and fatal overdoses are an excellent example of an issue where a wide range of interventions at the individual, public health, and public policy levels have been implemented to reduce harm. As with many public health issues, prevention of opioid overdose can be thought of in terms of (1) primary prevention, focused on the reduction of use or misuse of opioids; (2) secondary prevention, focused on the reduction of overdose; and (3) tertiary prevention, focused on the reduction of deaths from overdose (**Box 2**).

Despite these various efforts, it is difficult to attribute any observed benefits to a given intervention as, in many cases, multiple interventions were in effect simultaneously.[18,25,26] It is also important to point out that the success of many primary prevention initiatives in reducing the availability and misuse of prescription opioids may have played a role in the unintended result of increased use of heroin and related overdose seen in the United States beginning around 2010,[27–29] though this is far from a universally held belief.[29] Similarly, it is not clear how many patients with pain are negatively impacted by these same efforts as they have increased difficulty accessing opioids for appropriate use.[30]

Primary prevention

Largely as a response to the increase in prescription opioid misuse and overdose starting in the late 1990s, a number of efforts have focused on reducing the prescribing, obtaining, and use and misuse of these medications. Although some efforts have been in existence for decades, there has been a significant increase in local, state, and federal efforts since the early to mid-2000s. Across these categories, there are efforts focused both on the individual patient and entire populations. Some of these interventions (increased provider education, prescription guidelines, quantity limits, Risk Evaluation and Mitigation Strategy, and so forth) are an attempt to increase the use of evidence-based medicine in the management of pain and would not generally be seen as typical "harm reduction" interventions. However, a primary goal is the reduction of the incidence of opioid use disorder and overdose.

Secondary prevention

Over the past 15 to 20 years, a growing amount of effort has been put into reducing/preventing opioid overdose and increasing help for those already meeting criteria for opioid use disorder. Many of these interventions can be thought of as being both secondary and tertiary prevention, focused on reducing overdose and reducing related fatalities. Most studies or evaluation efforts are unable to distinguish the relative effects of the two. As an example, various studies of SCSs have been shown to reduce fatal opioid overdoses.[31–33] However, a few studies found no significant reduction in overall overdoses.[34] Similarly, some studies of heroin-assisted treatment (HAT) have shown modest reductions in fatal and nonfatal overdoses but it is unclear if this can truly be attributed to the HAT.[20,22]

Box 2
Harm reduction measures for opioid overdose prevention

Primary Prevention (preventing opioid use/misuse)
- Prescriber education voluntary; mandated by the state licensure boards or other organizations (eg, food and drug administration (FDA) Risk Evaluation and Mitigation Strategy (REMS) for extended-release/long-acting opioid medications)
- Prescription guidelines (local and national, by specialty or procedure)
- Insurance company prescription monitoring (drug utilization review programs)
- Insurance company medication quantity limits/prior authorization requirements (may also create other harms like delays)
- Prescription drug identification laws (requiring photographic identification for controlled substances)
- Prescription drug monitoring programs[16,17]
- Electronic Prescriptions for Controlled Substances
- drug enforcement administration (DEA) changes in scheduling (eg, hydrocodone from Schedule III to Schedule II in 2014)
- FDA post-marketing surveillance of opioid safety and risk
- State "Pill Mill" and "Doctor Shopping" Laws[18]
- Increased law enforcement interdiction (eg, DEA "Operation Pill Nation" and "Operation Oxy Alley")
- Screening of patients with pain for risk of substance misuse (eg, Opioid Risk Tool)
- Prescription medication disposal and "take-back" (eg, The Secure and Responsible Drug Disposal Act; DEA-sponsored National Prescription Drug Take-Back Days; Patch-4-Patch Return Program in Canada)
- Public awareness/education about safe storage of medications and non-opioid pain management (eg, *Facing Addiction in America: The Surgeon General's Report on Alcohol, Drugs, and Health;* Partnership For A Drug-Free America's "Mind Your Meds" campaign)
- Abuse-deterrent formulations (eg, Embeda, Hysingla, Xtampza, Zohydro)

Secondary Prevention (preventing overdose)
- Prescriber education specifically focused on reducing overdose risk (eg, REMS; FDA Black box warning of combination of opioids and benzodiazepines)
- Public awareness/education specifically focused on reducing overdose risk; safe storage
- Overdose fatality review team members of various agencies meeting
- Increased treatment of opioid use disorder (OUD) w/medications (methadone, buprenorphine, long-acting naltrexone; slow-release morphine & hydrocodone used in some other countries)[19–21]
- Use of "diverted" buprenorphine/methadone (shown to decrease overdose and fatal overdose in individuals not in treatment as well as increase acceptability and engagement in treatment)
- Safe injection facilities (aka supervised consumption centers/rooms/facilities/services; overdose prevention centers; drug consumption rooms) (Switzerland, the Netherlands, Germany, Spain, Denmark, Norway, Luxembourg, France, Canada, Australia, United States)
- Heroin-assisted treatment (aka polymorphine- or diacetylmorphine-assisted treatment or supervised injectable heroin (Canada, the United Kingdom, Switzerland, Germany, the Netherlands, Denmark)[20,22]
- Drug testing-fentanyl test strips (eg, Energy Control International)

Tertiary Prevention (preventing fatal overdose)
- Public education/awareness specifically focused on the recognition of overdose and the use of naloxone; International Overdose Awareness Day (August 31)
- Naloxone prescription/distribution (to illicit opioid users, patients taking opioids for pain, patients in treatment for opioid use disorder, "third parties")[23,24]
- Naloxone carried by law enforcement and other first responders
- Good Samaritan Laws/Overdose Immunity (from related charges for individual who has overdosed and individual providing aid)
- Overdose survivor outreach programs
- Mobile/wearable technology (eg, "Remote Egg Timer," Trek Medics, OD Help)

- Environmental manipulations (eg, reverse motion detectors in bathrooms that detect when someone has stopped moving and alert staff that an overdose may have occurred)
- Hydromorphone vending machines (eg, MySafe Project in Vancouver)

Tertiary prevention

As mentioned above, many initiatives focus on both prevention of overdose and prevention of fatal overdose. The use of naloxone is one example where the intervention is clearly geared at tertiary prevention, intervening once the individual has experienced an overdose. The provision of naloxone to individuals who use heroin was first discussed in the mid-1990s with small programs beginning distribution around 1996. Multiple U.S. professional societies and government agencies have also made naloxone distribution a key component to their recommendations for battling the opioid overdose epidemic. Programs now exist in more than 15 other countries in Europe, Asia, Africa, and Australia with more being added as the World Health Organization has added naloxone to its Model List of Essential Medicines.

Cannabis

Cannabis has proven itself to have a wide therapeutic index and to be relatively physiologically safe over the millennia of human use. The history of harm reduction as a public health policy, internationally, was first applied in the context of cannabis, when the Netherlands Public Prosecutor's guideline allowed for the establishment of "coffee shops," in an effort to separate cannabis from "harder" drugs. In North America today, broadening legalization in the United States and federal legalization in Canada has increased access to medical and recreational cannabis products, subject to rigorous testing to ensure a safe and uncontaminated supply. This policy decision represents a significant reduction in harm when compared with the previous policy of blanket prohibition and criminalization. Given the lengthy detection period of tetrahydrocannabinol (THC) on typically conducted drug screenings, with subsequent legal or vocational ramifications, individuals may be compelled to seek cannabis-adjacent products to avoid detection. This contributed to the popularity of synthetic cannabinoids (aka Spice or K2) which have been associated with increased psychotic episodes, agitation, and violence.[35]

The 2018 Farm Bill effectively legalized the sale of hemp-derived cannabinoids, aimed at increasing the availability of cannabidiol (CBD), but provided limited oversight, leading to an increasingly popular market for analogous molecules to delta-9 THC, such as delta-8-THC among others, which may provide favorable alternative cannabis high with the decreased risk of legal consequence.[36] There is a dearth of information about these compounds and their safety for medical or recreational use, warranting more research as these markets expand.[36]

Synthetic Stimulants and Hallucinogens

There are hundreds of illicitly available synthetic stimulant and hallucinogenic compounds that are used recreationally in nightlife or concert settings, the most widely known among them being lysergoc acid diethylamide (LSD),[3,4] methylenedioxymethamphetamine (MDMA), and methamphetamine. These substances are associated with serious physical health problems, in addition to the risks of harm related to risky or disinhibited behavior previously described with other intoxicants.[37] Some harm reduction strategies include regulating the quantity of drugs used, spacing out doses, and not combining stimulants with depressants.[38] Harm reduction outreach services focused on recreational drug use in the nightlife setting include *Energy Control* (1997) in Spain and the public health organization *DanceSafe* (1998), both of which disseminate objective information around recreational and responsible use of drugs.

Drug checking is a harm reduction intervention that allows for identification of drug composition and the chance to minimize exposure to unexpected adulterants, which have been found at high rates in illicit drugs.[37] The point-of-care testing technologies have been used for years in Europe but are only now starting to be used in this context in North America[37] (Testing kits may not only significantly reduce accidental overdoses and fatalities, but data gleaned from them may signal trends in the circulation of novel and potentially lethal substances[37].

Alcohol

The consumption of alcohol is widely associated with socialization, ceremony, and pleasure across cultures. Binge drinking (>5 drinks in a sitting for men, >4 for women), and chronic drinking patterns are more likely to lead to harm and should be categorically discouraged (**Box 3**).

Approaches to addressing problematic alcohol use range from complete abstinence from alcohol (ie, 12-step models or Alcoholics Anonymous [AA]) to managed or controlled drinking which aims to reduce negative consequences from drinking if abstinence is not attainable. Managed alcohol programs can decrease the number of alcohol beverages consumed per day, increase safety and quality of life, lower the incidence of alcohol-related harm, that is, reduced Extended Release (ER) visits or hospital admissions, fewer police or legal interactions, and provide potential cost savings to the health care and legal services.[39] However, a Cochrane review was unable to make conclusions about the efficacy of managed alcohol programs given lack of control or comparison interventions in the 22 studies reviewed.[40]

Alcohol, driving, and educational programs

A recent study from the National Center for Statistics and Analytics found that approximately one-third of fatal motor vehicle crashes involve a driver who had consumed any alcohol, including a total of 10,142 (28%) deaths in 2019. Drinkers tend to underestimate the rate of alcohol absorption and overestimate the rate of elimination.[41] Without training, drinkers are very poor estimators of blood alcohol concentration (BAC), which is especially pertinent to decisions about legal driving ability.[42]

Designated drivers have been shown to reduce alcohol-related fatalities when executed well, that is, designating the person before drinking begins, and typically connoting abstinence from alcohol during the night.[43] However, loose interpretation of this concept (ie, driver simply being the least intoxicated person in the group) can limit effectiveness.[43] One study, finding that the mean BAC for 66 designated drivers leaving campus bars was 0.06 g/dL, summarized that the "differences between the ideal of abstinence and the actual behavior of designated drivers may result in smaller public health benefits from designated driver use than would be expected under the assumption of abstinence[44]" (**Box 4**: Rideshare Services as Harm Reduction).

Alcohol is routinely cited as the most misused substance on college campuses, with 68% of students consuming alcohol in the past month and nearly 40% admitting to heavy drinking (ie, >5 drinks in a row for men, >4 for women).[47] Education programs for consumers can help shape better informed drinking behaviors and increase awareness around the risks and harms of excessive alcohol consumption, particularly important in the college population who may just be starting to experiment with alcohol. Server education programs may lead to the increased recognition of overly intoxicated patrons, which can lead to ceasing beverage service and may also

Box 3	
Alcohol-related harms that stand to benefit from harm reduction modalities	
Domain	Examples
Health	• Alcohol-related injury and death due to acute accidents
	• Alcohol-related morbidity and mortality due to chronic disease
	• Worsening of psychiatric outcomes, increased rates of suicide
	• Impulsive sexual behaviors, increased rates of sexually transmitted disease (STD) transmission
	• Costs to health care system, for example, emergency department, transplantation
Crime/Public Disorder	• Disinhibited and risky behaviors, impulsive decision-making
	• Drunk driving injuries and death
	• Alcohol-related domestic violence
	• Arrests for public intoxication or disorderly conduct
	• Costs imposed to the criminal justice system
Workplace	• Working days and productivity lost due to alcohol-related illness
	• Working days and productivity lost due to reduced rates of employment
	• Costs imposed on economy due to workplace absenteeism and illness/disability/death
Family/Social Network	• Increased rates of divorce or separation
	• Children or family impacted by parental alcohol use disorder
	• Risk for neglect and strain on social service systems
	• Higher rates of domestic abuse

increase the chances that the patron can be assisted in safely getting home (see **Box 4**: Harm reduction alcohol policy).

Tobacco

Tobacco remains one of the largest contributors to morbidity and mortality worldwide. Higher taxes generally lead to lower smoking rates[53] Manipulating and lowering the nicotine content in cigarettes may render them less reinforcing, leading to lower rates of initiation and more successful quit attempts. However, lower nicotine content may lead to compensatory increases in smoking or use of other combusted nicotine products which may worsen harms related to smoke inhalation, though this effect seems inconsistent.[54]

Graphic warning labels (GWLs) have been recommended as a cost-effective means to increase public awareness of the physical harms induced by tobacco use by increasing both risk perceptions and quit intentions[55] GWLs are implemented in over 100 countries and are currently being challenged in U.S. courts by the tobacco industry on the grounds of their effectiveness.[55]

A full discussion of nicotine replacement therapy (NRT) transcends the scope of this paper, but suffice it to say that research has shown increases in smoking cessation rates up to two times with the use of NRT compared with placebo or no additional aid as well as improvements in moderating or reducing use[56] It has also been shown that those with mental health conditions have a more difficult time with cessation, and treating comorbid mood disorders may improve cessation outcomes. This consideration may shift the use

Box 4		
Individual, public health, and public policy alcohol harm reduction interventions		
Individual	**Potential Harms Addressed**	**Interventions/Implementation/ Feasibility**
Medications for Alcohol Use Disorder	• Helping to reduce cravings for alcohol • Helping to reduce heavy drinking days even for those not abstinent	• Naltrexone for reducing pleasure related to drinking, addressing, and reducing cravings, has been shown to reduce heavy drinking days (ASAM text) • Antabuse as deterrent treatment, negative conditioning due to disulfiram reaction to deter ongoing drinking • Acamprosate to regular GABA/glutamate tone in those abstinent, mechanism still unclear
Thiamine Supplementation of Alcohol[45]	• High rates of poor nutrition, vitamin depletion with chronic alcohol use • Risk for progression to Wernicke's encephalopathy and Korsakoff's psychosis	• Thiamine has been verified to be stable when stored in alcoholic beverages with minimal to no alteration in taste • Clear cost savings when compared with costs of medical care and lost productivity related to high rates of Korsakoff's psychosis in Queensland, Australia
Glassware Bans	• Glass-related damage or injuries related to progressive intoxication and impairment of coordination, that is, glass containers thrown or dropped • Glass shards can be used as weapons in bar fights	• Glassware bans have been shown to reduce harmful events related to glass injuries, that is, using aluminum cans or plastic containers • Some pubs in Scotland use a special type of glass which shatters into very fine particles, preventing use of shards as weapons[46]
Public Health Initiatives	**Potential Harms Addressed:**	**Interventions/Implementation/ Feasibility:**
College Education Programs[47,48]	• Missed classes or other poor academic performance • Increased rates of emotional, physical, or sexual assault • Increased rates of STDs • Increased rates of vandalism or property damage on campus	• Infusing awareness and education into coursework or campus orientation events • Strong evidence found that education programs by themselves were ineffective in reducing student alcohol use and related problems • Two published, commonly implemented programs achieved National Institute on Alcohol Abuse and

		Alcoholism (NIAAA) Tier 1 intervention status that have resulted in significant reductions in harmful alcohol use on campus: ○ Alcohol Skills Training Program based on cognitive behavioral principles ○ Brief Alcohol Screening and Intervention for College Students based on motivational interviewing
Server or Vendor Education Programs[49]	• Increased rates of binge drinking episodes if given easy or cheap access to alcohol • Despite the idea that limiting beverage sales may impact venue profits, it has been shown that venues with more responsible serving practices attract more customers[46]	• Avoiding self-service models • Avoiding volume discounts, that is, extended happy hours • Restrictions on supply such as keg bans or keg registration may also serve to limit binge consumption[50] • Charging higher prices for higher proof alcohol products • Substituting higher proof beverages for lower proof selections • Offering a wider selection of light or nonalcoholic drinks to help reduce overall alcohol intake without impacting subjective perceptions about drinking volume[46]
Public Policy Initiatives	Potential Harms Addressed:	Interventions/Implementation/Feasibility:
Prices	• Lower prices increase consumption	• Increasing price of alcohol leads to decrease in consumption rates according to studies in the general population[48] • Effect seems mediated by culture and age as well as the types and quantities typically consumed[48] • Heavier drinkers appear less affected by variations in price than others, though younger heavy drinkers such as college students may be an exception[48]
Taxes/Addressing Unrecorded or Illegal Alcohol Consumption	• Increased rates of compensatory drinking of illegal or unrecorded products such as moonshine or other homemade preparations	• Tax hikes on approved alcohol products do not appear to lead to compensatory drinking

	• These carry the rare but well-described risks from methanol or other contaminants[51]	• Buy backs for homemade alcohol products to limit potential harms have been implemented in some countries, though this may not be efficacious or cost feasible in the United States
Advertising Bans	• Advertising alcohol broadly may lead to increased salience and increased consumption	• Research is limited, but available evidence from the general population suggests that banning alcohol advertising seems to reduce alcohol abuse in some circumstances[48]
Restricting Licenses for Retail Sales of Alcohol	• Significant relationships between density of alcohol licenses per population size, rates of consumption, and related issues such as violence or crime	• May be restricted by making licenses more difficult to attain that is, increasing cost, density of stores per area • Mixed conclusions regarding restrictions of days or hours of sale
Minimum Legal Drinking Age (MLDA)	• Increased risks of harm with youth drinking and inexperienced, intoxicated drivers	• By 1988, all states had established the minimum legal driving age to be 21, hence MLDA being the most well studied alcohol control policy[50] Studies have shown that higher legal drinking age is related to: • Reduced alcohol consumption • Decreased rates of traffic crashes • Decreased rates of suicide, homicide, vandalism
Lowered Blood Alcohol Concentration (BAC) Limits	• Higher BAC leading to increasingly impaired driving ability • People incorrectly estimating their BAC when deciding to drive	• States that lowered legal BAC limits from 0.10% to 0.08% experienced a 6% greater post-law decline in alcohol-related fatal crashes in which drivers had blood alcohol levels of >0.10% than states that retained the 0.10% standard"[48] • Providing BAC information to would be drivers did not influence perceptions of driving safety risk, with limitations including: ○ Minimal impact on risk-averse individuals who would abstain from driving regardless of BAC level ○ Potentially negative impact on risk-tolerant individuals who may use

		BAC information to justify driving while intoxicated, albeit under the legal .08 limit[52]
Administrative License Revocation	• Repeat offenders may be more likely to continue driving impaired	• Legally mandated license revocation for drinking-and-driving offenses and mandatory seat belt use have resulted in decreases in alcohol-related fatalities[48]
Rideshare Programs	• Increased rates of impaired driving if no other commuting options exist • Safety and convenience of rideshare services such as Uber or Lyft may tip the decision-making away from impaired driving, perhaps even to a greater extent than do conventional public transportation, that is, bus, taxi	• The density of active rideshare trips near a crash site was associated with decreased odds that the crash involved alcohol[53] • "Nez Rouge" ("Red Nose") program in Quebec—community-based service providing two drivers (one for the drinker and one for their car) to anyone who has had too much to drink at a party or licensed establishment to be able to drive home safely[46] • College campus free ride or shuttle services to nearby establishments in the area—decrease risks of drunk driving incidents on campus

of bupropion higher in the treatment algorithm for cessation attempts, with better data for the SR formulations compared with extended release (XL) formulations.[57]

Electronic nicotine delivery systems/vaping

The use of e-cigarettes or vapes, broadly referred to as electronic nicotine delivery systems (ENDS), remains controversial despite their increasing popularity and media attention. These devices not only address the physiologic dependence on nicotine but also potentially address the behavioral and sensory aspects of cigarette use that is lacking from most standard pharmacologic nicotine replacement therapies aside from the Nicotrol inhaler. Although a previous small review had found ENDS helpful with long-term cessation compared with placebo[58], a more recent systematic review concluded that there is very limited evidence regarding the impact of ENDS of smoking cessation, reduction, or adverse effects.[59,60] The benefits are considered in the context of relatively minimal rates of adverse effects associated with ENDS.[58,59]

There remains a lack of evidence about more specific questions such as the differences between high- and low-concentration nicotine ENDS products, differences between daily or non-daily users, or the differences between earlier generation ENDS with newer products. Issues around quality control, production, and manufacturing add to inconsistencies in described benefits and may pose risks to consumers. Differentiating the effects of nicotine dose from the effects of device type/preference, or related sensory aspects, is likely to be challenging. These represent new frontiers of research that need to be pursued for providers to be able to speak with patients about safe and responsible use of these new and emerging products and consider them as harm reduction strategies when treating patients with tobacco use disorder.

FDA approval
In an unexpected decision, the food and drug administration (FDA) recently (October 2021) granted its first market authorizations through the Premarket Tobacco Product Application pathway for three new ENDS products from RJ Reynolds, permitting the sale of these products but not conveying an official FDA approval or acknowledgment of safety. FDA concluded that the benefits of reduced cigarette smoking in current adult smokers, that is, reduction in exposure to harmful chemicals evidenced by urinary and blood biomarkers, outweighed the potential risks of exposing youth to these nicotine products. Existing data suggest that there is a low intention to purchase these products among adult nonusers and the most youth who use ENDS start with fruit or candy flavors and continue to prefer these products to the tobacco-flavored products that were approved in the recent announcement. The FDA implemented post-marketing restrictions on media advertisements to reduce youth exposure and retained the ability to suspend or withdraw the marketing order if the products are found to no longer be "appropriate for the protection of the public health, such as if there is a significant increase in youth initiation."

Integration of Harm Reduction with Traditional Addiction, Psychiatric, and Medical Treatment

The integration of harm reduction with other treatment services can be conceptualized in two main ways. One involves the genuine adoption of the principles (humanism, individualism, and so forth) and philosophy of low barrier access to care as well as the acceptance that total abstinence from all substance use is not the only acceptable goal/outcome of successful treatment. The other involves the actual inclusion of traditional harm reduction services (syringe exchange, overdose prevention, and so forth) into traditional medical, psychiatric, and addiction treatment settings as well as the integration of or easy access to medical, psychiatric, and addiction treatment services in traditional harm reduction settings.

Incorporating humanism, individualism, and autonomy can be achieved by speaking to patients in a nonjudgmental manner and taking the time to understand ongoing decision-making around their substance use, understanding that there may be perceived benefits from otherwise outwardly harmful behaviors. It is paramount to create a treatment space where patients feel comfortable speaking with their providers, feel safe making their needs known, and where they are encouraged to take agency in their treatment planning and decision-making.

The principle of pragmatism may stand in opposition to moral and abstinence-based programs, which may estrange those where complete abstinence may not be their personal goal. Abstinence-based programs which frown on medication-assisted treatments may also alienate those who truly do require pharmacologic assistance and subsequently diminish chances at ongoing engagement and support. It is worth noting that for some patients, abstinence and "perfect" health decisions are unattainable due to social determinants of health. This is where the divide between the two ideologies can best be bridged, whereby continued engagement with these patients affords the opportunity to address these social determinants (ie, provision of or referral to ancillary vocational and housing services) and may indeed help move someone toward complete abstinence. Incrementalism may also manifest itself in the form of motivational interviewing, where listening out for and encouraging change talk can lead to progress in their journey toward abstinence. By continuing to engage with those who cannot immediately or easily achieve complete abstinence, providers can position themselves to help make ongoing use as safe as possible until abstinence is attainable or realistic for the individual.

Syringe services programs, supervised consumption facilities, and managed alcohol programs that make treatment providers available in their settings allow for increased psychoeducation and engagement in treatment. Individuals who continue to use substances may fluctuate between different stages of motivation at different times, and providing consistent access to a mental health or addiction professional can help reduce ambivalence and reinforce incremental positive changes toward less harmful use. These endeavors implement similar approaches, namely aiming for objective provision of information and engagement to the extent that individuals are willing. Drawing similarities to management of other chronic illnesses with behavioral components such as obesity also serves to reduce the stigma accompanying the use of harm reduction principles to address substance use disorders.

Until recently, the provision of harm reduction services or messaging within traditional medical, psychiatric, and addiction treatment programs was seen as "enabling" of substance use and a violation of the "Hippocratic Oath." A gradual shift over recent years has resulted in many traditional treatment settings now providing easy access to naloxone and overdose education. Similarly, many more providers are providing information on SSPs and safer injection techniques with some addiction treatment programs even offering syringe services within the program. Although these examples of integration are promising, it is imperative that all providers work to increase this integration in the settings in which they work. It is also important that providers advocate with local and national policy makers to help make harm reduction a routine part of all medical care.

CLINICS CARE POINTS

- The principles of harm reduction should be integrated in to all medical, psychiatric, and addiction treatment programs.

- The basic philosophy that total abstinence from all substance use is not the only acceptable goal/outcome of successful treatment has become much more acceptable in the current addiction treatment world.

- Efforts should be made to reduce the barriers to accessing care and for individuals using substances.

- Providers should familiarize themselves with local harm reduction services and refer patients to them readily.

DISCLOSURE

None of the authors have any conflicts of interest. There was no external funding used in the creation of this article.

REFERENCES

1. Lopez G. Covid-19's big public health lesson: ask people to be careful, not perfect harm reduction works. Covid-19 has proved it. Vox. Available at. https://www.vox.com/22315478/covid-19-coronavirus-harm-reduction-abstinence. Accessed January 24, 2022.

2. Reduction International Harm. Global state of harm reduction 2020 2020. p. 7. Available at. https://www.hri.global/files/2021/03/04/Global_State_HRI_2020_BOOK_FA_Web.pdf.

3. Harm Reduction Coalition. Principles of Harm Reduction. Available at. https://harmreduction.org/about-us/principles-of-harm-reduction/. Accessed January 15, 2022.

4. Hawk M, Coulter RWS, Egan JE, et al. Harm reduction principles for healthcare settings. Harm Reduct J 2017;14(1):70.

5. See I, Gokhale RH, Geller A, et al. National public health burden estimates of endocarditis and skin and soft-tissue infections related to injection drug use: a review. J Infect Dis 2020;222(Supplement_5):S429–36.

6. Szalavitz M. Undoing drugs: the untold story of harm reduction and the future of addiction. First edition. Hachette Go; 2021.

7. Des Jarlais DC. Harm reduction in the USA: the research perspective and an archive to David Purchase. Harm Reduct J 2017;14(1):51.

8. Patel MR, Foote C, Duwve J, et al. Reduction of injection-related risk behaviors after emergency implementation of a syringe services program during an HIV outbreak. J Acquir Immune Defic Syndr 2018;77(4):373–82.

9. Rogers H. Congress ends ban on federal funding for needle exchange programs. 2016. Available at. https://www.npr.org/2016/01/08/462412631/congress-ends-ban-on-federal-funding-for-needle-exchange-programs. Accessed January 21, 2022.

10. Sanchez DP, Tookes H, Pastar I, Lev-Tov H. Wounds and skin and soft tissue infections in people who inject drugs and the utility of syringe service programs in their management. Adv Wound Care 2021;10(10):571–82.

11. Lupick T. Fighting for space: how a group of drug users transformed one city's struggle with addiction. Arsenal Pulp Press; 2017.

12. Semaan S, Fleming P, Worrell C, Stolp H, Baack B, Miller M. Potential role of safer injection facilities in reducing HIV and Hepatitis C infections and overdose mortality in the United States. Drug Alcohol Depend 2011;118(2–3):100–10.

13. Mays J, Newman A. Nation's first supervised drug-injection sites open in New York. New York Times. 2021. Available at. https://www.nytimes.com/2021/11/30/nyregion/supervised-injection-sites-nyc.html. Accessed January 21, 2022.

14. Guta A, Perri M, Strike C, Gagnon M, Carusone SC. With a PICC line, you never miss": The role of peripherally inserted central catheters in hospital care for people living with HIV/HCV who use drugs. Int J Drug Policy 2021;96:103438.

15. Veve MP, Patel N, Smith ZA, Yeager SD, Wright LR, Shorman MA. Comparison of dalbavancin to standard-of-care for outpatient treatment of invasive Gram-positive infections. Int J Antimicrob Agents 2020;56(6):106210.

16. Patrick SW, Fry CE, Jones TF, Buntin MB. Implementation of prescription drug monitoring programs associated with reductions in opioid-related death rates. Health Aff (Millwood) 2016;35(7):1324–32.

17. Paulozzi LJ, Kilbourne EM, Desai HA. Prescription drug monitoring programs and death rates from drug overdose. Pain Med 2011;12(5):747–54.

18. Johnson H, Paulozzi L, Porucznik C, Mack K, Herter B. Hal Johnson consulting and division of disease control and health promotion, florida department of health. decline in drug overdose deaths after state policy changes-Florida, 2010-2012. MMWR Morb Mortal Wkly Rep 2014;63(26):569–74.

19. Jegu J, Gallini A, Soler P, Montastruc JL, Lapeyre-Mestre M. Slow-release oral morphine for opioid maintenance treatment: a systematic review: Slow-release

oral morphine for opioid maintenance treatment. Br J Clin Pharmacol 2011;71(6): 832–43.

20. Oviedo-Joekes E, Brissette S, Marsh DC, et al. Diacetylmorphine versus methadone for the treatment of opioid addiction. N Engl J Med 2009;361(8):777–86.

21. Sordo L, Barrio G, Bravo MJ, et al. Mortality risk during and after opioid substitution treatment: systematic review and meta-analysis of cohort studies. BMJ 2017;j1550. Published online April 26.

22. Ferri M, Davoli M, Perucci CA. Heroin maintenance for chronic heroin-dependent individuals. In: Cochrane Drugs and Alcohol Group, editor. Cochrane database syst rev. 2011.

23. Gaston R, Best D, Manning V, Day E. Can we prevent drug related deaths by training opioid users to recognise and manage overdoses? Harm Reduct J 2009;6(1):26.

24. Walley AY, Xuan Z, Hackman HH, et al. Opioid overdose rates and implementation of overdose education and nasal naloxone distribution in Massachusetts: interrupted time series analysis. Bmj 2013;346.

25. Franklin G, Sabel J, Jones CM, et al. A comprehensive approach to address the prescription opioid epidemic in washington state: milestones and lessons learned. Am J Public Health 2015;105(3):463–9.

26. Paone D, Tuazon E, Kattan J, et al. Decrease in rate of opioid analgesic overdose deaths—Staten Island, New York City, 2011–2013. MMWR Morb Mortal Wkly Rep 2015;64(18):491.

27. Ciccarone D. Fentanyl in the US heroin supply: a rapidly changing risk environment. Int J Drug Policy 2017;46:107–11.

28. Cicero TJ, Ellis MS, Surratt HL, Kurtz SP. The changing face of heroin use in the united states: a retrospective analysis of the past 50 years. JAMA Psychiatry 2014;71(7):821.

29. Compton WM, Jones CM, Baldwin GT. Relationship between nonmedical prescription-opioid use and heroin use. In: Longo DL, editor. N Engl J Med 2016;374(2):154–63.

30. Jones CM, Lurie P, Woodcock J. Addressing prescription opioid overdose: data support a comprehensive policy approach. JAMA 2014;312(17):1733.

31. Fry Dolan JK Craig, McDonald David, Fitzgerald John, Trautmann Franz, Kate. Drug consumption facilities in Europe and the establishment of supervised injecting centres in Australia. Drug Alcohol Rev 2000;19(3):337–46.

32. Addiction EMC for D and D. Drug consumption rooms: an overview of provision and evidence. European Monitoring Centre for Drugs and Drug Addiction Lisbon; 2018.

33. Marshall BD, Milloy MJ, Wood E, Montaner JS, Kerr T. Reduction in overdose mortality after the opening of North America's first medically supervised safer injecting facility: a retrospective population-based study. Lancet 2011;377(9775): 1429–37.

34. Davies G. A critical evaluation of the effects of safe injection facilities. J Glob Drug Policy Pract 2007;1(3).

35. Featherstone S. Cheap, unpredictable and hard to regulate, synthetic marijuana has emergency responders scrambling to save lives. N Y Times.2015:6.

36. Kruger JS, Kruger DJ. Delta-8-THC: Delta-9-THC's nicer younger sibling? J Cannabis Res 2022;4(1):4.

37. Fregonese M, Albino A, Covino C, et al. Drug checking as strategy for harm reduction in recreational contests: evaluation of two different drug analysis methodologies. Front Psychiatry 2021;12:596895.

38. Fernández-Calderón F, Díaz-Batanero C, Barratt MJ, Palamar JJ. Harm reduction strategies related to dosing and their relation to harms among festival attendees who use multiple drugs: Dosing-related harm reduction strategies. Drug Alcohol Rev 2019;38(1):57–67.
39. Pauly B, Brown M, Evans J, et al. There is a Place": impacts of managed alcohol programs for people experiencing severe alcohol dependence and homelessness. Harm Reduct J 2019;16(1):70.
40. Muckle W, Muckle J, Welch V, Tugwell P. Managed alcohol as a harm reduction intervention for alcohol addiction in populations at high risk for substance abuse. Cochrane drugs and alcohol group. Cochrane Database Syst Rev 2012. https://doi.org/10.1002/14651858.CD006747.pub2.
41. Martin CS, Rose RJ, Obremski KM. Estimation of blood alcohol concentrations in young male drinkers. Alcohol Clin Exp Res 1991;15(3):494–9.
42. Aston ER, Liguori A. Self-estimation of blood alcohol concentration: a review. Addict Behav 2013;38(4):1944–51.
43. Ditter SM, Elder RW, Shults RA, Sleet DA, Compton R, Nichols JL. Effectiveness of designated driver programs for reducing alcohol-impaired driving. Am J Prev Med 2005;28(5):280–7.
44. Timmerman MA, Geller ES, Glindemann KE, Fournier AK. Do the designated drivers of college students stay sober? J Safety Res 2003;34(2):127–33.
45. Price J, Theodoros MT. The Supplementation of alcoholic beverages with thiamine—a necessary preventive measure in queensland? Aust N Z J Psychiatry 1979;13(4):315–20.
46. Single E. Harm reduction as an alcohol-prevention strategy. Alcohol Health Res World 1996;20(4):239–43.
47. US Department of Health and Human Services. National institutes of health; national institute on alcohol abuse and alcoholism task force of the national advisory council on alcohol abuse and alcoholism. a call to action: changing the culture of drinking at. U.S. Colleges; 2002. Published online.
48. Nelson TF, Toomey TL, Lenk KM, Erickson DJ, Winters KC. Implementation of NIAAA college drinking task force recommendations: how are colleges doing 6 years later?: implementation of NIAAA college drinking task force recommendations. Alcohol Clin Exp Res 2010;34(10):1687–93.
49. McKnight AJ. Server intervention. Alcohol Health Res World 1993;17(1):76–84.
50. Toomey TL, Wagenaar AC. Environmental policies to reduce college drinking: options and research findings. J Stud Alcohol Suppl 2002;(14):193–205.
51. Rehm J, Neufeld M, Room R, et al. The impact of alcohol taxation changes on unrecorded alcohol consumption: a review and recommendations. Int J Drug Policy 2022;99:103420.
52. Johnson MB, Voas RB, Kelley-Baker T, Furr-Holden CDM. The consequences of providing drinkers with blood alcohol concentration information on assessments of alcohol impairment and drunk-driving risk. J Stud Alcohol Drugs 2008;69(4):539–49.
53. Morrison CN, D'Ambrosi G, Kamb A, MacManus K, Rundle AG, Humphreys DK. Rideshare trips and alcohol-involved motor vehicle crashes in Chicago. J Stud Alcohol Drugs 2021;82(6):720–9.
54. Bader P, Boisclair D, Ferrence R. Effects of tobacco taxation and pricing on smoking behavior in high risk populations: a knowledge synthesis. Int J Environ Res Public Health 2011;8(11):4118–39.
55. Donny EC, White CM. A review of the evidence on cigarettes with reduced addictiveness potential. Int J Drug Policy 2022;99:103436.

56. Strong DR, Pierce JP, Pulvers K, et al. Effect of graphic warning labels on ciga-rette packs on us smokers' cognitions and smoking behavior after 3 months: a randomized clinical trial. JAMA Netw Open 2021;4(8):e2121387.

57. Logan DE, Marlatt GA. Harm reduction therapy: a practice-friendly review of research. J Clin Psychol 2010;66(2):201–14.

58. Ries RK, Fiellin DA, Miller SC, Saitz R. The ASAM principles of addiction medi-cine. Lippincott Williams & Wilkins; 2014.

59. McRobbie H, Bullen C, Hartmann-Boyce J, Hajek P. Electronic cigarettes for smoking cessation and reduction. In: The Cochrane collaboration, editor. Co-chrane database of systematic reviews. John Wiley & Sons, Ltd; 2014. p. CD010216, pub2.

60. El Dib R, Suzumura EA, Akl EA, et al. Electronic nicotine delivery systems and/or electronic non-nicotine delivery systems for tobacco smoking cessation or reduc-tion: a systematic review and meta-analysis. BMJ Open 2017;7(2):e012680.

Individual Paths to Recovery from Substance Use Disorder (SUD)

What Are the Implications of the Emerging Recovery Evidence Base for Addiction Psychiatry and Practice?

David Best, PhD*, Mulka Nisic, MSc

KEYWORDS

• Addiction • Recovery • Recovery capital

KEY POINTS

• Recovery is a process that is generally mediated by access to social and community resources.
• Those resources are a part of "recovery capital" that can be broken down into personal, social, and community components that are dynamically linked.
• Recovery capital provides us with a metric that can improve assessment, measurement, and recovery care planning and allows improved scientific modeling of recovery pathways.
• There are multiple pathways to recovery that may involve specialist treatment, mutual aid, community recovery organizations, and access to jobs, friends, and satisfactory housing.

INTRODUCTION/HISTORY/DEFINITIONS/BACKGROUND

Although recovery is a decade-old term, with a central role of peers and grassroots organizations[1] in supporting well-being and reintegration, recently it has become a core theme for policymakers in the substance misuse field and a subject for academic research and debate in the United Kingdom[2,3] and the United States.[4,5] This has resulted in a significant shift in our understanding of substance use problems and their effective resolution. Key elements have been captured by the Betty Ford Institute Consensus Panel[6] definition of recovery as a "voluntarily maintained lifestyle characterized by sobriety, personal health and citizenship." The UK Drug Policy Commission[7]

Business, Law and Social Sciences, University of Derby, One Friar Gate Square, Derby, Derbyshire DE1 1DF, United Kingdom
* Corresponding author.
E-mail address: D.Best@derby.ac.uk

Psychiatr Clin N Am 45 (2022) 547–556
https://doi.org/10.1016/j.psc.2022.04.006
0193-953X/22/© 2022 Elsevier Inc. All rights reserved.

psych.theclinics.com

characterizes recovery as " voluntarily sustained control over substance use which maximizes health and well-being and participation in the rights, roles, and responsibilities of society." There has also been a growth in interest in the idea that long-term recovery requires effective engagement in meaningful activities and involvement in prosocial groups that are supportive of recovery. The new UK Drugs Strategy "From harm to hope"[3] perceives recovery as a process that often takes time to achieve and effort to maintain, highlighting the need for people to have access to meaningful activities, housing, and a support system within the community.

The Betty Ford Institute Consensus Panel[6] has also conceptualized recovery as a process that has temporal dimensions and identified three stages: (1) early recovery (the first year), (2) sustained recovery (between 1 and 5 years), and (3) stable recovery (more than 5 years in recovery). The evidence base suggests that relapse risk reduces for up to 5 years after achieving abstinence. The risk plateaus after this point[8] in line with the longitudinal research by Dennis, Scott, and Laudet[9] who claim that recovery becomes "self-sustaining" after 5 years, while before that, external support is needed. The first area on which we will focus addresses the question of the forms that external support should take. This article aims to outline some of the ways that this can be conceptualized and provides an overview of the practical implications for addiction treatment and sustaining the gains made in specialist treatment services.

KEY CONCEPTS

There are three core components and conceptual underpinnings that will be used to provide the foundations for recovery models. These are all predicated on the idea that there are many paths to recovery (that do not necessarily require specialist treatment) and the focus needs to be shifted from resolving pathologies to building strengths, using social and societal resources as the triggers for these transitions.

Multiple Paths to Recovery

The dominant approach to addressing addiction has been an acute model of care shaped by an addiction treatment system and oversight and support by a multidisciplinary professional team. The concept of recovery has for a long time been dominated by two very distinct approaches that represent two powerful traditions of recovery with fundamentally different philosophies drawn from the 12-step fellowships and the Therapeutic Communities tradition. Recently, however, Humphreys and Lembke[10] identified what they regarded as the three areas of recovery intervention that have a strong and supportive research evidence base. These are (1) mutual aid groups such as AA and Narcotics Anonymous (NA), (2) peer-delivered interventions, and (3) recovery housing. What is in common for all those models is a central role for peer-delivered, rather than professionally delivered services, positive role modeling and the active engagement, and significance of peer champions. The phenomenon of peer transmission of recovery was also described as a "recovery cascade"[11] in which each step of growth in recovery "lowers the kindling point for initiation of future change—at personal, family, community, and cultural levels." In other words, recovery is a social contagion that not only transmits from peer to peer but also has a residual (and beneficial) effect on the community in which it occurs.

To map paths to recovery and provide evidence on multiple mechanisms that help to initiate and support recovery, the Recovery Pathways (REC-PATH) study was undertaken in Europe,[12] examining five candidate pathways (12-step mutual aid, other peer-based support, residential treatment, community treatment, and natural recovery). This study has shown[13] that engaging in multiple pathways to recovery is associated with significantly improved outcomes across multiple domains, including housing, substance use, offending, and engagement in meaningful activities, particularly employment. There are, however, marked differences in typical pathways for men and women, with men more actively involved in visible recovery communities and women more likely to engage in wider community activities. There were also marked variations across countries, with residential treatment more common in Belgium and 12-step mutual aid playing a much more prominent role in the United Kingdom.

One of the key findings was that those who engaged in specialist treatment services and in mutual aid groups had significantly better outcomes than those who engaged in only one of these pathways, but the study did not suggest that there were gender differences in engagement with different types of peer and specialist processes.

Social Model for Understanding and Explaining Recovery

This model relies on the evidence, belonging to recovery-focused groups and associating with other people who have made the same journey plays a crucial role in supporting the transition from active addiction to recovery and maintaining and predicting a long-term recovery.[14] Best and colleagues[15] also asserted that two critical predictors of well-being in recovery are engagement with other people in recovery and participation in meaningful activities, such as employment. This is consistent with the evidence from Project MATCH where Longabaugh and colleagues[16] have argued that transitioning from social networks supportive of drinking to networks supportive of recovery is an essential component of recovery success.

This is also consistent with the work of Litt and colleagues[17] who randomly assigned problem drinkers who had recently completed alcohol detoxification to either standard aftercare or to "network support," which involved attempting to add at least one person [generally recruited from Alcoholics Anonymous (AA)] to their social network. Those in the Network Support condition were 27% less likely to have relapsed to drinking at the 1-year follow-up assessment.

In an Australian cohort study, based on 300 individuals entering residential Therapeutic Communities, it was not only changes in social groups but also changes in the underpinning sense of social identity that was associated with positive recovery outcomes. Their latter study was designed to test the application of Social Identity Theory to addiction recovery. What it attempts to explain are the beneficial effects of group membership[8,18] that has resulted in the development of the Social Identity Model of Recovery.[19–21] This model has the primary objective of explaining the processes of transitioning from groups that are supportive of addiction to groups that are supportive of recovery using 12-step groups as an example and highlights that pathways to sustainable recovery are generally characterized by a change in social identity. This happens not only as an active choice but also as a more subtle process of building social bonds and social capital that, in turn, results in gradual transitions in personal roles, values, norms, orientations, and beliefs that act as conditions for active participation in the group.[22]

Creating these attachments related to active participation in group activities results in a form of informal social control that strengthens the motivation for recovery as well as increases access to support to sustain it.[23] This has been described by Moos[24] as a combination of social learning and social control as the group provides not only role modeling but also corrective direction and advice to support recovery progress. In his work on the effective and active mechanisms of AA, Kelly[25] has argued that not only is active engagement in AA-associated with positive recovery outcomes but that this peer-delivered mutual aid approach works primarily through its impact on social networks for men and changes in self-efficacy for women. Although spiritual awakening happens on occasion, this is relatively rare as a mechanism of action for AA members.

Attending AA meetings is not sufficient—it is active participation and the impact of that participation that is central to a sense of belonging and to social identification with AA (and with other groups) and the norms and values they adhere to. The authors of this article[26] have also demonstrated, using the retrospective accounts of a large sample of people in recovery from across Europe that the higher the proportion of people in recovery and the lower the proportion of those who use drugs in one's social network, the greater the total number of current strengths and the smaller the number of current barriers.

These findings are also consistent with the idea of "recovery contagion,"[27,28] and previous publication on the Strengths And Barriers Recovery Scale (SABRS),[29] which was a part of the REC-PATH study, that was undertaken in Europe.[12] Findings from this study show that having as few as two different kinds of close relationships (an intimate partner and children) is associated with greater positive changes in recovery strengths and greater reductions in barriers to recovery. Each positive relationship predicted greater strengths and well-being in recovery and reduced experienced barriers to recovery (such as ongoing psychological health problems and involvement with the justice system). Similarly, having larger social networks of people in recovery, as well as more people in whom to confide, are associated with more positive growth in recovery strengths and reductions in barriers to recovery.[26] This is especially the case if the network does not consist exclusively of people in recovery, which is congruent with Jetten, Haslam, and Haslam's "social cure" concept which claims that the effects of belonging to multiple groups are more beneficial.[23] Central to the "social cure" concept is the idea that group membership confers a sense of belonging and pride to belonging the group is salutogenic in that it actively promotes health and is beneficial to positive life changes.

This is consistent with a review of the key elements of *mental health* recovery, summarized in the acronym CHIME. What Leamy and colleagues[30] showed was that supporting recovery was best served through providing *C*onnections, *H*ope, *I*dentity, *M*eaning, and *E*mpowerment. In translating this to the *addictions* recovery space, Best[27] has argued that positive *C*onnections (through social learning and social control) provide a feeling of *H*ope that change is possible which motivates and inspires engagement in *M*eaningful activities that, in turn, generates a positive sense of *I*dentity and a resulting internal experience of *E*mpowerment.

Recovery Capital

Evaluating and assessing addiction problem severity and complexity, such as co-occurring medical or psychiatric problems, have been done with reasonable success by traditional addiction assessment instruments. However, the focus on resolving pathologies of addiction needs to shift to building strengths with the overall goal of wellness is at the heart of long-term care.[31] This is a key part of the strength-based approach, which presupposes that long-term recovery is fundamentally relational and happens in the community and not in the clinic and it relies on the acceptance of recovery by the community and family. Recovery Capital was first described by Granfield and Cloud[32] as the breadth and depth of resources available to a person to support their recovery pathway.

Best and Laudet[33] then categorized these resources into three dynamically related domains:

I. Personal Recovery Capital (internal qualities and skills such as communication skills and resilience)

II. Social Recovery Capital (positive social support and the individual's commitment to those individuals and groups as outlined above under social identity theory)

III. Community Recovery Capital (resources available and accessible in the community, including jobs, education, and safe housing).

The assumption is that recovery capital is both quantifiable and dynamic and so it can be used as the foundation for recovery care planning and measuring progress in a recovery journey.

Dennis and colleagues[34] asserted that recovery is an ongoing process that can last several years post-acute treatment and relies on accessing supports and resources in the community including but not restricted to mutual aid groups and community recovery organizations. Once acute harms have been addressed, progress is most likely to be evidenced in continued growth and strengths among people in the post-acute treatment period. Hence, the metrics that measure growth and community integration are very much needed, and this has led to a gradual emergence of a science of recovery capital.[35]

The first measure in this process was the Assessment of Recovery Capital,[36] a 50-item scale, which assesses key dimensions of personal and social recovery capital. A second measure is the Recovery Group Participation Scale,[37] which assesses one dimension of community capital in relation to engagement with peer recovery support groups. Both of these scales have been embedded into a holistic approach to care planning and measurement tool called the REC-CAP.[38] The REC-CAP has acceptable psychometrics and is designed to be used in a range of treatment and recovery group settings to not only capture the growth of recovery strengths but also to support recovery care planning and growth.

More recently, Best and colleagues[29] developed innovative work on the use of the SABRS. The scale is based on the Life in Recovery (LiR) survey, first reported by Laudet,[39] which retrospectively assesses respondents' experiences in active addiction and in recovery using five life domains (work, finances, legal status, family and social relations, and citizenship). The LiR Scale assesses changes in recovery resources and barriers to recovery over time and provides a method for assessing the extent of recovery growth in a cross-sectional survey. Results from the use of this scale further support the idea that recovery capital grows over time beyond acute treatment support and that recovery barriers diminish during this period, although they are typically not completely eradicated.

As Best and Hennessy[35] point out, recovery capital remains a young science with much more conceptual development and empirical testing required to create adequate predictive validity of scales and applications for practitioners and peer champions. However, recovery capital creates a metric that allows recovery to move from something that is seen as vague, individual, and unstable over time to something that can be measured, mapped, and tested with exceptionally promising results to date. It also offers a transition to a strength-based approach more suited to testing long-term reintegration and quality of life than the traditional outcomes assessments based on the amelioration of pathologies.

DISCUSSION

The three areas discussed in this article—social foundations for change, multiple pathways to recovery, and the development of recovery capital measurement tools—are all part of an emerging science and evidence base on the process of growth and societal reintegration that characterizes the post-acute period of treatment which can be used to complement it. However, there is no reason to assume that the methods and logics of recovery capital building cannot be applied successfully to those whose recovery journeys involve ongoing engagement in treatment. This is particularly applicable for those people who are taking substitution opioid medications on an open-ended time frame. The transition from acute treatment to sustained recovery in the community is typically characterized[40] as the transition from a deficit to a strengths model, from a clinic to the community, from professional patient to partnership working, and from a past to a future focus.

The collection of resources at the disposal of recovering individuals aids in the long-term growth and maintenance of their recovery.[33] Recovery capital as a conceptual framework reflects a paradigmatic shift toward long-term personal, family, and community recovery. As Best and Hennessy[35] found in their recent review of recovery capital science, the field currently relies on self-report questionnaires for the development of the theory and quantification of recovery capital rigorous and systematic conceptual and empirical development of recovery capital are urgently needed. Although its theoretic development is not complete and has been insufficiently researched empirically, the possibilities and usefulness of its application are clear.

The concept of recovery capital provides a valuable analytical framework for identifying, describing, and analyzing resources available to individuals who are seeking recovery. It also provides a framework for operationalizing and actioning the CHIME framework by emphasizing the importance of social connections and meaningful activities as key catalysts in generating and sustaining the key internal qualities—self-esteem, self-efficacy, resilience, and coping skills—that will sustain recovery over time. In studies in both the United Kingdom (Best and colleagues, 2011; Best and colleagues, 2013) and the United States (Cano and colleagues, 2017), the combination of engaging in meaningful activities and connecting with pro-social groups was most strongly associated with recovery well-being and recovery capital.

This reflects the ecosystem perspective and a strength-oriented approach and is consistent with the Social Identity Model of Recovery, in which there is a "double echo" of both the social (in the sense of immediate access to positive individuals and groups) and the societal (in the sense of access to resources that are accessible in the community). A social identity model of recovery needs to be inclusive of multiple paths to recovery and support recovery service provision. Such a model should also create positive psychological benefits by generating trust through discussing growth and well-being rather than pathology and illness and challenging stigma by building on personal and social capabilities.[35] Thus, recovery within this approach relies not only on drive, commitment, and motivation but also on access to the social and community resources that will often act as the catalysts for positive change. For this reason, recovery support services will typically be much more outward- looking than their treatment equivalents.

- This will require a body of emerging research using multiple methods and is why the 'Life In Recovery' studies are important. They provide a way of showcasing and celebrating how many people recover, how diverse their pathways are to recovery, and how important is the support from other people. It is also of note that in several Life in Recovery (LIR) studies internationally,[41,42] around half of the participating sample was female, something rarely achieved in treatment studies of problem drinkers and drug users. This approach is also a way of demonstrating to families, communities, and professionals that people can and do recover and that they play an active role in their recovery journeys. In addition, these studies challenge stereotype ideas held by the general public as well as negative expectations about how people with addictions can change. They highlight the ways in which people in recovery make huge contributions to society and give back in many ways, including family involvement, employment, and volunteering in the community.

SUMMARY

If there is anything modern research on recovery is teaching us, it is two critical lessons: People with alcohol and drug problems—even the most severe of such problems—are not a homogenous population, and there are many pathways and styles of long-term recovery.[43]

Recovery is a complex and dynamic process influenced by individual, interpersonal, and community factors, as well as their interactions. Often, people with addiction have completely different recovery journeys. Some recover naturally, without formal treatment. Others enter the treatment cycle, usually repeatedly and use multiple mechanisms for change before they achieve long- term recovery. Some, unfortunately, never achieve sustained recovery. But what we know is that there are multiple paths to recovery and that 58%[44] of those with lifetime addiction do recover and achieve a satisfactory quality of life as contributing members of society. And what is clear about those who recover and what they have in common is that no one does it alone and long-term recovery does not happen in the clinic—it happens in the community.

What is the recovery agenda and movement going to provide? It is going to bring an agenda both for challenging the exclusion of addicted individuals and also for policy and research about how we can build on those successful recovery stories. Those unique stories of inspiration show that these people change—they grow and develop and become valuable citizens. This work is not about negating negative things but building positive things, starting from individuals and spreading and growing more generally. Within a social model for explaining and understanding recovery, we aim to develop a body of work around recovery that allows us to understand much more deeply the fundamental social processes that promote recovery and to understand that recovery is not just something that happens in people's heads or in clinics. It's something that happens between people and within people and allows society to grow and develop by reintegrating and allowing people to develop their potential and experience full human growth.

CLINICS CARE POINTS

- Addiction is complex but treatable, and people can and do recover—according to SAMHSA,[44] 58% of those with a lifetime substance use disorder (SUD) will eventually recover.

- No single recovery mechanism is right for everyone, but what applies to everyone is that people need to have quick access to recovery services that address their needs in a holistic way. Although more research is needed, there seems to be gender differences in recovery pathways and the LiR studies would also suggest that contextual and structural factors shape recovery pathways.

- We need to understand recovery from a psychosocial perspective as the person transitions in identity and network from those proscribed by using networks to networks that allow access to new resources and identities in the community. To sustain the gains made in specialist treatment services, continuing care service models must be holistic and provide strength-based connections and multiple pathways to support effective participation in and engagement with the community groups and activities and provide effective transitions to social and societal resources to continue the personal journey of growth beyond the clinic.

- Recovery capital depends on personal, interpersonal, and social factors. Clinicians and administrators are important actors in offering services beyond acute care and in building continuity of care and effective community integration aiming to improve recovery outcomes as well as the well-being and quality of life of people struggling with addiction.

DISCLOSURE

The authors have no conflicts of interest to declare.

REFERENCE

1. White WL. Recovery: Old wine, flavor of the month or new organizing paradigm? Subst Use Misuse 2008;43(12–13):1987–2000.
2. Strategy D. Reducing demand, restricting supply, building recovery: Supporting people to live a drug-free life. London: HM Government; 2010.
3. From harm to hope: A 10-year drugs plan to cut crime and save lives. UK Government. 2022. Available at: https://www.gov.uk/government/publications/from-harm-to-hope-a-10-year-drugs-plan-to-cut-crime-and-save-lives/from-harm-to-hope-a-10-year-drugs-plan-to-cut-crime-and-save-lives. Accessed January 30, 2022.
4. SAMHSA's working definitions of recovery. SAMHSA. 2022. Available at: https://store.samhsa.gov/sites/default/files/d7/priv/pep12-recdef.pdf.   Accessed January 23, 2022.
5. The Biden-Harris Administration's Statement of Drug Policy Priorities for Year One. Office of National Drug Control Policy. 2022. Available at: https://www.whitehouse.gov/wp-content/uploads/2021/03/BidenHarris-Statement-of-Drug-Policy-Priorities-April-1.pdf. Accessed January 30, 2022.
6. Panel TBFIC. What is recovery? A working definition from the Betty Ford Institute. J Subst Abuse Treat 2007;33(3):221–8.
7. Commission UDP. The UK policy Commission recovery Consensus group. A vision of recovery. London: UK Drug Policy Commission; 2008.
8. Best D, Bamber S, Battersby A, et al. Recovery and straw men: An analysis of the objections raised to the transition to a recovery model in UK addiction services. J Groups Addict Recovery 2010;5(3–4):264–88.
9. Dennis ML, Scott CK, Laudet A, et al. Beyond bricks and mortar: recent research on substance use disorder recovery management. Curr Psychiatry Rep 2014; 16(4):1–7.
10. Humphreys K, Lembke A. Recovery-oriented policy and care systems in the UK and USA. Drug alcohol Rev. 2014;33(1):13-18.
11. Recovery Cascades (Bill White and David Best). williamwhitepapers. 2021. Available at: http://www.williamwhitepapers.com/blog/2019/05/recovery-cascades-bill-white-and-david-best.html. Accessed December 12, 2021.
12. Best D, Vanderplasschen W, Van de Mheen D, et al. REC-PATH (Recovery Pathways): Overview of a four-country study of pathways to recovery from problematic drug use. Alcohol Treat Q 2018;36(4):517–29.
13. Martinelli TF, van de Mheen D, Best D, et al. Are members of mutual aid groups better equipped for addiction recovery? European cross-sectional study into recovery capital, social networks, and commitment to sobriety. Drugs Educ Prev Policy 2021;28(5):389–98.

14. Best D, Day E, Homayoun S, et al. Treatment retention in the Drug Intervention Programme: Do primary drug users fare better than primary offenders? Drugs Educ Prev Pol 2008;15(2):201–9.
15. Best D, Gow J, Knox T, et al. Mapping the recovery stories of drinkers and drug users in Glasgow: Quality of life and its associations with measures of recovery capital. Drug Alcohol Rev 2012;31(3):334–41.
16. Longabaugh R, Wirtz PW, Zywiak WH, et al. Network support as a prognostic indicator of drinking outcomes: The COMBINE study. J Stud Alcohol Drugs 2010; 71(6):837–46.
17. Litt MD, Kadden RM, Kabela-Cormier E, et al. Changing network support for drinking: Network support project 2-year follow-up. J Consult Clin Psychol 2009;77(2):229.
18. Zywiak WH, Neighbors CJ, Martin RA, et al. The Important People Drug and Alcohol interview: Psychometric properties, predictive validity, and implications for treatment. J Subst Abuse Treat 2009;36(3):321–30.
19. Best D, Beckwith M, Haslam C, et al. Overcoming alcohol and other drug addiction as a process of social identity transition: The social identity model of recovery (SIMOR). Addict Res Theor 2016;24(2):111–23.
20. Best D, Beswick T, Hodgkins S, et al. Recovery, ambitions, and aspirations: an exploratory project to build a recovery community by generating a skilled recovery workforce. Alcohol Treat Q 2016;34(1):3–14.
21. Best D, Lubman DI, Savic M, et al. Social and transitional identity: Exploring social networks and their significance in a therapeutic community setting. Ther Communities 2014;35(1):10–20.
22. Bliuc AM, Best D, Iqbal M, et al. Building addiction recovery capital through online participation in a recovery community. Social Sci Med 2017;193:110–7.
23. Jetten J, Haslam SA, Haslam C, et al. The case for a social identity analysis of health and well-being. The social cure: Identity, health and well-being. 2012:3-19.
24. Moos RH. Theory-based active ingredients of effective treatments for substance use disorders. Drug Alcohol Depend 2007;88(2–3):109–21.
25. Kelly JF. Is Alcoholics Anonymous religious, spiritual, neither? Findings from 25 years of mechanisms of behavior change research. Addict 2017;112(6):929–36.
26. Best D, Sondhi A, Brown L, et al. The strengths and barriers recovery scale (SABRS): relationships matter in building strengths and overcoming barriers. Front Psychol 2021. https://doi.org/10.3389/fpsyg.2021.663447. 12663447.
27. Best D. Pathways to recovery and desistance. Brighton, UK: Policy Press; 2019.
28. Best D, Ivers J-H. Inkspots and ice cream cones: A model of recovery contagion and growth. Addict Res Theor 2021;1–7.
29. Best D, Vanderplasschen W, Nisic M, et al. Measuring capital in active addiction and recovery: The development of the strengths and barriers recovery scale (SABRS). Substance Abuse Treat Prev Policy 2020;15(1):40.
30. Leamy M, Bird V, Le Boutillier C, et al. Conceptual framework for personal recovery in mental health: Systematic review and narrative synthesis. Br J Psychiatry 2011;199(6):445–52.
31. Laudet AB. The road to recovery: Where are we going and how do we get there? Empirically driven conclusions and future directions for service development and research. Subst Use Misuse 2008;43(12–13):2001–20.
32. Granfield R, Cloud W. Social context and "natural recovery": The role of social capital in the resolution of drug-associated problems. Subst Use Misuse 2001; 36(11):1543–70.
33. Best D, Laudet A. The potential of recovery capital. London: RSA; 2010.

34. Dennis ML, Foss MA, Scott CK, et al. An eight-year perspective on the relationship between the duration of abstinence and other aspects of recovery. Eval Rev 2007;31(6):585–612.

35. Best D, Hennessy EA. The science of recovery capital: Where do we go from here? Addiction 2022;117(4):1139–1145..

36. Groshkova T, Best D, White W, et al. The Assessment of Recovery Capital: Properties and psychometrics of a measure of addiction recovery strengths. Drug Alcohol Rev 2013;32(2):187–94.

37. Groshkova T, Best D, White W, et al. Recovery Group Participation Scale (RGPS): Factor structure in alcohol and heroin recovery populations. J Groups Addict Recovery 2011;6(1–2):76–92.

38. Cano I, Best D, Edwards M, et al. Recovery capital pathways: Modelling the components of recovery wellbeing. Drug Alcohol Depend 2017;181:11–9.

39. Laudet A. "Life in recovery": report on survey findings. Washington, DC: Faces & Voices of Recovery; 2013.

40. White WL. Peer-based addiction recovery support: history, theory, practice, and scientific evaluation executive summary. Madison, WI: Great Lakes Addiction Technology; 2009.

41. Best D, Savic M, Bathish R, et al. Life in Recovery in Australia and the United Kingdom: Do Stages of Recovery Differ Across National Boundaries? Alcohol Treat Q 2018;36(4):530–41.

42. Best D, Albertson K, Irving J, et al. The UK life in recovery survey 2015: The first national UK survey of addiction recovery experiences. 2015.

43. Topical Quotes from William White and Co-authors' Recovery Writings. William White Papers. 2022. Available at: http://williamwhitepapers.com/pr/Quotes%20from%20William%20White%20%26%20Co-authors%202015.pdf. Accessed January 23, 2022.

44. Sheedy CK, Whitter M. Guiding principles and elements of recovery-oriented systems of care: What do we know from the research? J Drug Addict Educ Eradication 2013;9(4):225.

The Protective Wall of Human Community

The New Evidence on the Clinical and Public Health Utility of Twelve-Step Mutual-Help Organizations and Related Treatments

John F. Kelly, PhD

KEYWORDS

- Alcoholics anonymous • 12-step • Mutual-help • Self-help • Twelve-step facilitation
- Addiction • Recovery

KEY POINTS

- Substance use disorders are often chronic conditions conferring a prodigious burden of disease, disability, and premature mortality in most middle- and high-income countries.
- Ubiquitous mutual-help organizations (MHOs), such as AA, despite being community-based and peer-led, are a de facto part of most societies' response to addressing the endemic problems caused by substance use disorders and are the most commonly sought source of help for alcohol and other drug (AOD) problems.
- Until recently little was known from a rigorous scientific standpoint about the clinical and public health utility of these organizations or about the efficacy of the clinical interventions (twelve-step facilitation [TSF]) designed to facilitate their use during and following treatment.
- Following a call for more research from the Institute of Medicine of the National Academy of Sciences in 1990, a flurry of rigorous randomized controlled trials (RCT), cost-effectiveness analyses, and studies of the mechanisms through which the largest recovery MHOs, AA, confers benefit, has revealed that AA and TSF interventions are valuable empirically supported, highly cost-effective, interventions that confer benefit through dynamically mobilizing a variety of therapeutic mechanisms.
- AA and similar freely available community-based 12-step and non-12-step (eg, SMART Recovery) MHOs may be the closest thing public health has to a "free lunch."

MGH Recovery Research Institute, Massachusetts General Hospital and Harvard Medical School, 151 Merrimac Street, 6th Floor, Boston, MA 02114, USA
E-mail address: jkelly11@mgh.harvard.edu

Psychiatr Clin N Am 45 (2022) 557–575
https://doi.org/10.1016/j.psc.2022.05.007
0193-953X/22/© 2022 Elsevier Inc. All rights reserved.

psych.theclinics.com

INTRODUCTION

For those with severe forms of alcohol and other drug (AOD) use disorders the duration of the clinical course of illness tends to be a lengthy one before initial (one year), and stable (five or more years), remission is achieved. **Boxes 1** and **2** As shown in **Fig. 1** for instance, studies show that it can take up to 8 years and around 4 to 5 treatment/ mutual-help participation episodes before adults treated for alcohol or other drug use disorders achieve initially sustained remission.[1-4] Furthermore, as shown on the right of this figure, it can take another roughly 5 years of continuing remission before the risk of meeting criteria for alcohol/drug use disorder in the ensuing year drops less than 15%—the annual rate in the general population of meeting criteria for an alcohol or other drug use disorder.[5-8]

Most countries respond to these endemic and often enduring problems by providing a system of professionally directed and delivered care and through a more unplanned reliance on freely available community-based services such as recovery-focused mutual-help organizations (MHOs). There are dozens of these organizations of varying size, scope, availability, accessibility, emphasis, philosophy, and practices.[9-11] The oldest and by far the most ubiquitous and influential of these is alcoholics anonymous (AA).

Beginning in 1930s Akron Ohio, in the United States, AA has expanded from 2 to roughly 2 million, members at any given time and has spread to more than 150 countries around the world. Its rapid growth and 12-step program and literature inspired the founding of myriad other 12-step organizations addressing other drug use disorders

---

Box 1
Clarifying 12-step terminology and concepts

- There is often confusion regarding the evidence on "AA" vs "12-step treatment." Also, within 12-step "treatments," there can be additional confusion. Most of the scientifically rigorous research evidence to date comes from outpatient rather than inpatient delivered models of care. The outpatient models which have provided most of the RCT evidence for AA have provided the most rigorous tests of so-called, "Twelve-Step Facilitation" (TSF) interventions which have been developed and tested in various formats (**Fig. 2**) including as a fully independent multi-session 12-step focused treatments (eg, Project MATCH TSF;[22]; see **Fig. 2A**); as a combined and integrated treatment (TSF infused with CBT elements; eg,[23]; see **Fig. 2B**); as part of an intensive outpatient program whereby one of the groups is dedicated to TSF (eg, Making AA Easier [MAAEZ];[24]; see **Fig. 2C**); or as a specific TSF modular add-on that is added on to the end of usual treatment—typically taking the form of a clinically facilitated "warm handoff" linkage to existing members (eg,[25-27]; see **Fig. 2D**).

- In contrast, "12-step treatment" as it is usually described, is delivered in residential facilities whereby it is harder to conduct RCTs (very high-quality quasi-experimental studies have been conducted; see,[28,29] but includes intensive immersion in 12-step philosophy and practices in preparation for linkage with community-based AA following discharge to help prevent relapse. Obviously, in both instances, these differing formal levels of care delivery are not direct tests of AA, per se. Rather, they are tests of clinical preparation, initial exposure (eg, through onsite 12-step meetings), and active linkage to these community-based organizations. To test the ability of AA itself to confer these benefits, additional tests of mediation are conducted under the auspices of these RCTs of TSF to uncover why it is that TSF treatments tend to produce better outcomes than comparison conditions such as cognitive-behavioral therapies (CBTs) (see,[30] and later in discussion). Such studies have shown that the reason why TSF confers this additional benefit in terms of sustaining remission is due to the fact that it engages more patients with AA and thereby, enhances outcomes.[23,31,32]

Box 2
Summary of the efficacy and effectiveness research on treatment step facilitation treatments

• Confusion regarding the clinical and public health utility of AA, other 12-Step mutual-help organizations (MHOs), and related 12-Step treatments, has persisted until relatively recently.

• Findings now reveal that, when AA and TSF interventions for alcohol use disorder are subjected to exactly the same scientific standards as other clinical interventions, AA/TSF performs at least as well on most outcomes, but better regarding helping patients achieve continuous abstinence and remission over time, and at a substantially reduced health care cost.

• For other drug use disorders, less high-quality research is available. Yet, this body of research shows a similar and highly promising pattern of results supporting the utility of groups such as cocaine anonymous, crystal methamphetamine anonymous, and narcotics anonymous for patients suffering from a variety of drug use disorders.

• Given the long-clinical course to initial and stable remission for addiction patients (see **Fig. 1**), these community-based recovery support resources have strong clinical and public utility that seem well matched the undulating course of addiction recovery.

as well as help for distraught family members who are trying to cope with the grave and enduring unpredictability of addiction (eg, Al Anon).

While growth, size, and longevity, offer one type of observational evidence for potential benefit—at least for some—it has not been until recently that the scientific picture regarding the verifiable clinical and public health utility of AA and 12-step clinical treatments that are designed to introduce and systematically encourage and provide linkage to AA (so-called, "Twelve-Step Facilitation" [TSF] treatments) has been clarified from a rigorous empirical standpoint.

This chapter reviews the background, significance, and scientific evidence on AA and TSF treatments in the treatment of AOD use disorders. In addition, the cost-effectiveness and mechanisms of behavior change through which AA has been shown to confer recovery benefits are reviewed revealing some intriguing findings that may bode well for the clinical and public utility of other types of recovery-focused mutual organizations.

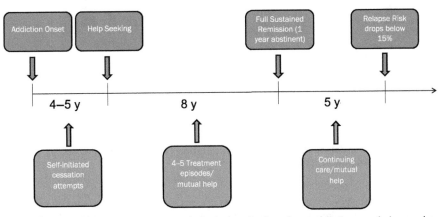

Fig. 1. Timeline of the clinical course of alcohol and other drug addiction remission and recovery for adult clinical cases.

Background and Significance

AA is a highly ubiquitous, indigenous, community recovery support resource. By design, the noncentralized and fully self-governing and financially self-supporting structure of AA outlined in its group guidance manual "Twelve Traditions,"[12] gave free authorization to anyone who wanted to start an AA group to do so, provided they generally kept to these AA traditions.[13] This meant, of course, that AA was less able to have much "quality control" over the week-to-week operation of AA groups, with the tradeoff being uninhibited dissemination which facilitated widespread adoption wherever people felt they needed it. This expansion was accelerated also by what might be considered an evangelical AA spirit of "carrying the message" of recovery to others in need that was embodied in AA's 12th step ("Having had a spiritual awakening as the result of these steps, we tried to carry the message to other alcoholics and to practice the principles in all of our affairs")[14]. This aspect of 12-step practice that potentially emanated from its Christian origins in the Oxford Group movement[15,16] was later supported therapeutically from a clinical standpoint in the construction of the "helper principle"—that helping others helps yourself[17] and in AA research itself.[18] The fact that AA adopted a law of "corporate poverty," never to own any property, declining any outside financial contributions to its operations, and even declining donations from its own members above a small annual amount (currently no more than $5000 per year;[19]) was, and remains, so highly unusual of any organization—even religious ones—that it gained favorable press and media coverage that helped the public gain awareness of AA and its methods.[20]

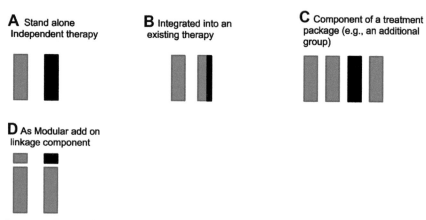

Fig. 2. Methods of delivery of twelve-step facilitation (TSF) techniques as compared with other types of treatments (TSF in black).

AA's accessibility and presumed positive impact were acknowledged and awarded over the years since its beginning. In 1956, AA was awarded the Lasker Award from the America Public Health Association (America's own version of the Nobel prize);

renowned Secretary of State, Henry Kissinger, described AA as "America's gift to the world"; and AA's main text was published in 1939 ("the Big Book"[14]; has a place among just 88 books in the US Library of Congress in the category of "books that have shaped America").

AA was winning and has won many accolades, but popularity and even public recognition and awards are not always commensurate with scientifically verifiable clinical and public health impacts. Nonetheless, AA and its philosophy made their way into nearly every addiction treatment program in the US and by the 1980s was the predominant model of US care for addiction.[16] The next section reviews the growing quantity and quality of evidence that has emerged during the past 70 years regarding AA.

Current Evidence

As reviewed in detail later in discussion, whereas the scientific picture of the true effectiveness of AA and related 12-step treatments has now been clarified, it was not until 1990 that an influential report from the US Institute of Medicine[21] of the National Academy of Sciences was published that highlighted the need for greater study in the of MHOs. "Broadening the Base of Treatment for Alcohol Problems"[21] explicitly requested more 12-step research be conducted and specifically on the mechanisms through which AA conferred benefit. For the first time, this legitimized serious scientific investigation into AA and 12-step treatment that brought with it funding support from the US National Institutes of Health (NIH), the Department of Veterans Affairs, and numerous private foundations. In the 30 years since, there has been a flurry of federally funded clinical trials, studies of health care cost offsets and cost-benefits analyses, and dozens of investigations of its mechanisms of behavior change, which has finally and convincingly revealed AA's clinical and public health utility, cost-benefits, and clarity on how it helps people into remission.

This section reviews the most rigorous scientific evidence on AA participation, 12-step clinical treatments designed to link patients with AA, and cost-effectiveness studies. It also reviews the mechanisms of behavior change research that has begun to uncover the therapeutic factors that are dynamically mobilized by AA participation over time.

Systematic Reviews and Meta-Analyses of the Evidence on Alcoholics Anonymous and 12-Step Treatments

The first systematic quantitative review of scientific research on AA was published in 1993.[33] At that time, it included studies conducted during the 1960s, 70s, and 80s, concluding that AA conferred a moderate beneficial effect on alcohol use outcomes. Yet, it also noted that the quality of the research up until the time of the review was generally methodologically poor, comprised of nearly all correlational, nonexperimental, investigations; low follow-up rates; and use of poorly validated measures with low content validity.[33,34] It also noted that the AA variable associated most strongly with future alcohol use reductions and abstinence was having an AA mentor known in AA terminology as an AA "sponsor" (ie, having a more experienced member with more sobriety duration who provides ongoing recovery coaching, advice, support, accountability, and role-modeling). As noted previously, as the initial request from the IOM,[21] dozens of clinical trials have been conducted to test the clinical utility and benefits and cost-benefits of introducing patients with alcohol use disorder to the 12-step philosophy and practices of AA and proactively linking patients with this free community-based resource.

By far the most rigorous review of the best evidence was summarized and published in the Cochrane Library in 2020.[30] The Cochrane library of systematic reviews is regarded worldwide as the gold standard in scientific rigor and is the organization that national governments and health agencies look to for informing and helping to guide decisions of health care protocol delivery for addressing a variety of high volume and high burden disorders including AOD use disorders.

The Cochrane review[30] included 27 studies published across 35 peer-reviewed papers and included almost 11,000 patients with mostly severe alcohol use disorder. In terms of included study designs, they had to be either randomized controlled trials (RCTs), or high-quality comparative effectiveness studies that followed patients prospectively over time. Any reported outcome was permissible with most of the studies reporting various types of abstinence-related outcomes (eg, proportion of patients who were completely abstinent at various follow-ups; the longest average period of abstinence; the percentage of days on which patients in the different treatment conditions were abstinent); the average intensity of alcohol use on days on which patients consumed alcohol (drinks per drinking day); or average heavy drinking days (usually 5 or more drinks); as well as combined indices of addiction severity measured typically via the Addiction Severity Index.[35] Despite all outcomes of any type being permissible for inclusion in the review, there were no measures included on quality of life or functioning in the published reports.

Economic analyses that examined the cost-effectiveness of different treatments were also included and examined for health care offset potential given that linking patients to freely available AA community resources was anticipated not only to help patients maintain remission but also to reduce the use of more expensive professional counseling and health care services (eg, emergency departments; overnight hospital stays).

The Cochrane review was coded also for studies that used manualized treatment approaches because having, and adhering to, a manual in treatment studies ensures that the presumed active ingredients of the therapy are actually delivered in an explicitly articulated way and are presumed to be a more scientifically rigorous test of the treatment. Also, manualized interventions can be replicated by others in different contexts to ensure that the effects of the therapy itself (ie, TSF) are not due to other factors.

Quite strikingly, compared with other active and theoretically well-grounded interventions to which TSF was compared, such as manualized and well-articulated cognitive-behavioral therapies (CBTs) and motivational enhancement therapies (METs), the TSF intervention linkage conditions to which patients had been randomly assigned were found to do as well as active comparison treatments on every single outcome measured except 2 whereby TSF outperformed such active comparison treatments: randomization to TSF resulted in substantially higher rates of continuous abstinence and remission from alcohol use disorder for up to 3 years following treatment; and TSF produced much greater health care cost savings of approximately $10,000 per patient over a 2 year period. When extrapolated to the US population of alcohol addiction patients treated annually in the United States, this resulted in a health care cost reduction in the region of $15 billion per year (in 2019 dollars) if all similar patients in the US were linked to AA.[30]

The magnitude of these differences in clinical outcomes and health cost savings is even more striking when one considers that many patients in the active comparison treatments who received CBT, MI/MET, or other interventions, also elected to attend AA in the posttreatment follow-up period making these effect size estimates more conservative with regard to the true effect of AA/TSF.

Additional research using sophisticated instrumental variable analyses that used randomization as the instrumental variable to rule out self-selection bias (Boef, Cessie, Dekkers, 2013), also provides additional strong scientific support for the benefit of TSF to AA linkages in improving patients' outcomes.[36]

Evidence on 12-Step Treatments and Community 12-Step Participation for Other Drug Use Disorders

Given the size and influence of alcohol use disorder in the substance use disorder (SUD) epidemiologic landscape, accounting for 75% of addiction cases nationally,[37] and thus the corresponding size and influence of AA, the vast majority of research on MHOs and related professional TSF linkage treatments have been conducted on patients with alcohol use disorder. A sizable scientific literature exists also, however, on RCTs and naturalistic observational studies for other drug use disorders.

Most of the more rigorous RCT studies of drug use disorders included patients who were addicted to cocaine (eg,[38]) or methamphetamine (eg,[39]). Naturalistic follow-up studies have included patients with a variety of drug use disorders (eg, opioids, cocaine, amphetamine/methamphetamine, cannabis) many of whom also had either a primary or secondary cooccurring alcohol use disorder.[40] A number of the more rigorous trials were summarized in another rigorous systematic review published by the Campbell Collaboration.[41] This systematic review found that TSF interventions performed as well on every outcome measured and found some advantage of TSF at shorter-term follow-ups. The evidence base for this review was much smaller, however, compared with that of patients with AA and alcohol use disorder, consisting of only 10 studies and only about 1000 total patients.

The quality of these drug use disorder-focused studies in the Bog and colleagues[41] review was judged to be generally of low quality. Consequently, more high-quality research is needed on TSF interventions and use of mutual-help groups (eg, NA, CA, Crystal Methamphetamine Anonymous [CMA], Marijuana Anonymous [MA]) for drug use disorders. That said, the Bog and colleagues[41] review did not include some landmark RCTs, such as the Cocaine Collaborative Study comparing three different psychosocial treatments for cocaine use disorder, one of which was a 12-step oriented counseling ("Individual Drug Counseling" [IDC] which was compared with a psychodynamically oriented "Supportive Expressive Therapy," as well as to a "Cognitive Therapy" specifically catering to drug use disorders;[38]); and the STAGE-12 study[39] for treating methamphetamine use disorder. It is possible that the cocaine collaborative investigation was not included because it may have not seemed in searches of "12-Step" because it did not explicitly mention that terminology in the titles or abstracts of the published studies. It is possible also that the STAGE-12 study was not included because it compared the experimental manualized intervention (STAGE-12) to "treatment-as-usual [TAU]" that also included 12-step elements. That said, the Cochrane Review on AA/TSF did include such studies and found a bigger benefit for the more well-articulated manualized AA/TSF interventions compared with TAU which often included elements of TSF. Both the Cocaine Collaborative study and the STAGE-12 RCTs found significant advantages for the manualized TSF treatments for cocaine[38] and methamphetamine use disorder,[39] respectively.

Regarding opioid use disorder, specifically, there have been numerous studies published on the effects of Narcotics Anonymous (NA), but none of these studies are of high quality from a rigorous scientific standpoint that allows for clear causal attributions to be made.[42,43] Emerging evidence from statistically controlled prospective observational studies do show positive salubrious relationships between NA participation and better opioid use disorder outcomes, particularly increased abstinence and enhanced adherence to medications for the treatment of opioid use disorder.[44,45]

NA attendance has been shown associated with better opioid outcomes among those with opioid use disorder in buprenorphine treatment,[44] in buprenorphine or extended-release naltrexone treatment, or over the long-term independent of buprenorphine or methadone engagement.[45] In a long-term follow-up of participants in the Prescription Opioid Addiction Treatment Study, NA mutual-help attendance was associated with twice the rate of abstinence independent of buprenorphine or methadone engagement more than 3 years after entering the trial.[45] Professionally delivered behavioral treatment in that study, on the other hand, was not associated with opioid abstinence.

During a 24-week RCT comparing buprenorphine to extended-release naltrexone,[46] whereby all participants were offered individual and group therapy, and could attend 12-Step MHOs in the community, both self-selected 12-Step MHO attendance and individual therapy, but not group therapy, were associated with significantly greater opioid abstinence at the end of the trial controlling for treatment arm, baseline heroin use, and other clinical and demographic characteristics.[47] Each additional 1 hour (ie, 1 NA meeting) was uniquely associated with 5% increased odds of abstinence. Interestingly, individual therapy and NA attendance had multiplicative benefits on opioid abstinence, suggesting that the combination may offer unique recovery benefits.

Also, in a 6-month randomized trial comparing standard to intensive outpatient treatment, in which all participants received buprenorphine, self-selected attendance at NA meetings was associated with both treatment retention and abstinence during the 6-month study.[44] Controlling for demographic characteristics, treatment site, group therapy attendance, and counselor requirements to attend NA, each additional NA meeting attended was uniquely associated with 2% increased odds of treatment retention and 1% increased odds of abstinence.

These positive effects are perhaps somewhat surprising given NA's official, more negative, stance on agonist medication use in the treatment of opioid use disorder (buprenorphine, methadone), in particular, as such individuals are sometimes viewed as still being under the influence of opioids and therefore not yet in "real" recovery.[48] The Monico and colleagues[44] provide some helpful insights from extensive qualitative work as to how patients on medications for opioid use disorder are able to nevertheless use NA and benefit from participation. On the whole, however, much more research is needed on NA given its size, influence, accessibility, as well as its potential to assist many with opioid and other drug use disorders to achieve and sustain remission over the longer term.

How Do 12-Step Mutual-Help Organizations Confer Benefit: Research on the Mechanisms of Behavior Change?

As noted above, since the request for more rigorous research on the clinical and public health utility of AA and related professional treatments and greater understanding of its mechanisms, dozens of rigorous clinical trials have been conducted along with dozens of sophisticated mechanisms of behavior change studies. Largely funded by the National Institutes of Health (NIH) and the Department of Veterans Affairs, these studies have uncovered some of the many mechanisms through which AA confers benefit over time. Although the following review of such mechanism's research pertains specifically to AA participation, it is likely that many of these same mechanisms are mobilized by participation in other 12-Step, as well as non–12-Step, MHOs (eg, SMART Recovery, LifeRing, and so forth) as many of the same broad-based therapeutic dynamics are likely common to all types of groups.[49]

Of note, 12-Step organizations' own theory about how recovery is purportedly achieved is through what it terms a "spiritual awakening." Although this was conceived initially to take the form of a sudden quantum shift in outlook and functioning (a new "God consciousness,"[50] that facilitated the ability to recover from deadly alcohol addiction, this notion was later expanded to include many member's recovery experiences that were characterized by more of a gradual change in outlook and functioning of the "educational variety"[50]. While much remains to be investigated regarding the examination of AA's mechanisms, most of the existing body of research has revealed that AA confers relapse prevention and recovery benefit mostly by successfully mobilizing changes across multiple domains simultaneously; notably helping participants exclude heavy drinking/drug using individuals from their social networks and adopting abstaining and recovering individuals into their social networks.[51–53] It also been shown to enhance recovery motivation and abstinence self-efficacy[54–58] as well boost cognitive-behavioral relapse prevention skills,[55,58] reduce impulsivity,[59] and reduce craving.[60] Empirical tests of some of its other central purported mechanisms such as spirituality[61,62]; J. S.[63] have demonstrated that enhancing spiritual practices is one of the mechanisms through which AA also confers relapse prevention benefit. Other tests of AA's central theoretic mechanisms through which the organization itself purports to prevent relapse (ie, through decreasing anger/resentment; and reducing self-centeredness),[14,50] have also been tested but have not been supported as mechanisms of behavior change (eg, anger;[64] self-centeredness.[63];) Reductions in symptoms of negative affect (depression symptoms) as a potential mechanism through which AA prevents relapse have also been rigorously tested showing that AA does reduce negative affect, but this reduction by itself may not relate to reductions in relapse risk in rigorously controlled analyses.[52]

Given that each of these studies almost without exception tested only a single mediating variable (eg, abstinence self-efficacy alone or social networks alone), finding support for each one's ability to explain at least some of AA's beneficial recovery effects, a question has remained as to what are the most salient and important mechanisms through which AA confers a benefit.

The answer to this question was elucidated in several published studies testing multiple mechanisms simultaneously.[52,65,66] In these tests of "multiple mediation," we incorporated six different mediators simultaneously that had been shown previously in individual mediator analyses to explain, at least in part, AA's beneficial effects on increasing abstinence and reducing relapse risk (see schematic in **Fig. 3**). Of note, we also examined variables that may have influenced the degree to which these multiple mechanisms helped AA participants reduce relapse risk (ie, we conducted tests of moderated multiple mediations). These sets of analyses, thus, examined questions such as: 1. What are the most important mechanisms through which AA confers benefit? 2. Do the various ways in which patients benefit from AA differ by addiction severity ([66]; **Fig. 4A**) by gender[52]; (**Fig. 4B**) or by age ([65]; **Fig. 4C**).

Intriguingly, the mechanisms through which AA is shown to reduce relapse risk differ in nature and magnitude and also across different characteristics (ie, addiction severity; gender; age). As highlighted in **Fig. 4A**, for more severely addicted "aftercare" patients, AA was shown to increase abstinence (percent days abstinent [PDA]) and reduce the intensity of alcohol use (drinks per drinking day [DDD]) mostly by the mobilization of adaptive changes in patients' social networks, but also by boosting spirituality which in turn reduced relapse risk. Of note, spirituality was not found to be a mediator for the less severely addicted "outpatient" patients. Instead, the vast majority of the effect of the way that AA participation helped the less severely addicted patients recover, was through facilitating adaptive changes in their social networks and by boosting confidence in their ability to cope with high-risk social situations without drinking (ie, by enhancing abstinence social self-efficacy).

When testing whether men and women differ in the ways that AA aids their addiction recovery (see **Fig. 3**), analyses demonstrated that men and women both derived equal overall relapse prevention benefits from participation in AA, but the ways in which they

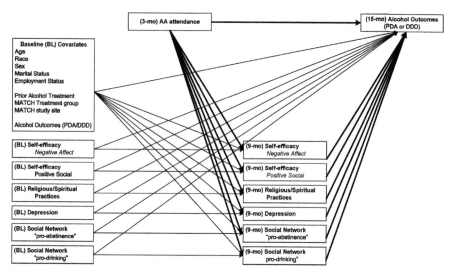

Fig. 3. Schematic of the mechanisms of behavior change studies testing the relative importance of six mediators of relapse prevention effects from AA participation. Note: "Pro-drinking" is measured to assess AA's ability to *reduce* pro-drinking social network members. DDD, drinks per drinking day; PDA, percent days abstinent. (Figure reproduced from Kelly, Hoeppner, Stout, Pagano (2012), Determining the relative importance of the mechanisms of behavior change within Alcoholics Anonymous: A multiple mediator analysis. *Addiction 107(2):289-99.*)

benefitted differed significantly and dramatically.[52] Among women, for example, by far the most significant way that AA helped them to prevent relapse was by boosting their confidence in their ability to cope with negative affect without drinking (ie, by enhancing their negative affect-specific abstinence self-efficacy) and by reducing depression symptoms. Interestingly, men showed a strikingly different picture. Among men, by far the most salient way that AA helped them prevent relapse was by boosting their confidence in their ability to cope with high-risk social situations whereby alcohol was present without drinking and by helping men shift their social networks toward recovery-oriented ones.

The magnitude of these differences was stark and highlights the different types of biobehavioral and social context relapse risk factors facing men and women with alcohol addiction during the mid-stage of the life course: for men, the biggest risk for relapse seems to involve direct and indirect alcohol cue exposure in social contexts; for women, it is the experience of negative affect.[52]

A further analysis compared young adults (18–29 years old) to older adults (30+ years old) again to investigate whether the mechanisms through which AA helped prevent youth relapse were different from those aiding older addicted patients ([67]; see **Fig. 3**).

Noteworthy in these moderated multiple mediation analyses, was that young adults derived the same degree of relapse prevention benefit as older adults but once again the ways that this occurred differed in nature and magnitude across the 2 cohorts.

First, the set of 6 mediators (see **Fig. 3**) was only able to account for about 25% of the direct effect of AA in preventing relapse — this was half of that explained by these same 6 mediators for older adults. Second, the most striking way that AA helped young adults recover was by helping them exclude heavy drinking/drug using

Aftercare (PDA)

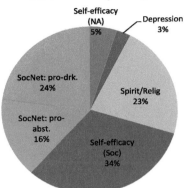

Aftercare (DDD)

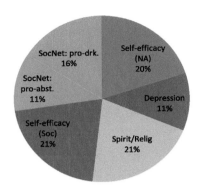

Outpatient (PDA)

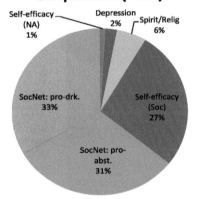

Outpatient (DDD)

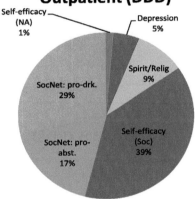

Fig. 4. (*A*) Figure reproduced from Kelly, Hoeppner, Stout, Pagano (2012), Determining the relative importance of the mechanisms of behavior change within Alcoholics Anonymous: A multiple mediator analysis. *Addiction 107(2):289-99.* (*B*) Figure reproduced from Kelly and Hoeppner (2013), Does Alcoholics Anonymous work differently for men and women? A moderated multiple-mediation analysis in a large clinical sample. *Drug and Alcohol Dependence, 130*(1–3), 186-193. (*C*). Figure based on data from Hoeppner, Hoeppner, Kelly (2014), Do young people benefit from AA as much, and in the same ways, as adult aged 30+? A moderated multiple mediation analysis. *Drug and Alcohol Dependence.* 143, 181-188. DDD, average drinks per drinking day; PDA, average percentage of days on which participants were abstinence from alcohol.

individuals from their social networks. The magnitude of this mediated effect was about twice that of their older adult counterparts (see **Fig. 4**A "pro-drink" segment). Interestingly, unlike the older adults, who benefitted from AA also by it helping them adopt abstainers and recovering individuals into their social networks, AA was not found to work through this mechanism for young adults. The exact reason for this big difference remains unclear, but one plausible explanation is the relative dearth of young adults in AA compared with older adults,[68,69] making it simply more challenging for young adults to find new significant social network members in AA with whom such members can associate.

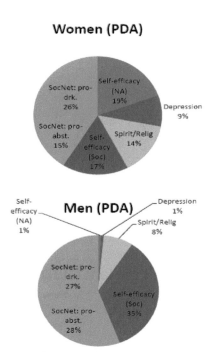

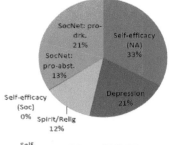

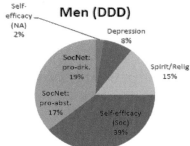

Fig. 4. (*continued*).

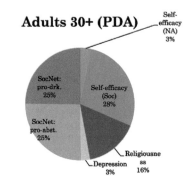

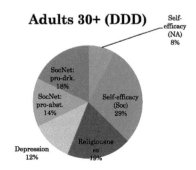

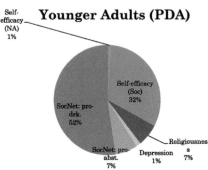

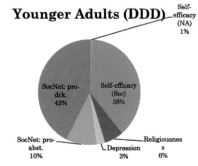

Fig. 4. (*continued*).

It is also noteworthy, that the 6 mediators that explained 50% of the direct of AA in preventing relapse for older adults, only explained 25% of this direct effect among young adults, despite young adults deriving the same degree of recovery benefit as their older adult counterparts. This means that we still have a lot to learn and investigate regarding how young adults, in particular, are benefiting from groups such as AA.

Summary of the Mechanisms of Behavior Change Research and Related Implications

In sum, this rigorous body of research on mechanisms of behavior change highlights a number of empirically supported mechanisms through which AA has been shown to confer benefit (**Fig. 5**). The findings have some potentially significant implications for how exactly AA and possibly other 12-step MHOs work to initiate and support addiction recovery.

The set of findings suggests the way AA works may have a closer fit with the broader pragmatic social, cognitive, and behavioral aspects of how its members stay sober documented in its later publications[70] than with its principle and original text, the *Big Book*[14,50] first published in 1935 when the fellowship numbered only about 100 and consisted mostly of very severely addicted male patients (only 4 women), and based on the relatively little accumulation of sober experience (ie, most had short lengths of sobriety with a maximum of 3 to 4 years at the time of writing). The Big Book, first published in 1939[14]—with the main text remaining almost completely unchanged in the intervening years—relies heavily on the supposition that the liberating and curative active ingredients of recovery are explicitly spiritual as noted in its 12th step—"Having had a spiritual awakening as the result of these steps we tried to carry

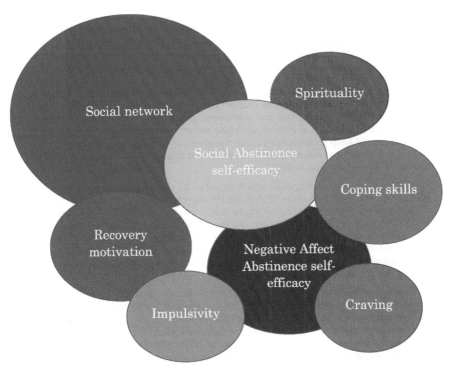

Fig. 5. Empirically supported mechanisms of behavior change through which alcoholics anonymous has been shown to confer recovery benefit.

the message to other alcoholics and practice the principles in all our affairs." Interestingly, we have found support for "spirituality" being an important mechanism of behavior change in relapse prevention and recovery for AA participants, but only for those with more severe addiction.[66,71] Consequently, given the clear severity of the documented addiction cases on which the Big Book[14,50] and its 12-Step program is based, the reflections of the AA founders and early members that highlighted spirituality as an essential component of recovery may have been consistent with their actual observations at that time of these very severe cases (ie, spirituality was the answer). As the organization grew in size to several million;[9]), however, and become more demographically and clinically inclusive in the following decades (that is, about one-third are women and AA participants exhibit a broad range of clinical severity,[72,73] it facilitated entry for less severe cases who seem to benefit from a variety of additional therapeutic elements that support recovery; and, for most, these benefits need not always include an explicit spiritual component.[71] This, of course, may mean that irrespective of spiritual beliefs, or the degree of engagement with 12-Step specific spiritual philosophy or practices, many prospective AA participants can still benefit to a large degree from engagement with AA or other recovery specific 12-Step organizations.

For clinical providers, there are now numerous manualized, empirically supported TSF intervention protocols available that if adopted and implemented in clinical care settings are likely to produce higher rates of continuous remission or otherwise as good clinical outcomes as delivering other kinds of commonly used clinical interventions (eg, MET, CBT), while simultaneously providing greater reductions in health care costs.

CLINICS CARE POINTS

- For individuals with SUD who have also received professional treatment, clinicians' opinions about mutual-help organizations (MHOs) such as AA, can have an impact on whether or not patients will attend.[74] Some clinicians may be unfamiliar with or object to particular aspects of 12-step (eg, spirituality). Some clinicians may not realize the potential of available community support networks to help sustain and complement professional treatment efforts and may even actively dissuade patients from participating in groups such as AA. Because of the increasingly compelling evidence base in favor of the use of MHOs, particularly, AA, for alcohol use disorder, and the fact that professionals have been found to substantially influence the likelihood that patients with SUD will attend such groups (for example,[74] clinicians should keep an open mind about the potential of these free, community-based resources to serve as a useful adjunct to treatment or as a form of continuing care after professional treatment has ended.

- Patients may oppose participation in AA or other 12-step organizations on grounds of spiritual incompatibility or other 12-step-specific aspects. In such cases, it can be helpful to inquire if such patients would be willing to sample other non-12 step alternatives such as SMART Recovery or LifeRing. There are also more religious alternatives to 12-step organizations, such as Celebrate Recovery (based on Christianity) and Refuge Recovery (based on Buddhist principles and practices). Some of these may be more palatable for certain patients. Also, some patients use a combination of mutual-help alternatives to help achieve and sustain remission.

- For reluctant individuals who may be willing nonetheless to at least sample some AA or other types of mutual-help meetings without investing too much effort or travel time, there are numerous online portals (eg, In The Rooms) that provide opportunities to observe, listen, and experience the nature and content of such meetings without the need to travel long distances or actively talk or otherwise participate. These might be prescribed as a way to introduce mutual-help practices to prospective patients who stand to benefit.

SUMMARY

A flurry of federally funded rigorous randomized clinical trials, cost-effectiveness, and mechanisms of behavior change studies during the past 30 years have now clarified the clinical and public utility and cost-benefits of AA, and also elucidated how AA confers benefits over time. In sum, a number of different modalities of professionally delivered TSF treatments demonstrate that these fairly unsophisticated linkages work at least as well as other empirically supported treatments such as cognitive-behavioral treatments on most outcomes, but TSF is able to produce superior outcomes when it comes to continuous abstinence and remission for alcohol use disorder. TSF also results in substantially reduced health care costs as patients are being admitted less frequently to the hospital or ED and also are relying more on peers with lived experience of active addiction and successful long-term recovery from it to remedy a variety of psychological challenges free of charge. AA and other ubiquitous, freely accessible and flexible, recovery-focused MHOs seem to be well-suited to the ongoing undulating course of addiction recovery risk. Given the burden of disease, disability, premature mortality, and economic costs, attributable to AOD use disorders annually in the United States and most other middle- and high-income countries globally, their ubiquity and utility may well be the closest thing public health has to a "free lunch."

DISCLOSURE

Dr J.F. Kelly has received research funding from the National Institutes of Health (NIAAA, NIDA, NIMH), the Substance Abuse and Mental Health Services Administration (SAMHSA), the Department of Veterans Affairs, as well as state governments, and charitable foundations to conduct research on addiction, treatment, and recovery support services.

REFERENCES

1. De Soto CB, O'Donnell WE, et al. Long-term recovery in alcoholics. Alcohol Clin Exp Res 1989;13(5):693–7.
2. Dennis ML, Scott CK, Funk R, et al. The duration and correlates of addiction and treatment careers. J Subst Abuse Treat 2005;28(Suppl 1):S51–62.
3. Nathan PE, Skinstad AH. Outcomes of treatment for alcohol problems: current methods, problems, and results. J Consult Clin Psychol 1987;55(3):332–40.
4. Wang PS, Berglund P, Olfson M, et al. Failure and delay in initial treatment contact after first onset of mental disorders in the National Comorbidity Survey Replication. Arch Gen Psychiatry 2005;62(6):603–13.
5. Dawson DA. Correlates of past-year status among treated and untreated persons with former alcohol dependence: United States, 1992. Alcohol Clin Exp Res 1996; 20(4):771–9.
6. Dennis ML, Foss MA, Scott CK. An eight-year perspective on the relationship between the duration of abstinence and other aspects of recovery. Eval Rev 2007; 31(6):585–612.
7. Jin H, Rourke SB, Patterson TL, et al. Predictors of relapse in long-term abstinent alcoholics. J Stud Alcohol 1998;59(6):640–6.
8. Schutte KK, Byrne FE, Brennan PL, et al. Successful remission of late-life drinking problems: a 10-year follow-up. J Stud Alcohol 2001;62(3):322–34. Available at: http://www.ncbi.nlm.nih.gov/pubmed/11414342.

9. Humphreys K. Circles of recovery: self-help organizations for addictions. Cambridge, UK: Cambridge University Press; 2004.

10. Kelly JF, White WL. Broadening the base of addiction mutual-help organizations. J Groups Addict Recover 2012;7(2–4):82–101.

11. Kelly JF, Yeterian JD. Mutual-help groups for alcohol and other substance use disorders. In: McCrady BS, Epstein EE, editors. Addictions: a comprehensive guidebook. Oxford, UK: Oxford University Press; 2013. p. 500–25.

12. Alcoholics Anonymous. Twelve steps and twelve traditions. Center City, MN: Alcoholics Anonymous World Services; 1952.

13. Kurtz, E. (1991). Not-God: A History of Alcoholics Anonymous. Hazelden.

14. Alcoholics. Anonymous. Alcoholics Anonymous: The story of how thousands of men and women have recovered from alcoholism. New York, NY: Alcoholics Anonymous World Services; 1939.

15. Oxford Group. What is the Oxford group? Oxford, England: Oxford University Press; 1933.

16. White WL. Slaying the dragon: The history of addiction treatment and recovery in America. 2nd edition. Normal, IL: Chestnut Health Systems/Lighthouse Institute; 2014.

17. Riessman F. The 'helper therapy' principle. Soc Work 1965;10:27–32.

18. Pagano ME, Friend KB, Tonigan JS, et al. Helping other alcoholics in alcoholics anonymous and drinking outcomes: findings from project MATCH. J Stud Alcohol 2004;65(6):766–73. Available at: https://www.ncbi.nlm.nih.gov/pubmed/15700515.

19. Alcoholics Anonymous. Alcoholics Anonymous Contributions - FAQs. 2022. Retrieved March 21, 2022 from. https://contribution.aa.org/sca-dev-2020-1/checkout.ssp?is=checkout&lang=en_US#/frequently-asked-questions.

20. Alcoholics Anonymous. (1957). Alcoholics Anonymous Comes of Age. AA World Services.

21. Institute of Medicine. Broadening the base of treatment for alcohol problems. New York, NY: The National Academies Press; 1990. Available at: http://www.nap.edu/catalog/1341/broadening-the-base-of-treatment-for-alcohol-problems.

22. Nowinski, J., Baker, S., & Carroll, K. (1992). Twelve Step Facilitation Therapy Manual: A Clinical Research Guide for Therapists Treating Individuals with Alcohol Abuse and Dependence.

23. Walitzer KS, Dermen KH, Barrick C. Facilitating involvement in Alcoholics Anonymous during out-patient treatment: a randomized clinical trial. Addiction 2009;104(3):391–401.

24. Kaskutas LA, Subbaraman MS, Witbrodt J, et al. Effectiveness of Making Alcoholics Anonymous Easier: a group format 12-step facilitation approach. J Subst Abuse Treat 2009;37(3):228–39.

25. Sisson RW, Mallams JH. The use of systematic encouragement and community access procedures to increase attendance at Alcoholic Anonymous and Al-Anon meetings. Am J Drug Alcohol Abuse 1981;8(3):371–6. Available at: https://www.ncbi.nlm.nih.gov/pubmed/7340507.

26. Timko C, Debenedetti A, Billow R. Intensive referral to 12-Step self-help groups and 6-month substance use disorder outcomes. Addiction 2006;101(5):678–88.

27. Tonigan Rynes K, Toscova R, et al. Do changes in selfishness explain 12-step benefit? A prospective lagged analysis. Substance Abuse 2013;34(1):13–9.

28. Humphreys K, Moos R. Can encouraging substance abuse patients to participate in self-help groups reduce demand for health care? A quasi-experimental study.

Alcohol Clin Exp Res 2001;25(5):711–6. Available at: https://www.ncbi.nlm.nih. gov/pubmed/11371720.

29. Humphreys K, Moos RH. Encouraging posttreatment self-help group involvement to reduce demand for continuing care services: two-year clinical and utilization outcomes. Alcohol Clin Exp Res 2007;31(1):64–8.

30. Kelly JF, Humphreys K, Ferri M. Alcoholics Anonymous and other 12-step programs for alcohol use disorder. Cochrane Database Syst Rev 2020. https://doi. org/10.1002/14651858.CD012880.pub2.

31. Litt MD, Kadden RM, Kabela-Cormier E, et al. Changing network support for drinking: network support project 2-year follow-up. J Consult Clin Psychol 2009;77(2):229–42.

32. Longabaugh R, Wirtz PW, Zweben A, et al. Network support for drinking, Alcoholics Anonymous and long-term matching effects. Addiction 1998;93(9): 1313–33. Available at: https://www.ncbi.nlm.nih.gov/pubmed/9926538.

33. Emrick CD, Tonigan JS, Montgomery H, et al. Alcoholics anonymous: what is currently known?. In: McCrady BS, Miller WR, editors. Research on alcoholics anonymous: opportunities and alternatives. New Brunswick, NJ: Rutgers Center of Alcohol Studies; 1993. p. 41–76.

34. Tonigan JS, Toscova R, Miller WR. Meta-analysis of the literature on Alcoholics Anonymous: sample and study characteristics moderate findings. J Stud Alcohol 1996;57(1):65–72. Available at: https://www.ncbi.nlm.nih.gov/pubmed/8747503.

35. McLellan AT, Kushner H, Metzger D, et al. The Fifth Edition of the Addiction Severity Index. J Subst Abuse Treat 1992;9(3):199–213.

36. Humphreys K, Blodgett JC, Wagner TH. Estimating the efficacy of Alcoholics Anonymous without self-selection bias: an instrumental variables re-analysis of randomized clinical trials. Alcohol Clin Exp Res 2014;38(11):2688–94.

37. Substance Abuse and Mental Health Services Administration. Key substance use and mental health indicators in the United States: Results from the 2020 National Survey on Drug Use and Health (Vol. HHS Publication No. PEP21-07-01-003, NSDUH Series H-56)). Cent Behav Health Stat Qual 2021. Available at: https:// www.samhsa.gov/data/sites/default/files/reports/rpt35325/NSDUHFFRPDFWHT MLFiles2020/2020NSDUHFFR1PDFW102121.pdf.

38. Crits-Christoph P, Siqueland L, Blaine J, et al. Psychosocial treatments for cocaine dependence: National Institute on Drug Abuse Collaborative Cocaine Treatment Study. Arch Gen Psychiatry 1999;56(6):493–502. https://doi.org/10. 1001/archpsyc.56.6.493.

39. Donovan DM, Daley DC, Brigham GS, et al. Stimulant abuser groups to engage in 12-step: a multisite trial in the National Institute on Drug Abuse Clinical Trials Network. J Substance Abuse Treat 2013;44(1):103–14.

40. Gossop M, Stewart D, Marsden J. Attendance at Narcotics Anonymous and Alcoholics Anonymous meetings, frequency of attendance and substance use outcomes after residential treatment for drug dependence: a 5-year follow-up study. Addiction 2008;103(1):119–25.

41. Bog M, Filges T, Brannstrom L, et al. 12-step programs for reducing illicit drug-use: A systematic review. Campbell Syst Rev 2017.

42. White W, Galanter M, Humphreys K, et al. The paucity of attention to narcotics anonymous in current public, professional, and policy responses to rising opioid addiction. Alcohol Treat Q 2016;34(4):437–62.

43. White W, Galanter M, Humphreys K, et al. "We Do Recover": Scientific Studies on Narcotics Anonymous. 2020. Available at: http://www.williamwhitepapers.com/pr/ dlm_uploads/2020-Review-of-Scientific-Studies-on-NA.pdf.

44. Monico LB, Gryczynski J, Mitchell SG, et al. Buprenorphine Treatment and 12-step Meeting Attendance: Conflicts, Compatibilities, and Patient Outcomes. J Subst Abuse Treat 2015;57:89–95.

45. Weiss RD, Griffin ML, Marcovitz DE, et al. Correlates of opioid abstinence in a 42-month posttreatment naturalistic follow-up study of prescription opioid dependence. J Clin Psychiatry 2019;80(2):18m12292.

46. Lee JD, Nunes EV Jr, Novo P, et al. Comparative effectiveness of extended-release naltrexone versus buprenorphine-naloxone for opioid relapse prevention (X: BOT): a multicentre, open-label, randomised controlled trial. Lancet 2018; 391(10118):309–18.

47. Harvey LM, Fan W, Cano M, et al. Psychosocial intervention utilization and substance abuse treatment outcomes in a multisite sample of individuals who use opioids. J Subst Abuse Treat 2020;112:68–75.

48. Narcotics Anonymous. Wolrd service board of trustees bulletin #29: regarding methadone and other drug replacement programs. 1996. Retrieved March 21, 2022 from https://na.org/?ID=bulletins-bull29. .

49. Kelly JF, Magill M, Stout RL. How do people recover from alcohol dependence? A systematic review of the research on mechanisms of behavior change in Alcoholics Anonymous. Addict Res Theor 2009;17(3):236–59.

50. Alcoholics Anonymous. Alcoholics anonymous: the story of how thousands of men and women have recovered from alcoholism. 4th edition. New York, NY: Alcoholics Anonymous World Services; 2001.

51. Kaskutas LA, Bond J, Humphreys K. Social networks as mediators of the effect of Alcoholics Anonymous. Addiction 2002;97(7):891–900.

52. Kelly JF, Hoeppner BB. Does Alcoholics Anonymous work differently for men and women? A moderated multiple-mediation analysis in a large clinical sample. Drug Alcohol Depend 2013;130(1–3):186–93.

53. Witbrodt J, Kaskutas LA. Does diagnosis matter? Differential effects of 12-step participation and social networks on abstinence. Am J Drug Alcohol Abuse 2005;31(4):685–707. Available at: http://www.ncbi.nlm.nih.gov/entrez/query.fcgi?cmd=Retrieve&db=PubMed&dopt=Citation&list_uids=16320441.

54. Bogenschutz MP, Tonigan JS, Miller WR. Examining the effects of alcoholism typology and AA attendance on self-efficacy as a mechanism of change. J Stud Alcohol 2006;67(4):562–7. Available at: http://www.ncbi.nlm.nih.gov/entrez/query.fcgi?cmd=Retrieve&db=PubMed&dopt=Citation&list_uids=16736076.

55. Kelly JF, Myers MG, Brown SA. A multivariate process model of adolescent 12-step attendance and substance use outcome following inpatient treatment. Psychol Addict Behav 2000;14(4):376–89.

56. Kelly JF, Myers MG, Brown SA. Do adolescents affiliate with 12-step groups? A multivariate process model of effects. J Stud Alcohol 2002;63(3):293–304. Available at: https://www.ncbi.nlm.nih.gov/pubmed/12086130.

57. Kelly JF, Urbanoski KA, Hoeppner BB, et al. Ready, willing, and (not) able" to change: young adults' response to residential treatment. Drug Alcohol Depend 2012;121(3):224–30.

58. Morgenstern J, Labouvie E, McCrady BS, et al. Affiliation with Alcoholics Anonymous after treatment: a study of its therapeutic effects and mechanisms of action. J Consult Clin Psychol 1997;65(5):768–77. Available at: https://www.ncbi.nlm.nih.gov/pubmed/9337496.

59. Blonigen DM, Timko C, Moos RH. Alcoholics Anonymous and reduced impulsivity: a novel mechanism of change [Research Support, N.I.H., Extramural

Research Support, U.S. Gov't, Non-P.H.S.]. Substance Abuse 2013;34(1):4–12. https://doi.org/10.1080/08897077.2012.691448.

60. Kelly JF, Greene MC. The twelve promises of alcoholics anonymous: psychometric validation and mediational testing as a 12-step specific mechanism of behavior change. Drug Alcohol Depend 2013;133(2):633–40.

61. Kelly JF, Stout RL, Magill M, et al. Spirituality in recovery: a lagged mediational analysis of alcoholics anonymous' principal theoretical mechanism of behavior change. Alcohol Clin Exp Res 2011;35(3):454–63.

62. Krentzman AR, Cranford JA, Robinson EA. Multiple dimensions of spirituality in recovery: a lagged mediational analysis of Alcoholics Anonymous' principal theoretical mechanism of behavior change. Substance Abuse 2013;34(1):20–32.

63. Tonigan JS, Rynes KN, McCrady BS. Spirituality as a change mechanism in 12-step programs: A replication, extension, and refinement. Subst Use Misuse 2013; 48(12):1161–73. https://doi.org/10.3109/10826084.2013.808540. Available at:.

64. Kelly JF, Stout RL, Tonigan JS, et al. Negative affect, relapse, and Alcoholics Anonymous (AA): does AA work by reducing anger? [Research Support, N.I.H., Extramural]. J Stud Alcohol Drugs 2010;71(3):434–44. Available at: https://www.ncbi.nlm.nih.gov/pubmed/20409438.

65. Hoeppner B, Hoeppner S, Kelly JF. Does AA work differently for younger people? A moderated multiple mediation analysis. Int J Behav Med 2014;21:S215 <Go to ISI>://WOS:000209816100746.

66. Kelly JF, Hoeppner B, Stout RL, et al. Determining the relative importance of the mechanisms of behavior change within Alcoholics Anonymous: a multiple mediator analysis. Addiction 2012;107(2):289–99.

67. Hoeppner BB, Hoeppner SS, Kelly JF. Do young people benefit from AA as much, and in the same ways, as adult aged 30+? A moderated multiple mediation analysis. Drug Alcohol Depend 2014;143:181–8.

68. Alcoholics Anonymous World Services. 2014 Membership Survey. A.A. World Services Inc. 2014. Retrieved March 21, 2022 from. http://www.aa.org/assets/en_US/p-48_membershipsurvey.pdf.

69. American Psychiatric Association. Diagnostic and statistical manual of mental disorders. 5th edition. Washington, DC: American Psychiatric Association; 2013.

70. Alcoholics Anonymous. Living Sober. Alcoholics Anonymous World Services 1975.

71. Kelly JF. Is Alcoholics Anonymous religious, spiritual, neither? Findings from 25 years of mechanisms of behavior change research. Addiction 2017;112(6): 929–36.

72. Moos RH, Moos BS. The interplay between help-seeking and alcohol-related outcomes: divergent processes for professional treatment and self-help groups. Drug Alcohol Depend 2004;75(2):155–64.

73. Moos RH, Moos BS. Participation in treatment and Alcoholics Anonymous: a 16-year follow-up of initially untreated individuals. J Clin Psychol 2006;62(6):735–50.

74. Manning V, Best D, Faulkner N, et al. Does active referral by a doctor or 12-Step peer improve 12-Step meeting attendance? Results from a pilot randomised control trial. Drug Alcohol Depend 2012. https://doi.org/10.1016/j.drugalcdep.2012.05.004.

Technological Addictions

James Sherer, MD[a],*, Petros Levounis, MD, MA[b]

KEYWORDS

- Internet gaming disorder (IGD) • Online shopping addiction (OSA)
- Social media addiction (SMA) • Cybersex

KEY POINTS

- Given the rapidly changing nature of technology, definitions and inclusion criteria for the technological addictions must remain somewhat fluid. Having a working understanding of the technology itself is crucial to separating healthy engagement from addiction.
- Certain technological addictions can already be found in the 5th Edition of the Diagnostic and Statistical Manual, such as Internet gaming disorder and in the 11th Revision of the International Classification of Diseases (ICD-11), such as gaming disorder.
- There are proposed therapies and medications to address many of the TAs, with more research and literature developing at a rapid pace.

INTRODUCTION

Cravings, loss of control, and continued use despite serious consequences are the three elements all addictions share.[1] Stigma, which reinforces addictive behaviors,[2] may soon be considered a fourth. Behavioral addictions (BAs) are no different—the cravings, loss of control, escalation, and stigma that result from them is just as devastating as any substance use disorders (SUDs). BAs can cause irreparable harm and may worsen treatment outcomes for those struggling with mood, anxiety, and psychotic disorders.[3,4]

Despite their potential harm, BAs receive far less media attention and research funding compared with SUDs.[5] Although it is true that more people struggle with SUDs than BAs, BAs are on the rise, with incidence numbers skyrocketing as the coronavirus SARS-CoV-2 (COVID) pandemic lingers on.[6] A recently described subset of BAs, the technological addictions (TAs), is taking the stage in 2022 and beyond.[7] The reason for this is plain to see: the technology we rely on every day, which makes our lives easier and connects us to a global community, may also be slowly laying the groundwork for new types of addiction. Although the core elements of TAs may be similar, the devil is in the details. It may take years of further research to understand

[a] New York University Grossman School of Medicine, 462 1st Avenue, #NB20N11, New York, NY 10016, USA; [b] Rutgers New Jersey Medical School, 357 West 29th Street, #3A, New York, NY 10001, USA
* Corresponding author. 10 Joanna Way, Summit, NJ 07901-3111.
E-mail address: James.Sherer@NYULangone.org

Psychiatr Clin N Am 45 (2022) 577–591
https://doi.org/10.1016/j.psc.2022.04.007
0193-953X/22/© 2022 Elsevier Inc. All rights reserved.
psych.theclinics.com

TAs to the same extent we understand SUDs, but the problem is here now, in clinics, on inpatient units and in the news. Luckily, there are effective interventions available today as well, and all psychiatrists can benefit from a working understanding of the most recent research and literature on the subject.

Technological Addictions: A Diagnostic Dilemma

Despite their rise, many providers consider TAs a "blind spot." Identifying and diagnosing TAs are a nuanced exercise, requiring a working knowledge of the technology itself and its role in society. Diagnosing and treating TAs are further complicated by a confusing and, at times, conflicting set of definitions outlined in the 11th Revision of the International Classification of Diseases (ICD-11) and 5th Edition of the Diagnostic and Statistical Manual (DSM-5). Many TAs outlined in the literature simply have not been clearly defined.

The difficulty of defining TAs stems from the central role that technology plays in all our lives. We rely on our smartphones, laptops, and other devices for everything from maintaining our social circles to banking and getting work done. Drawing the line between healthy engagement and dependence becomes difficult when so much of our daily routine is impossible without technology. This highlights a central issue—what constitutes normal use for some people may amount to addiction in others. Where, then, do we as clinicians draw the line? Is the line worth drawing in the first place?

It has been argued that "Internet and smartphone addicts are no more addicted to the Internet or their smartphones than alcoholics are addicted to bottles. "[8] However, as tech companies spend countless dollars to make the "user experience" surrounding their products more enticing,[9] the "bottle" becomes a topic of serious consideration. As companies such as Facebook leverage virtual reality (VR) and augmented reality to propose digital ecosystems such as the "metaverse" that can rival the real world in scope and engagement,[10] ignoring the technology itself may lead to clinical misunderstandings.

Neurobiological Correlates

Similarly to the neurobiology of SUDs, TAs hijack the dopaminergic pleasure-reward pathways of the brain[11] centering around the nucleus accumbens (NAc), a focal point in reward neurocircuitry.[12] D1 and D2 receptor activation play an important role in reinforcing behaviors.[13,14] Neurons with D1 receptors project to areas including the cortex, striatum, hippocampus, and amygdala ensconcing addiction in the brain. Glutamatergic projections to the NAc play a secondary role in boosting addictive behaviors.[15]

A growing body of research, using fMRI and PET scanning techniques, shows that TAs affect the brain in much the same way.[16] TAs are typified by abnormal connectivity between additional dopaminergic pathways that begin in deeper structures in the striatum and project to the cortex, as described above.[17] More specifically, engagement with technology such as online games can reduce the availability of the dopamine active transporter in the brain and desensitize the brain to dopamine overall.[18] What are the broader implications of these neurobiological changes? Although each TA will affect the brain somewhat differently, studies show that in adolescents who meet the criteria for Internet gaming disorder (IGD) have reduced gray matter volume in regions associated with executive function and attention as well as lower white matter in regions involved in impulse control and decision-making.[19] These changes not only perpetuate addictive behavior but also predispose patients to comorbidities such as Attention-deficit/hyperactivity disorder (ADHD) and depression.[20]

INTERNET GAMING DISORDER/GAMING DISORDER
Nature of the Problem

Video games sales and hours played have skyrocketed since their introduction to the American home in the 1970s and 1980s.[21] Today, games are available on seemingly every electronic device from smartwatches and phones to desktops, laptops, and consoles, and they have easily eclipsed other forms of media. As an industry, video games are more profitable than movies and traditional sports combined.[22]

The ongoing COVID-19 pandemic only lengthened the amount of time children in the United States and the United Kingdom spent gaming.[23] In some studies, more than half of young people interviewed believed they may be addicted to video games, and a quarter of them used video games to alter their mood.[24] Many children spend hours gaming daily, and parents are often unaware.[25] Time spent gaming is high for adults as well, with many spending hours a day on the hobby, and it likely contributing to medical comorbidities such as metabolic syndrome.[26] It is now estimated the average gamer spends over 8 hours weekly playing.[27]

How much is too much? There is a subset of patients (14% of girls and 5% of boys) who spend between 4 and 10 hours gaming every day.[28] Video games displace healthy behaviors such as socializing and exercise, meaning that the more hours spend gaming, the worse patient's feel overall.[29] The distinction between healthy engagement and addiction is murky when it comes to video games. Playing 2 hours nightly may be debilitating for some patients but may be normal (or even a healthy means of maintaining social connectedness) in others. Ultimately, it comes down to the provider to decide when the patient has become addicted to games.

As new diagnoses, much remains unknown about IGD and GD. Even identifying prevalence rates has remained difficult, with some studies claiming rates as low as 0.7% and others reporting rates as high as 27%.[30] Looking globally, it seems the prevalence may be similar to that of obsessive compulsive disorder.[31] Cultural attitudes toward video games play a large role in determining prevalence. In China, where video games are considered a public health crisis and the government has limited the hours that adolescents are allowed to play daily, even a moderate amount of gaming may be seen as problematic.[32]

Before discussing the inclusion criteria for IGD and GD—a word of caution, the social importance (or even necessity) of video games today, especially in the lives of young people, cannot be overlooked. Young people feel pressured to excel at video games, with potentially disastrous social consequences if they cannot.[33] Even if the patients do not experience this pressure, video games have become a crucial social lifeline as the COVID pandemic persists and socializing in-person is often not a possibility.[34] In many, if not most instances, video games may be helping more than harming, but it will fall to the provider to make the distinction.

Evaluation

Table 1 shows the comparison of the definitions of IGD in the DSM-5 and GD in the ICD-11. Each definition has its strengths and weaknesses, and both will almost assuredly be revised in the future as our understanding of these disorders grows.

There are several striking differences between the definitions presented above. It should be noted that the DSM-5 definition is labeled as "requiring further research." The relatively high number of associated symptoms required to meet criteria for IGD ensures that prevalence rates will remain relatively low and perhaps more realistically

Table 1
Internet gaming disorder versus gaming disorder

Defining Body	Diagnostic and Statistical Manual, 5th Edition (DSM-5)	The International Classification of Diseases, 11th Edition
Disorder Name	Internet gaming disorder	Gaming disorder
Definition fully Ratified?	No, currently appears in the section of the DSM-5 (requiring further research)	Yes
General Definition	Persistent and recurrent use of the Internet to engage in games, often with other players, leading to clinically significant impairment or distress, requiring five of the following:	Characterized by a pattern of persistent or recurrent gaming behavior ("digital gaming" or "video gaming") which may be online (ie, over the Internet) or offline, manifested by the following:
Time Frame	Five of the symptoms below must be concurrent within 1 year.	Gaming behavior must persist at least 1 year.
Number of Symptoms Required	Five of nine required	Not specified
Symptoms	1. Preoccupation or obsession with Internet games 2. Withdrawal symptoms when not playing Internet games 3. A build-up of tolerance—more time needs to be spent playing the games. 4. The person has tried to stop or curb playing Internet games but has failed to do so. 5. The person has had a loss of Interest in other life activities, such as hobbies. 6. A person has had continued overuse of Internet games even with a knowledge of how much they impact a person's life 7. The person lied to others about his or her Internet game usage. 8. The person uses Internet games to relieve anxiety or guilt—it is a way to escape 9. The person has lost or put at risk an opportunity or relationship because of Internet games	1. Impaired control over gaming (eg, onset, frequency, intensity, duration, termination, context); 2. Increasing priority given to gaming to the extent that gaming takes precedence over other life interests and daily activities; and 3. Continuation or escalation of gaming despite the occurrence of negative consequences. This pattern results in significant impairment in personal, family, social, educational, occupational, or other important areas of functioning

Data from American Psychiatric Association. (2013). Diagnostic and statistical manual of mental disorders (5th ed.); World Health Organization. (2018). International classification of diseases for mortality and morbidity statistics (11th Revision). Retrieved from https://icd.who.int/browse11/l-m/en

embraces the normality and ubiquity of video games in society today. The WHO seems to be casting a wider net in its definition of GD, defining GDs associated symptoms more broadly, and not specifying any number of symptoms required for the diagnosis.

Treatment Options

Research into medications for IGD has expanded greatly in recent years, but there is still a lack of rigorous, large-scale randomized control trials (RCTs), and many of these studies look at short-term effects only.[35] Many of these studies look at readily available medications used to treat ADHD, depression, and anxiety, such as methylphenidate, atomoxetine, bupropion, and escitalopram. Although early results are promising, further research is needed.

Looking at the RCTs first, one study found that bupropion and escitalopram were both superior to no treatment,[36] and another found that bupropion was better than placebo for IGD symptoms.[37] One study using a pretest-posttest design showed that IGD symptoms were reduced with an 8-week course of methylphenidate.[38] Two other studies using a pretest-posttest design found that 6-week and 12-week courses of bupropion were effective in reducing IGD symptoms.[39,40] Two additional studies did head-to-head comparisons of different medications, one of atomoxetine and methylphenidate[41] and another of bupropion and escitalopram.[42] Neither of these studies included a placebo group. In each of these two studies, no medication was found to be superior and all were efficacious—further signaling that atomoxetine, methylphenidate, bupropion, and escitalopram can all reduce IGD symptoms.[41,42]

Many types of psychotherapy have been researched and found effective for treating IGD. Given the ubiquity of video games today, reducing use rather than abstinence should be the treatment goal, and these therapies were targeted toward IGD with that in mind. A recent meta-analysis of 12 independent studies found that cognitive behavioral therapy (CBT) is highly effective for reducing IGD symptoms in the short term, but did not reduce time spent gaming and the effects did not last beyond the initial treatment window.[43] Standard CBT as well as CBT for Internet addiction (CBT-IA) are both effective.[44] Providers versed in CBT need not retrain in CBT-IA, as standard CBT is equally successful.[45] Motivational interviewing (MI) for IGD has also been proven effective, although progress may be somewhat slowed compared with CBT.[46]

Special Considerations

One important consideration is the link between video games and violent behavior. Although violent video games are a perennial source of political outrage,[47] the relationship between violent games and violent behavior remains unclear, with no clear connection linking video game and real-world violence.[48] However, it is generally accepted in the literature that patients with a serious history of violence should be encouraged to play less violent games.[49,50]

CYBERSEX AND ONLINE PORN
Nature of the Problem

The Internet had transformed pornography into a multibillion dollar industry responsible for a disproportionately large amount of Internet traffic as high as 30% by some measures.[51] The industry has its own lobby, called the Free Speech Coalition, and has exerted influence in the realms public health and politics over the last few decades. As Internet pornography has exploded, side industries such as "teledildonics" have flourished as well, allowing people to use technologies like VR to engage in cybersex over long distances.[52]

Cybersex is an amorphous term that encompasses acts from online sexual talk[53] to using VR to engage in sexual activity or games.[54] Researchers classify cybersex as a type of online sexual activity, which can be a solitary or shared experience, involves technologies such as webcams and may be part of healthy relationships.[55] Reasons for the popularity of cybersex are many—it allows users to explore aliases and engage in novel acts[56] or engage in riskier sexual activity than they are willing to in real life.[57] Perhaps, then, it is no surprise that the prevalence of problematic cybersex and Internet porn use may be as high at 10% of the general population.[54]

Evaluation

Given the widespread use of cybersex and online porn, three use types have emerged in the literature: recreational, compulsive, and at-risk use.[58] Recreational users can maintain control, only engage in cybersex or online porn intermittently, and may lose interest and stop altogether—this population does not require clinical intervention.[59] Compulsive users have an underlying sexual preoccupation or dysfunction, such as a paraphilic disorder, and continue using despite some problems. Cybersex may provide a validation for these patients, so clinical intervention may warrant depending on the case.[60] Unlike compulsive users, at-risk users may not experience symptoms at all were it not for the Internet. In addition to preoccupation, increased time spent use, and serious consequences of using online porn, these users continue, even despite mounting depressive and anxiety symptoms. These patients may require clinical intervention.[59]

In the ICD-11, a new diagnosis of compulsive sexual behavior disorder (CSBD) is now included. CSBD is a "persistent pattern of failure to control intense, repetitive sexual impulses, or urges resulting in repetitive sexual behavior" and is perhaps more in line with current research.[61]

In addition to being classified as a BA, problematic cybersex use has also been classified as secondary to other psychiatric conditions, an impulse-control disorder and also simply as a sexual disorder.[62] In the end, a familiar triad emerges when evaluating problematic cybersex and pornography usage: spending more time, losing control, and continuing to use despite serious consequences. Using this as a cornerstone, Wery and Billeux proposed the following criteria in 2017 (**Table 2**).

The Internet Sex Screening Test (ISST) can further help providers screen for problematic use.[63] Developed in 2003, it consists of 25 yes or no questions. Compulsivity, social cybersex use, isolated cybersex use, money spent on cybersex, and interest in online sexual behavior are the five elements evaluated by the ISST.[64]

Treatment Options

Although there is a good body of research regarding treatments for sex addiction, treatments for cybersex addiction have a relatively scant but growing research

Table 2 Problematic cybersex, a definition	
Uncontrolled and Excessive Use of Online Sexual Activities Associated with	
1.	A persistent desire or unsuccessful efforts to stop, reduce, or control cybersexual behaviors
2.	Cognitive salience (persistent and intrusive cybersex-related thoughts and obsessions pertaining to cybersex)
3.	Use of cybersexual behavior for mood regulation purposes
4.	Withdrawal (occurrence of negative mood states when cybersex is unavailable)
5.	Tolerance (need for more hours of use or for new sexual content)
6.	Negative consequences

Data from Wéry A, Billieux J. Problematic cybersex: Conceptualization, assessment, and treatment. Addict Behav. 2017;64:238-246. https://doi.org/10.1016/j.addbeh.2015.11.007

base. Several studies have investigated psychotherapeutic options for cybersex addiction. One study looked at a 16-week course of psychoeducation, CBT, MI, and readiness to change training in 35 men. They found that, at the end of the course of treatment, depressive symptoms had improved by cybersex activity remained the same.[54] A study with six men found that eight, 90-min sessions of acceptance and commitment therapy (ACT) led to durable reductions in cybersex behavior 3 months after treatment in four of the participants.[65] This study design was later repeated with 26 patients. At 3 months posttreatment, 35% of participants showed complete cessation, with 74% of participants showing at least 70% reduction in viewing.[66] The largest study reviewed involved 138 men and found that 10 courses of CBT led to reductions in obsessive sexual thoughts, pornography use, masturbation, and improvements in affect, self-control, culpability, management of temptation/craving, and relationship skills.[67]

There are no large scale studies investigating pharmacotherapeutic options for cybersex addiction but case reports indicate that paroxetine[68] and naltrexone[63] may be of use here. Naltrexone has been used off-label for hypersexual behavior, as well as other BAs, and reports indicate that it leads to reduced pornography use.[69] Antidepressants are known to decrease libido, and given that paroxetine is a somewhat sedating antidepressant, it may be effective in reducing problematic cybersex and online porn.[63] Given the relative paucity of evidence here, therapeutic interventions such as CBT and ACT appear first line, with medications serving as a second line of defense.

Special Considerations

Sexual health is a large component of mental and physical health overall.[70] Most people who engage in cybersex are not addicted to the behavior—their use may contribute to, rather than detract from, their overall mental health.

SOCIAL MEDIA ADDICTION
Nature of the Problem

Social media platforms, including Facebook, Twitter, Grindr, Bumble, LinkedIn, YouTube, Snapchat, and Instagram, enable users to share and create content, participate in social networking, help people stay connected over vast distances, date, explore their sexuality, apply for jobs, and follow the news. In other words, social media is whatever the user wants it to be. It is a one-stop-shop for our busy modern lives. When social media is unavailable, even for a few minutes, the ramifications for society are tremendous and often catastrophic.[71] Importantly, social media fosters dependence, because constant engagement is rewarded and sparing use is punished.[72]

Evaluation

Currently, social media addiction (SMA) is not outlined in the DSM-5, and working definitions from the literature reflect a rapidly progressing understanding of the tremendous impact social media has, especially on pediatric populations. Generally, SMA is defined as problematic and compulsive use of social media platforms resulting in significant impairment in functioning over an extended period.[73] An important note is that time spent on social media does not necessarily equate to addiction—it is the nature of the use itself which may cause impairment.[74] Social media engagement generally falls into four categories useful for providers: casual, habitual, compulsive, and obsessive use. Using a rating scale, such as the Social media disorder (SMD) scale presented by van Eijinden and colleagues, can help providers distinguish among these groups.[73] It consists of 27 items intended to screen for preoccupation, tolerance, withdrawal, displacement, escape, problems, deception, displacement, and conflict and was validated in a large-scale Dutch study.[73]

Treatment Options

Treatment options for SMA specifically are limited. To get a sense of the treatments available, the search must be broadened to include treatments for Internet addiction (IA). IA is defined as excessive or poorly controlled preoccupation, urges, and/or behaviors regarding Internet use that lead to impairment or distress in several life domains.[75] It is generally accepted that CBT can help reduce time spent on social media as well as the depression and anxiety that stems from overuse.[76] A meta-analysis by Zajac and colleagues validated the efficacy of CBT for IA across six studies using a range of CBT techniques but identified some methodological flaws in each.[77] Wölfling and colleagues designed and investigated a form of CBT for IA (CBT-IA) and found that it may be more efficacious than standard CBT.[78] Several studies from China indicate that family therapy may play a substantial role.[79,80] Only one study investigated pharmacotherapy for IA and found escitalopram to be effective.[81]

Special Considerations

Unlike the Internet in general, it has come to light that social media platforms aim to foster dependence in pediatric populations specifically.[82] Social media capitalizes on the "fear of missing out" which leads to feelings of loneliness and frantic attempts to guard against the anxiety and fear that comes with it.[83] Social media may also lead to "information overload" as well as misinformation.[84]

ONLINE SHOPPING
Nature of the Problem

Ecommerce is a multibillion-dollar industry, accounting for $205 billion in US sales in the third quarter of 2021 alone, an increase from the previous year.[85] This comes as no surprise given that 60% of US adults are Amazon Prime members.[86] Ecommerce platforms buy and sell consumer data, so targeted advertisements "follow" buyers across the web.[87]

The neurobiological basis of problematic shopping is an active focus of current research. It seems that cue-related responses in areas of the brain such as the dorsal and ventral striatum may play predispose certain individuals to buying-shopping disorder.[88] When online shoppers see aggregates of product ratings, there is Electroencephalogram (EEG) and behavioral evidence to show this has a substantial impact on buying habits, which may disproportionately affect impulsive shoppers.[89]

Evaluation

Online shopping addiction (OSA) does not have a clear, consistent definition. It is perhaps more clinically useful to think of OSA as a constellation of predisposing factors and resulting behaviors, rather than a set of inclusion criteria. Rose and colleagues described the following contributing factors: low self-esteem, low self-regulation, negative emotional states, psychological enjoyment, social anonymity, and cognitive overload.[90] Evaluating patients in these terms could inform a psychotherapeutic approach to OSA. Other assessment tools include the short version of the IT Test modified for online shopping sites and the pathologic buying screener.[91]

Treatment Options

A harm reduction approach is warranted when treating OSA,[92] and CBT has been shown to be effective.[93] Other therapies with limited evidence include cue-exposure therapy, in which the patient is exposed to cues (such as opening a shopping application on their phone), and response is prevented with monitoring from the therapist, which proved useful in two case studies.[94] Psychodrama is another option which involves role playing and dramatization to investigate patient's buying behavior and foster insight.[95]

Special Considerations

It is important to keep in mind that online shopping is a necessity for many, especially for those of low socioeconomic status or those living in urban food deserts.[96] For such patients, limiting online shopping to only certain types of items may be an effective treatment goal. For example, for a patient who compulsively buys shoes, deleting the Amazon app but keeping the Fresh Direct app may be beneficial.

SUMMARY

As companies like Facebook and Microsoft drive consumers into the "metaverse," cryptocurrency, and non-fungible tokens become legitimate alternatives to the dollar, and "gamification" continues to change the way we engage with the Internet, the TAs are becoming a pressing concern for mental health providers the world over. Although our knowledge base is growing and effective treatments are already being used, there is still much to learn in this burgeoning field.

CLINICS CARE POINTS

- As with all use disorders, most of the people who use technology regularly do not qualify as having a technological addiction.
- Cognitive behavioral therapy (CBT), bupropion, and methylphenidate are effective treatments for Internet gaming disorder.
- Motivational interviewing, CBT, and acceptance, and commitment therapy are effective treatments for cybersex and online porn addiction.
- Problematic social media usage may decrease with CBT and CBT for Internet addiction.
- Exposure and response therapy can help reduce excessive online spending.

DISCLOSURE

There are no commercial or financial conflicts of interest and any funding sources to report for either author.

REFERENCES

1. Pallanti S, Marras A, Makris N. A Research Domain Criteria Approach to Gambling Disorder and Behavioral Addictions: Decision-Making, Response Inhibition, and the Role of Cannabidiol. Front Psychiatry 2021;12:634418.
2. Levounis P. Addiction: Not a Hangnail, But Not Poverty Either. Acad Psychiatry 2018;42(2):277–8.
3. Coles AS, Knezevic D, George TP, et al. Long-Acting Injectable Antipsychotic Treatment in Schizophrenia and Co-occurring Substance Use Disorders: A Systematic Review. Front Psychiatry 2021;12:808002.
4. Berny LM, Tanner-Smith EE. Differential Predictors of Suicidal Ideation and Suicide Attempts: Internalizing Disorders and Substance Use in a Clinical Sample

of Adolescents. J Dual Diagn 2022;1–11. https://doi.org/10.1080/15504263.2021. 2016343.

5. Yau YHC, Potenza MN. Gambling Disorder and Other Behavioral Addictions: Recognition and Treatment. Harv Rev Psychiatry 2015;23(2):134–46.

6. Li Y, Sun Y, Meng S, et al. Internet Addiction Increases in the General Population During COVID-19: Evidence From China. Am J Addict. 2021;30(4):389-397. doi:

7. Levounis P, Sherer J, editors. Technological addictions. 1st edition. Washington, DC: American Psychiatric Association Publishing; 2022.

8. Griffiths MD. Conceptual Issues Concerning Internet Addiction and Internet Gaming Disorder: Further Critique on Ryding and Kaye (2017). Int J Ment Health Addict 2018;16(1):233–9. https://doi.org/10.1007/s11469-017-9818-z.

9. Gibson, Caitlin. The Next Level. The Washington Post. 2016. Available at: https://www.washingtonpost.com/sf/style/2016/12/07/video-games-are-more-addictive-than-ever-this-is-what-happens-when-kids-cant-turn-them-off/. Accessed January 6, 2022.

10. Analysis | In 2021, tech talked up 'the metaverse.' One problem: It doesn't exist. Washington Post. Available at: https://www.washingtonpost.com/technology/2021/12/30/metaverse-definition-facebook-horizon-worlds/. Accessed January 23, 2022.

11. Potenza MN. The neurobiology of pathological gambling. Semin Clin Neuropsychiatry 2001;6(3):217–26.

12. Volkow ND, Wang GJ, Fowler JS, et al. Addiction: Beyond dopamine reward circuitry. Proc Natl Acad Sci 2011;108(37):15037–42.

13. Uhl GR, Koob GF, Cable J. The neurobiology of addiction. Ann N Y Acad Sci 2019;1451(1):5–28.

14. Baik JH. Dopamine Signaling in reward-related behaviors. Front Neural Circuits 2013;7. https://doi.org/10.3389/fncir.2013.00152.

15. Yu J, Ishikawa M, Wang J, et al. Ventral Tegmental Area Projection Regulates Glutamatergic Transmission in Nucleus Accumbens. Sci Rep 2019;9(1):18451.

16. Den Ouden L, Suo C, Albertella L, et al. Transdiagnostic phenotypes of compulsive behavior and associations with psychological, cognitive, and neurobiological affective processing. Transl Psychiatry 2022;12(1):10.

17. Carpita B, Muti D, Nardi B, et al. Biochemical Correlates of Video Game Use: From Physiology to Pathology. A Narrative Rev Life 2021;11(8):775.

18. Ariatama B, Effendy E, Amin MM. Relationship between Internet Gaming Disorder with Depressive Syndrome and Dopamine Transporter Condition in Online Games Player. Open Access Maced J Med Sci 2019;7(16):2638–42.

19. Weinstein AM. An Update Overview on Brain Imaging Studies of Internet Gaming Disorder. Front Psychiatry 2017;8:185.

20. Sussman CJ, Harper JM, Stahl JL, et al. Internet and Video Game Addictions: Diagnosis, Epidemiology, and Neurobiology. Child Adolesc Psychiatr Clin N Am 2018;27(2):307–26.

21. Rideout V, Robb M. The Common Sense Consensus: Media Use by Tweens and Teens. Common Sense Media. Published online 2019. Available at: https://www.commonsensemedia.org/sites/default/files/uploads/research/2019-census-8-to-18-full-report-updated.pdf. Accessed January 16, 2021.

22. Witkowski,Wallace. Video games are a bigger industry than movies and North American sports combined, thanks to the pandemic. MarketWatch. Published January 2, 2021. Available at: https://www.marketwatch.com/story/videogames-are-a-bigger-industry-than-sports-and-movies-combined-thanks-to-the-pandemic-11608654990. Accessed January 10, 2022.

23. Mullan K, Hofferth SL. A Comparative Time-Diary Analysis of UK and US Children's Screen Time and Device Use. Child Indic Res 2021. https://doi.org/10.1007/s12187-021-09884-3.

24. Ramírez S, Gana S, Garcés S, et al. Use of Technology and Its Association With Academic Performance and Life Satisfaction Among Children and Adolescents. Front Psychiatry 2021;12:764054.

25. Yalçın SS, Çaylan N, Erat Nergiz M, et al. Video game playing among preschoolers: prevalence and home environment in three provinces from Turkey. Int J Environ Health Res 2021;1–14. https://doi.org/10.1080/09603123.2021.1950653.

26. Macías N, Espinosa-Montero J, Monterrubio-Flores E, et al. Screen-Based Sedentary Behaviors and Their Association With Metabolic Syndrome Components Among Adults in Mexico. Prev Chronic Dis 2021;18:210041.

27. Combs,Veronica. 8 hours and 27 minutes. That's how long the average gamer plays each week. TechRepublic. Available at: https://www.techrepublic.com/article/8-hours-and-27-minutes-thats-how-long-the-average-gamer-plays-each-week/. Accessed January 20, 2022.

28. Perrin A. 5 facts about Americans and video games. Pew Research Center. Available at: https://www.pewresearch.org/fact-tank/2018/09/17/5-facts-about-americans-and-video-games/. Accessed January 16, 2022.

29. Twenge JM. Have Smartphones Destroyed a Generation? The Atlantic. 2017. Available at: https://www.theatlantic.com/magazine/archive/2017/09/has-the-smartphone-destroyed-a-generation/534198/. Accessed January 16, 2022.

30. Mihara S, Higuchi S. Cross-sectional and longitudinal epidemiological studies of Internet gaming disorder: A systematic review of the literature. Psychiatry Clin Neurosci 2017;71(7):425–44.

31. Stevens MW, Dorstyn D, Delfabbro PH, et al. Global prevalence of gaming disorder: A systematic review and meta-analysis. Aust N Z J Psychiatry 2021;55(6):553–68.

32. Li J. China's crackdown on video games is getting more serious. Quartz. Available at: https://qz.com/2056875/chinas-crackdown-on-video-games-is-getting-more-serious/. Accessed January 17, 2022.

33. Robertson E. I don't want to get good at gaming, I want to escape the relentless pressure to improve myself. The Guardian. 2018. Available at: https://www.theguardian.com/commentisfree/2018/oct/11/i-dont-want-to-get-good-at-gaming-i-want-to-escape-the-relentless-pressure-to-improve-myself. Accessed January 16, 2022.

34. Khan I. Why animal crossing is the game for the coronavirus moment. The New York Times; 2020. Available at: https://www.nytimes.com/2020/04/07/arts/animal-crossing-covid-coronavirus-popularity-millennials.html. Accessed January 16, 2022.

35. Zajac K, Ginley MK, Chang R. Treatments of internet gaming disorder: a systematic review of the evidence. Expert Rev Neurother 2020;20(1):85–93.

36. Song J, Park JH, Han DH, et al. Comparative study of the effects of bupropion and escitalopram on Internet gaming disorder. Psychiatry Clin Neurosci 2016;70(11):527–35.

37. Han DH, Renshaw PF. Bupropion in the treatment of problematic online game play in patients with major depressive disorder. J Psychopharmacol Oxf Engl 2012;26(5):689–96.

38. Han DH, Lee YS, Na C, et al. The effect of methylphenidate on Internet video game play in children with attention-deficit/hyperactivity disorder. Compr Psychiatry 2009;50(3):251–6.

39. Han DH, Hwang JW, Renshaw PF. Bupropion sustained release treatment decreases craving for video games and cue-induced brain activity in patients with Internet video game addiction. Exp Clin Psychopharmacol 2010;18(4):297–304.

40. Bae S, Hong JS, Kim SM, et al. Bupropion Shows Different Effects on Brain Functional Connectivity in Patients With Internet-Based Gambling Disorder and Internet Gaming Disorder. Front Psychiatry 2018;9:130.

41. Park JH, Lee YS, Sohn JH, et al. Effectiveness of atomoxetine and methylphenidate for problematic online gaming in adolescents with attention deficit hyperactivity disorder. Hum Psychopharmacol 2016;31(6):427–32.

42. Nam B, Bae S, Kim SM, et al. Comparing the Effects of Bupropion and Escitalopram on Excessive Internet Game Play in Patients with Major Depressive Disorder. Clin Psychopharmacol Neurosci 2017;15(4):361–8.

43. Stevens MWR, King DL, Dorstyn D, et al. Cognitive-behavioral therapy for Internet gaming disorder: A systematic review and meta-analysis. Clin Psychol Psychother 2019;26(2):191–203.

44. Young KS, Brand M. Merging Theoretical Models and Therapy Approaches in the Context of Internet Gaming Disorder: A Personal Perspective. Front Psychol 2017;8:1853.

45. Torres-Rodríguez A, Griffiths MD, Carbonell X, et al. Treatment efficacy of a specialized psychotherapy program for Internet Gaming Disorder. J Behav Addict 2018;7(4):939–52.

46. Kuss DJ, Griffiths MD, Karila L, et al. Internet addiction: a systematic review of epidemiological research for the last decade. Curr Pharm Des 2014;20(25):4026–52.

47. Draper Kevin J. Video Games Aren't Why Shootings Happen. Politicians Still Blame Them. - The New York Times. N Y Times 2019;5.

48. Coyne SM, Stockdale L. Growing Up with Grand Theft Auto: A 10-Year Study of Longitudinal Growth of Violent Video Game Play in Adolescents. Cyberpsychology Behav Soc Netw 2021;24(1):11–6.

49. Greitemeyer T, Mügge DO. Video Games Do Affect Social Outcomes: A Meta-Analytic Review of the Effects of Violent and Prosocial Video Game Play. Pers Soc Psychol Bull 2014;40(5):578–89.

50. Suziedelyte A. Is it only a game? Video games and violence. J Econ Behav Organ 2021;188(C):105–25.

51. Infographic. How Much of the Internet Consists of Porn? Statista Infographics. Available at: https://www.statista.com/chart/16959/share-of-the-internet-that-is-porn/. Accessed January 17, 2022.

52. LoveWriting C. Teledildonics gave me the gift of long-distance sex with a stranger. Christopher Trout. Available at: https://www.christophertrout.com/teledildonics-gave-me-the-gift-of-long-distance-sex-with-a-stranger/2018/12/04. Accessed January 17, 2022.

53. Barrada JR, Ruiz-Gómez P, Correa AB, et al. Not all Online Sexual Activities Are the Same. Front Psychol 2019;10:339.

54. Wéry A, Billieux J. Problematic cybersex: Conceptualization, assessment, and treatment. Addict Behav 2017;64:238–46.

55. Döring N, Daneback K, Shaughnessy K, et al. Online Sexual Activity Experiences Among College Students: A Four-Country Comparison. Arch Sex Behav 2017; 46(6):1641–52.

56. Berg RC, Ross MW, Weatherburn P, et al. Structural and environmental factors are associated with internalised homonegativity in men who have sex with men: findings from the European MSM Internet Survey (EMIS) in 38 countries. Soc Sci Med 1982 2013;78:61–9.

57. Hertlein KM, Stevenson A. The Seven "As" Contributing to Internet-Related Intimacy Problems: A Literature Review. Cyberpsychology J Psychosoc Res Cyberspace 2010;4(1). Available at: https://cyberpsychology.eu/article/view/4230. Accessed January 17, 2022.

58. Derbyshire KL, Grant JE. Compulsive sexual behavior: a review of the literature. J Behav Addict 2015;4(2):37–43.

59. Cooper A, Putnam DE, Planchon LA, et al. Online sexual compulsivity: Getting tangled in the net. Sex Addict Compulsivity 1999;6(2):79–104.

60. Cooper A, Delmonico D, Griffinshelley E, et al. Online Sexual Activity:An Examination of Potentially Problematic Behaviors. Sex Addict Compulsivity 2004;11: 129–43.

61. Kraus SW, Krueger RB, Briken P, et al. Compulsive sexual behaviour disorder in the ICD-11. World Psychiatry 2018;17(1):109–10.

62. Courtice EL, Shaughnessy K, Blom K, et al. Young Adults' Qualitative Self-Reports of Their Outcomes of Online Sexual Activities. Eur J Investig Health Psychol Educ 2021;11(2):303–20.

63. de Alarcón R, de la Iglesia JI, Casado NM, et al. Online Porn Addiction: What We Know and What We Don't-A Systematic Review. J Clin Med 2019;8(1):E91.

64. Chen L, Jiang X. The Assessment of Problematic Internet Pornography Use: A Comparison of Three Scales with Mixed Methods. Int J Environ Res Public Health 2020;17(2):E488.

65. Twohig MP, Crosby JM. Acceptance and commitment therapy as a treatment for problematic internet pornography viewing. Behav Ther 2010;41(3):285–95.

66. Crosby JM, Twohig MP. Acceptance and Commitment Therapy for Problematic Internet Pornography Use: A Randomized Trial. Behav Ther 2016;47(3):355–66.

67. Hardy SA, Ruchty J, Hull TD, et al. A Preliminary Study of an Online Psychoeducational Program for Hypersexuality. Sex Addict Compulsivity 2010;17(4):247–69.

68. Gola M, Potenza MN. Paroxetine Treatment of Problematic Pornography Use: A Case Series. J Behav Addict 2016;5(3):529–32.

69. Dhuffar MK, Griffiths MD. A Systematic Review of Online Sex Addiction and Clinical Treatments Using CONSORT Evaluation. Curr Addict Rep 2015;2(2):163–74.

70. Navarro-Sánchez A, Luri-Prieto P, Compañ-Rosique A, et al. Sexuality, Quality of Life, Anxiety, Depression, and Anger in Patients with Anal Fissure. A Case–Control Study. J Clin Med 2021;10(19):4401.

71. Isaac M, Frenkel S. Gone in Minutes, Out for Hours: Outage Shakes Facebook. The New York Times. 2021. Available at: https://www.nytimes.com/2021/10/04/technology/facebook-down.html. Accessed January 20, 2022.

72. Andreassen CS, Pallesen S, Griffiths MD. The relationship between addictive use of social media, narcissism, and self-esteem: Findings from a large national survey. Addict Behav 2017;64:287–93.

73. van den Eijnden RJJM, Lemmens JS, Valkenburg PM. The Social Media Disorder Scale. Comput Human Behav 2016;61:478–87.

74. Griffiths M, Pontes H, Kuss D. Clinical psychology of Internet addiction: a review of its conceptualization, prevalence, neuronal processes, and implications for

treatment. Neurosci Neuroeconomics 2015;11. https://doi.org/10.2147/NAN. S60982.

75. Weinstein A, Curtiss Feder L, Rosenberg KP, et al. Internet Addiction Disorder. In: Rosenberg KP, Feder LC, editors. Behavioral addictions. Cambridge, MA: Elsevier; 2014. p. 99–117.

76. Pontes HM, Kuss DJ, Griffiths MD. Clinical psychology of Internet addiction: a review of its conceptualization, prevalence, neuronal processes, and implications for treatment. Neurosci Neuroeconomics 2015;4:11–23.

77. Zajac K, Ginley MK, Chang R, et al. Treatments for Internet Gaming Disorder and Internet Addiction: A Systematic Review. Psychol Addict Behav 2017;31(8): 979–94.

78. Wölfling K, Beutel ME, Dreier M, et al. Treatment outcomes in patients with internet addiction: a clinical pilot study on the effects of a cognitive-behavioral therapy program. Biomed Res Int 2014;2014:425924.

79. Liu QX, Fang XY, Yan N, et al. Multi-family group therapy for adolescent Internet addiction: exploring the underlying mechanisms. Addict Behav 2015;42:1–8.

80. Shek DTL, Tang VMY, Lo CY. Evaluation of an Internet addiction treatment program for Chinese adolescents in Hong Kong. Adolescence 2009;44(174): 359–73.

81. Dell'Osso B, Hadley S, Allen A, et al. Escitalopram in the treatment of impulsive-compulsive internet usage disorder: an open-label trial followed by a double-blind discontinuation phase. J Clin Psychiatry 2008;69(3):452–6.

82. Leaked Facebook Papers reveal social media giant targeted children as young as 6-years-old | Daily Mail Online. Available at: https://www.dailymail.co.uk/news/article-10146589/Leaked-Facebook-Papers-reveal-social-media-giant-targeted-children-young-6-years-old.html. Accessed January 21, 2022.

83. Anxiety, loneliness and Fear of Missing Out: The impact of social media on young people's mental health | Centre for Mental Health. Available at: https://www.centreformentalhealth.org.uk/blogs/anxiety-loneliness-and-fear-missing-out-impact-social-media-young-peoples-mental-health. Accessed January 21, 2022.

84. Horrigan JB. Information Overload. Pew Research Center: Internet, Science & Tech. 2016. Available at: https://www.pewresearch.org/internet/2016/12/07/information-overload/. Accessed January 21, 2022.

85. US ecommerce sales increase 6.8% in Q3 2021. Digital Commerce 360. Available at: https://www.digitalcommerce360.com/article/quarterly-online-sales/. Accessed January 21, 2022.

86. Are 70% of US Adults Amazon Prime Members? | Snopes.com. Available at: https://www.snopes.com/fact-check/amazon-prime-adults/. Accessed January 21, 2022.

87. Here's how ads are following you around on the internet | Business Insider India. Available at: https://www.businessinsider.in/tech/article/heres-how-ads-are-following-you-around-on-the-internet/articleshow/73272827.cms. Accessed January 21, 2022.

88. Trotzke P, Starcke K, Pedersen A, et al. Dorsal and ventral striatum activity in individuals with buying-shopping disorder during cue-exposure: A functional magnetic resonance imaging study. Addict Biol. 2021;26(6). doi:10.1111/adb.13073

89. Sun L, Zhao Y, Ling B. The Joint Influence of Online Rating and Product Price on Purchase Decision: An EEG Study. Psychol Res Behav Manag 2020;13:291–301.

90. Rose S, Dhandayudham A. Towards an understanding of Internet-based problem shopping behaviour: The concept of online shopping addiction and its proposed predictors. J Behav Addict 2014;3(2):83–9.

91. Müller A, Steins-Loeber S, Trotzke P, et al. Online shopping in treatment-seeking patients with buying-shopping disorder. Compr Psychiatry 2019;94:152120.
92. Carnes P, Carnes S, Bailey J. Facing addiction: starting recovery from alcohol and drugs. 0 edition. Carefree (AZ): Gentle Path Press; 2011.
93. Mitchell JE, Burgard M, Faber R, et al. Cognitive behavioral therapy for compulsive buying disorder. Behav Res Ther 2006;44(12):1859–65.
94. Bernik MA, Akerman D, Amaral JA, et al. Cue exposure in compulsive buying. J Clin Psychiatry 1996;57(2):90.
95. The psychodrama in the addiction treatment of pathological gambling and buying behavior | Revista Brasileira de Psicodrama. 2021. Available at: https://revbraspsicodrama.org.br/rbp/article/view/73. Accessed January 22, 2022.
96. HealthITAnalytics. Mobile App Data Reveals Prevalence of Urban Food Deserts. HealthITAnalytics. 2020. Available at: https://healthitanalytics.com/news/mobile-app-data-reveals-prevalence-of-urban-food-deserts. Accessed January 22, 2022.

Thirty Years of *The ASAM Criteria*: A Report Card

David R. Gastfriend, MD, DFASAM[a],*, David Mee-Lee, MD, DFASAM[b]

KEYWORDS

- ASAM criteria • Patient placement criteria • Medical necessity
- Substance use disorder • Addiction • Drug abuse treatment
- Utilization management

KEY POINTS

- *The ASAM Criteria* is the best-evidenced, most widely used approach in substance use disorder treatment for patient assessment, determination of needs, medical necessity criteria, and utilization management.
- The standard implementation of *The ASAM Criteria,* consisting of the textbook, the ASAM CONTINUUM software, and the ASAM–CARF Level of Care (LOC) Certification Program offers patients, providers, payers, and health care systems a common language and process for improving the quality of care.
- Providers and payers have made progress in operationalizing addiction as a multidimensional disease and tailoring treatment to each individual. However, more, systemic effort is needed to fully achieve these goals, including person-centered services with a focus on outcomes in the real-time delivery of care.

INTRODUCTION

The emergence and predominance of *The American Society of Addiction Medicine Criteria (ASAM)*[1] is a unique story in American health care, behavioral medicine, and health economics. The field of addiction treatment was historically buffeted by social stigma, politicization, underfunding, fragmentation, regulatory constraints, and inertia. Ultimately, the field responded by devising a sophisticated system for organizing treatment services and settings with patient care decision rules—*The ASAM Criteria*. These decision rules were initially consensus based, but they increasingly became informed by a growing body of science.[2] In addition, this system defined the infrastructure of addiction care, in the types and intensity of treatment, staffing, and service provision needed for each level of care (LOC). *The ASAM Criteria* and its ASAM CONTINUUM[3] structured interview and decision assistance software helped the field move

[a] DynamiCare Health, Inc., 6 Liberty Sq. #2102, Boston, MA 02109, USA; [b] DML Training and Consulting, 4228 Boxelder Place, Davis, CA 95618, USA
* Corresponding author.
E-mail address: drgastfriend@DynamiCareHealth.com

Psychiatr Clin N Am 45 (2022) 593–609
https://doi.org/10.1016/j.psc.2022.05.008
0193-953X/22/© 2022 Elsevier Inc. All rights reserved.

psych.theclinics.com

toward a national standard for addiction treatment and a leadership role in behavioral health. The ASAM Criteria led to widespread educational efforts, increased the differentiation of services to meet diverse patient needs, and introduced standardization of patient assessment. *The ASAM Criteria* influenced reimbursement reform,[4] federal court litigation,[5] and behavioral health care standardization (via the LOCUS Level of Care Utilization System[6]) and is poised to create the potential for measurement-based care, outcomes-based treatment, and value-based contracting in addiction treatment.

HISTORY

The American Society of Addiction Medicine Criteria Early Days

In the mid-1980s, a compelling need arose for objective standards for matching patients to treatments.[7] Conflict between 2 opposing forces created this need. One was the widespread treatment model in which most patients were expected to undergo 28-day inpatient rehabilitation—often at considerable expense—followed by discharge to an aftercare program, which often consisted of intermittent group meetings and referral to 12-step mutual support meetings. The second factor driving the need for standards was the rise of the managed care organization (MCO). In addiction treatment, the MCO challenged the 28-day model, steadily restricting this "one-size-fits-all" approach that lacked validation. This conflict ultimately led to *The ASAM Criteria* for the treatment of addictive, substance-related, and co-occurring conditions.

The ASAM first published the *Patient Placement Criteria for the Treatment of Psychoactive SUDs* in 1991 (ASAM PPC)[8] after a collaborative process with the National Association of Addiction Treatment Providers and the Northern Ohio Chemical Dependency Treatment Directors Association. An expanded second edition was published in 1996, *ASAM PPC-2*.[9] In 2001, a revision of PPC-2 was published, *ASAM PPC-2R*.[10] The much expanded third edition, *The ASAM Criteria*, was published in 2013.[1]

Research with The American Society of Addiction Medicine Criteria

Early abbreviated or incomplete attempts to study *The ASAM Criteria* met with mixed outcomes in research validation trials. At Harvard's Massachusetts General Hospital, however, Gastfriend and colleagues,[11] first demonstrated the feasibility of implementing *The ASAM Criteria* in a standardized, comprehensive fashion through computer-assisted technology. This facilitated a stream of controlled studies of *The ASAM Criteria* using a consistent research platform, which validated its feasibility,[8,12] inter-rater reliability,[13] convergent validity,[14,15] and predictive validity.[16–19] This evidence eventually encompassed diverse controlled study designs, outcome parameters, study populations, payer models, and even countries and languages.[2,20] A Harvard Business School study determined the financial readiness of the field for a standard software implementation of *The ASAM Criteria*.[21] This report led to the US Substance Abuse and Mental Health Services Administration contracting for the programming of the ASAM CONTINUUM software—the standard implementation of *The ASAM Criteria*.[22]

Over time, this evidence base led to a growing number of US states endorsing or requiring the use of *The ASAM Criteria* for their public treatment programs; by 2006, a majority required it.[23] In 2015, when the Centers for Medicare and Medicaid Services allowed state Medicaid programs to implement system reforms to improve substance use disorder (SUD) care *The ASAM Criteria* increasingly became highlighted in federal guidance[24] and states and counties began to respond.[25]

Thirty Years Later

By 2021, the 30th anniversary of ASAM's "Patient Placement Criteria for the Treatment of Psychoactive SUD," ASAM had developed a significant financial and staff infrastructure for explaining, training, and catalyzing systems change to implement the full spirit and content of the Criteria (**Table 1**).

On November 9, 2021, ASAM released a first-of-its kind, free, educational resource to assist interested states in using *The ASAM Criteria*, entitled, "Speaking The Same Language: A Toolkit for Strengthening Patient-Centered Addiction Care in the United States."[26] This comprehensive list of implementation strategies and tools, with examples from current state efforts, and model legislative, regulatory, and contractual language, establishes a common framework across all payers, providers, and patients for addiction care.

EVALUATION
Report Card on Progress with The American Society of Addiction Medicine Criteria

With 30 years of hindsight, it is now possible to construct a "report card" that grades the addiction treatment field on its improvements. The grades we have assigned are subjective, although partially data-driven. We ask the questions: Has the field addressed these fundamental guiding principles? How much?

Objective: moving from 1-dimensional to multidimensional assessment

Addiction is one of the most multifactorial conditions of all human diseases, making it essential to consider 6 different dimensions of assessment to determine treatment and level of care.

Before *The ASAM Criteria*, in the 1970s and the 1980s, treatment was unidimensional—the diagnosis alone was typically enough to gain admission into a residential program, only after which a stock "assessment and treatment planning week" occurred. In contrast, *The ASAM Criteria* first required a multidimensional assessment to then determine treatment needs and level of care. Because substance use and addictive and mental disorders are biopsychosocial in cause and expression, treatment and care management are most effective if they, too, are biopsychosocial. If the clinician can present a patient's needs and strengths concisely organized along the 6 assessment dimensions identified in *The ASAM Criteria*, the severity of the patient's illness and level of function—the basis of medical necessity—will be clear to both provider and payer (**Table 2**).[27]

Grade: Today, the vast majority of addiction treatment providers might seem to assess multiple needs of their clients; they get an *A grade* for the shift from focusing on diagnosis as the only criterion for admission to treatment to recognizing the need to assess SUD multidimensionally. Payers, although required by the majority of US states to abide by *The ASAM Criteria* for determining medical necessity,[23] get a *B-grade*, for inconsistency in their use or interpretation of *The ASAM Criteria*.[5,28] However, survey research indicates that with both payers and providers there is "a need to implement fidelity standards, enhance training, and create resources to help systems create and utilize assessment and patient placement tools that are consistent across the SUD treatment field."[28] Therefore, both payers and the treatment field deserve more of a *C grade* for inconsistently applying *The ASAM Criteria* in their assessments and placements.

Plans for improvement. Widespread training has raised consciousness, but not necessarily effective practice of multidimensional assessment. Adoption challenges include diverse training levels, service fragmentation, and high rates of staff turnover.

	Year	Type of Tool	Name
		Table 1	
		ASAM criteria toolkit: publications, guidelines, instruments, software, and programs	
1	1991	Text	*ASAM Patient Placement Criteria for the Treatment of Psychoactive SUDs*[8]
2	2004	Text	*Addiction Treatment Matching: Research Foundations of the American Society of Addiction Medicine (ASAM) Criteria*[2]
3	2010	Guideline	*ASAM Patient Placement Criteria: Supplement on Pharmacotherapies for Alcohol Use Disorders*[67]
4	2013	Text	*The ASAM Criteria: Treatment for Addictive, Substance-Related, and Co-Occurring Conditions*[1]
5	2016	Instrument	ASAM CONTINUUM[3]
6	2017	Instrument	CO-Triage[68]
7	2019	Program	ASAM CARF Level of Care Certification[35,36,50]
8	2021	Guideline	*The ASAM Criteria Powered by InterQual*[69]
9	2021	Instrument	Addiction Treatment Needs Assessment (ATNA)[39]
10	2021	Resource guide	"Speaking the Same Language: A Toolkit for Strengthening Patient-Centered Addiction Care in the United States"[26]

This need has led to the creation of "the standard implementation of *The ASAM Criteria*,"[1] the ASAM CONTINUUM—*The ASAM Criteria* Decision Engine.[3] This computer-guided, structured interview and clinical decision algorithm assures that interviewers perform the comprehensive 6-dimensional assessment, and then it executes all the adult admission decision rules of *The ASAM Criteria*.[11]

The decision engine uses research-quality questions and quantitative ratings (including tools such as the Addiction Severity Index, which supports the predictive validity of the system[29]; Clinical Institute Withdrawal Assessment; and Clinical Institute Narcotic Assessment) instruments to score an intricate algebraic algorithm and generate a comprehensive patient report, recommended level of care determinations, and problem list. More than 5000 counselors and other providers now use CONTINUUM tools for routine assessment and follow-up in nearly 40% (19) of all US states. The CONTINUUM database now generates more than 8000 new assessments each month, exceeding 200,000 records—the largest and most clinically intensive SUD dataset in existence. Empirical analysis indicates that it yields recommendations that are in agreement with ASAM's Practice Guidelines.[30,31] For example, most patients who show evidence of a diagnosis of opioid use disorder (OUD) receive a recommendation for medications for OUD, and many also receive recommendations for Biomedically Enhanced and Co-occurring Enhanced services (ASAM internal communication).

Payers still require assistance in interpreting patient clinical reports by providers and applying *The ASAM Criteria* decision rules. ASAM is developing specialized payer training and computer-guided tools to address these needs.

Objective: uphold individualized treatment and person-centered services

Several guiding principles of *The ASAM Criteria* encouraged payers and providers to do the following:

- Incorporate *patient-centered care*, that is, responsiveness, collaboration, and shared decision making.[32] Rapid engagement, meeting patients "where they're

Table 2
ASAM criteria assessment dimensions

Dimensions	Assessment and Treatment Planning Focus
1. Acute intoxication and/or withdrawal potential	Use objective measures. Consider both current status and impending course. Use recent and past history information. Manage withdrawal in a variety of levels of care. Plan for both safety and preparation for continued addiction services.
2. Biomedical conditions and complications	Assess and treat co-occurring physical health conditions or complications. Provide treatment within the level of care or through coordination of physical health services. Consider risks for impeding treatment follow-through and recovery effort.
3. Emotional, behavioral, or cognitive conditions and complications	Assess and treat whether diagnosed or subdiagnostic. Provide treatment within the level of care or through coordination of mental health services. Consider risks for impeding treatment follow-through and recovery effort.
4. Readiness to change	Assess the stage of readiness to change. If not ready to commit to full recovery, engage into treatment using motivational enhancement strategies. If ready for recovery, consolidate and expand action for change.
5. Relapse, continued use, or continued problem potential	Assess readiness for relapse prevention services, and teach where appropriate. Identify previous periods of sobriety or wellness and what worked to achieve this. At early stages of change, focus on raising awareness and salience of consequences of continued use or continued problems as part of motivational enhancement strategies.
6. Recovery environment	Assess in terms of support for, or distraction from/undermining of recovery. Determine needs for specific individualized family or significant other, housing, financial, vocational, educational, legal, transportation, childcare services. Identify any supports and assets in all these areas.

at," and embracing the stages of change model enhances treatment adherence and outcomes.[33] Shared decision making engages the adult, adolescent, legal guardian, and/or family member, assuring that they are aware of the proposed modalities of treatment, appropriate alternative treatment modalities, and the risks and benefits of treatments, including versus no treatment.

- Provide a broad and flexible continuum of care. Some payers have excluded coverages, for example, Level 3.1—Clinically Managed Low Intensity Residential Services, claiming this to be only a domiciliary-type service, whereas ASAM's specifications clearly delineate its professional staffing, hours, clinical care, assessment, and documentation. Providers may err if they do not move patients flexibly from an initial level, depending on needs and progress, to more or less intensive levels of care. For obvious financial reasons, the preferable level of care is the least intensive one, while still meeting treatment objectives and providing safety and security for the patient. However, 2 controlled studies have found that excessive intensity of care at a higher level than necessary may be associated with adverse clinical outcomes, too.[18,34]
- Eradicate "treatment failure" as an admission prerequisite (sometimes used to deny admission to intensive treatment). Comparison with other chronic diseases quickly illustrates this fallacy: for example, in diabetic ketoacidosis or hypertensive crisis, failure of outpatient treatment would never be a prerequisite for acute hospitalization.
- Move from program-driven to clinically driven, individualized, outcomes-driven treatment, rather than focusing on "placement" in fixed length of stay (LOS) programs with a monolithic program goals and uniform "graduation" phases (Table 3).

Grade: Rather than a seamless, flexible continuum of services, the treatment system still struggles with engagement of people who are not yet interested in full addiction recovery (which is a tension with the harm reduction model), long waiting times for an initial assessment, waiting lists for residential beds and supportive living environments, and inadequate funding for all levels of care.

In the 19 state or county systems across the United States where the ASAM CONTINUUM has been deployed, gaps in the continuum of service levels and intensities specified by The ASAM Criteria are the norm. Also, many states conflate the ASAM placement criteria with the specific SUD services, for example, thinking that medication for addiction treatment, counseling, and peer support can only be provided in outpatient treatment, whereas these should be available in combination with Level 3 care, as well. State Medicaid programs are changing this, fortunately, thanks to a federal waiver program.[4] Of 31 approved waivers, 21 states explicitly reference The ASAM Criteria continuum of care. Most will use the waiver specifically to add coverage of ASAM Levels 3 and 4, and some will make various withdrawal management (WM) levels of care available for the first time, regardless of delivery setting.

Payers are being challenged, including in a federal court class action lawsuit on behalf of 67,000 patients with mental health disorders and SUD, for arbitrary exclusions that obstruct coverage for the full continuum of the ASAM Levels of Care.[5]

Rigid bundling of WM services only at 4-WM or 3.7-WM remains common, driving up cost and allowing only brief LOSs in high-intensity settings. The frequent result is a rapid relapse when withdrawal has not been fully managed to completion. For some patients, ambulatory or residential care might be more clinically appropriate and less costly. With a continuum of WM, patients could receive more complete and effective care at lower cost. Programs will be expected to adhere to these

Table 3
ASAM criteria levels of care

Notes:
1. Can be Combined with Other Levels of Care
2. No Withdrawal Management Levels for Adolescents

ASAM Criteria Level Withdrawal Management Service for Adults	Level	
Ambulatory withdrawal management without extended on-site monitoring	1-WM	Mild withdrawal with daily or less than daily outpatient supervision; likely to complete withdrawal management and to continue treatment or recovery
Ambulatory withdrawal management with extended on-site monitoring	2-WM	Moderate withdrawal with all-day withdrawal management support and supervision; at night, has supportive family or living situation; likely to complete withdrawal management
Clinically managed residential withdrawal management	3.2-WM	Minimal to moderate withdrawal, but needs 24-h support to complete withdrawal management and increase the likelihood of continuing treatment or recovery
Medically monitored inpatient withdrawal management	3.7-WM	Severe withdrawal and needs 24-h nursing care and physician visits as necessary; unlikely to complete withdrawal management without medical or nursing monitoring
Medically managed inpatient withdrawal management	4-WM	Severe, unstable withdrawal and needs 24-h nursing care and daily physician visits to modify the withdrawal management regimen and manage medical instability
ASAM Criteria Levels of Care	**Level**	**Same Levels of Care for Adolescents Except Level 3.3**
Early intervention	0.5	Assessment and education for at-risk individuals who do not meet diagnostic criteria for SUD
Outpatient services	1	Adults: <9 h of service/week (adults) (adolescents: <6 h/wk) for recovery or motivational enhancement therapies/strategies
Intensive outpatient	2.1	Adults: 9 or more hours of service per week (adolescents: 6 or more hours per week) in a structured program to treat multidimensional instability
Partial hospitalization	2.5	20 or more hours of service per week in a structured program for multidimensional instability not requiring 24-h care
Clinically managed low-intensity residential	3.1	24-h structure with available trained personnel with emphasis on reentry to the community; at least 5 h of clinical service per week
Clinically managed population-specific high-intensity residential	3.3	24-h care with trained counselors for those with cognitive or chronic functional impairments requiring slower-paced, repetitive behavioral therapies

(continued on next page)

Table 3
(continued)

ASAM Criteria Levels of Care	Level	Same Levels of Care for Adolescents Except Level 3.3
Clinically managed high-intensity residential	3.5	24-h care with trained counselors to stabilize multidimensional imminent danger and prepare for outpatient treatment. Able to tolerate and use a full active milieu or therapeutic community
Medically monitored intensive inpatient	3.7	24-h nursing care with physician availability for significant problems in Dimensions 1, 2, or 3. 16 h/d counselor ability
Medically managed intensive inpatient	4	24-h nursing care and daily physician care for severe, unstable problems in Dimensions 1, 2, or 3. Counseling available to engage the patient in treatment
Opioid treatment program (OTP)/opioid treatment services (OTS)	OTP/OTS	Medication for opioid use disorder and counseling to maintain multidimensional stability. OTP: daily. Can be combined with any other level of care.

principles to certify for their Level of Care status, in the ASAM-endorsed program administered by CARF International.[35,36]

A similar, common problem is *restricting medications for opioid use disorder* (MOUD) to federally regulated Opioid Treatment Programs or outpatient treatment, which *The ASAM Criteria* specifies should be available in combination with all levels of care, including residential programs. An analysis of more than 5000 CONTINUUM cases during a single month found that more than a quarter of patients with an OUD should receive their MOUD along with residential or inpatient (Level 3 or 4) care (ASAM, internal communication). Yet, the latest federal data indicate that only 33% of residential programs can prescribe buprenorphine and 13% do not accept patients who are receiving MOUD.[37]

Finally, it is still common to find *fixed LOSs* in treatment plans, that is, not an individualized, outcomes-based approach. Often, LOSs may correspond to payer type, a sign of payment-driven rather than individualized care.

Overall, for delivering on individualized, person-centered treatment, in a continuum of care, providers, systems of care, and payers deserve a *B+ grade* for intention, but a *C grade* for execution and actualization.

Plans for improvement. *The ASAM Criteria* system offers opportunities for concrete, objective progress—for the provider, payer, patient, and system. Providers were notified in 2020 that the Joint Commission standards for appropriate level of care would reference *The ASAM Criteria,* specifically citing the optimal matching achieved with *The ASAM Criteria* software (CTS.02.03.13 EP1; p. 4).[38] Payers took note of the remedy order by the Federal District Court of Northern California against the nation's largest behavioral health payer, United Behavioral Health, specifically calling for compliance with *The ASAM Criteria* (even with a reversal by the Appeals Court).[5]

At the patient level, there is a need to go beyond technology-enhanced assessment (which can even be self-administered online at a rudimentary level[39]) and placement decision support (with ASAM CONTINUUM[3]), through the development of a standardized ASAM Criteria treatment planning tool. A patient-centered treatment plan would measure progress, individualize treatment objectives, help the choosing of treatment modalities to achieve these, and flexibly determine the timeframes for expected outcomes. At the system level, a standardized ASAM Criteria treatment plan tool would generate aggregate data regarding degree of individualization of services and LOS and case mix-adjusted outcomes and quantify the needs for services such as beds and slots within regions.

Objective: focus on outcomes, even in real time, to guide treatment

Addiction treatment is a field where outcomes have not been well measured, if at all. What outcomes have been recorded have not been consistent with the chronic disease model of addiction.[40] McLellan and colleagues[41] argued for a shift away from conventional methods of retrospective follow-up and posttreatment outcome evaluation to what they called Concurrent Recovery Monitoring. Treatment providers have been slow to incorporate measurement-based care or feedback-informed treatment using validated, reliable tools to aid in treatment planning and outcomes evaluation in real time.

Increasingly, funding for practitioners and programs will be based not on charges for the services provided, but on demonstrating value, and this will entail effective engagement and retention, using evidence-based practices (EBPs). Compared with the rest of health care, treatment programs in SUD have encountered extensive barriers to EBP implementation, for example, lack of administrative support, insufficient staff time, and lack of skills or knowledge.[42] The challenge for the field will be to adopt strongly evidentiary EBPs, such as measurement-based care, motivational interviewing,[43] establishing a helping alliance,[44] employing peer supports,[45] cognitive-behavioral therapy,[46] contingency management,[47,48] and community reinforcement approach.[49] ASAM Level of Care Certification site visits[35,50] will examine and document such offerings at a program; however, their mere presence will not be sufficient. Process measures will require programs to show whether they use EBPs, how often, for how many patients, and how individualized they are.

Finally, value-based contracting will require providers to document beneficial clinical outcomes. By the early 2000s, payers were expected to meet performance measures, such as the Washington Circle Measures,[51] which became adopted as the HEDIS measures[52] (Healthcare Effectiveness Data and Information Set) from the National Committee on Quality Assurance. It is likely that providers will be asked to submit to performance measures eventually, too, which will require documentation of patient retention, stabilization, abstinence, and functional health outcomes to obtain optimal reimbursement. These requirements will bring addiction treatment in line with trends in general health care, as with the management of hypertension or diabetes.[53] With these chronic illnesses, changes to the treatment plan are based on treatment outcomes and tracked by real-time, objective, quantitative measurement at every visit (eg, blood pressure or blood sugar levels are monitored to determine the success of the current treatment regimen).

In 2018, The Joint Commission modified its Standard CTS.03.01.09 (https://www.jointcommission.org/accreditation-and-certification/health-care-settings/behavioral-health-care/outcome-measures-standard/). The modification required that standardized patient outcomes be monitored to inform goals and objectives and inform individual treatment plans decisions (https://www.jointcommission.org/-/media/tjc/documents/accred-and-cert/bhc/rationale-cts030109-revised.pdf).

Grade: Addiction treatment gets a *C or D grade* if not an *F (Fail)* for this guiding principle. Very few programs are implementing measurement-based care. We lag far behind other chronic disease management services in implementing a focus on treatment outcomes to drive an individual's care.

Plans for improvement. Measurement-based care or feedback-informed treatment will require adoption of validated, reliable tools, such as the Brief Addiction Monitor[54,55] perhaps with biometric measures (eg, substance use testing, which is standard with health professional treatment programs). Follow-up assessment with CONTINUUM should afford opportunities to measure change over time, particularly in relation to dimensional needs that have been versus have not been addressed by specific treatments. These opportunities will serve real-time treatment planning, as well as, eventually, outcome prediction. When an oncologist tells a family their loved one's expected survival with a treatment, it engenders confidence. As statistician W. Edwards Deming famously stated, "In G-d we trust; all others must bring data." The addiction treatment field's absence of quantitative outcomes data, however, is an obstacle to both destigmatization and quality improvement. The challenge in improving quality is, as management guru Peter Drucker said, "If you can't measure it, you can't improve it." ASAM itself practices this preaching, in the empirically driven ability to continually refine *The ASAM Criteria* and CONTINUUM algorithmic equations, a key distinguishing feature from most other medical necessity Level of Care (LOC) criteria.

Other American Society of Addiction Medicine Criteria Principles and Objectives

Several other principles follow from *The ASAM Criteria* and highlight critical needs for the field that still await development.

Moving toward an interdisciplinary, team approach to care: With health reform, addiction care is increasingly delivered by staff from mental health, primary care, and community resources, including peer supports.[56] Physicians will remain essential in addiction treatment, never more so than during the opioid epidemic, thanks to the effectiveness of MOUD. Newer care delivery models, however, will use physician expertise via collaborative care,[57] integrative care, and incentivized care models[58] such as the Patient-Centered Health Care Home.[59] These approaches are essential for addressing the opioid epidemic, the stimulant epidemic, and for achieving diversity, equity, and inclusion needs.[60]

Identifying adolescent-specific needs: Adolescents who use alcohol, tobacco, and/ or other drugs differ from adults in significant ways,[61] including in their emotional, cognitive, physical, social, and moral development.[62] These adolescents differ in their interactions with family and peers, maturity of independent living skills, and by the fact that some testing of limits is a normative developmental task of adolescence. *The ASAM Criteria* distinguishes adolescent versus adult treatment, where appropriate, and the same dimensional model can be useful for measuring adolescent treatment outcomes.[63] A national survey of highly regarded adolescent treatment programs reported that *The ASAM Criteria* was the most commonly used SUD-related tool at intake and end of treatment.[64]

Grading The American Society of Addiction Medicine Criteria and Future Plans

As ASAM develops the fourth edition of *The ASAM Criteria*, the revision will involve rigorous review of systematic reviews, recent primary peer-reviewed studies, and clinical guidelines. The review will then use a formal modified Delphi process for developing expert consensus followed by field review from diverse stakeholders. The review will build on the following successes and needs:

- Success in establishing multidimensional criteria, the distributed Level of Care model, and accounting for co-occurring conditions, but increasing complexity raises the need for more salient trainings, for example, case-based learning.
- Success in launching standardized assessment via technology is encouraging, but this will require ongoing, empirically-driven quality improvement, which is underway thanks to the formation of ASAM's Quality and Science Team.
- Success in establishing standards for service intensities has been realized as ASAM launched the ASAM-CARF Level of Care Certification Program, but this is raising a need for greater clarity in the specifications for what exactly is a given level of care.
- *The ASAM Criteria* should continue to use technology to standardize, streamline, and make more objective the managed care, prior approval, and utilization management process.
- It is time for *The ASAM Criteria* to connect assessment with treatment planning and outcome measurement. If this can succeed, then *The ASAM Criteria* should become a vehicle for outcome data analysis, that is, pretreatment versus post-treatment patient assessment that yields objective measures of progress and need for further care.

SUMMARY

Over time, with technology and research, *The ASAM Criteria*, the ASAM CONTINUUM software, and the ASAM-CARF Certification Program are helping the field implement a national standard for addiction treatment. *The ASAM Criteria* have achieved substantial adoption by providers, states, courts, and payers, who increasingly use its concepts and principles, and are beginning to introduce its standards and technology tools into routine care.[25,65,66] As a result, the field has made considerable progress in evolving the quality of addiction treatment. Nationwide educational efforts have improved service differentiation, meeting diverse patient needs, improving assessment, and supporting payment reform, with the potential for measurement-based care, outcomes-based treatment, and value-based contracting in SUD treatment. More research and work are needed by the field, and by ASAM. For more than 30 years, however, addiction medicine and addiction treatment in general have embarked on a dramatic transition that is enviable in modern health care, with a forward trajectory that presages continued benefit for patients, their families, and society.

CLINICS CARE POINTS

- Coronavirus disease 2019 and the opioid and stimulant crises have increased public acceptance that addiction is "a treatable, chronic medical disease involving complex interactions among brain circuits, genetics, the environment, and an individual's life experiences." In response, providers and payers must surmount the limitations of legacy approaches by increasing adoption of *The ASAM Criteria* toolkit into routine care.

- Providers and payers can steadily improve access to care and quality of care by adoption of *The ASAM Criteria* toolkit. This toolkit is an evidence-based and expert consensus-driven set of software, processes, educational programs, and publications. *The ASAM Criteria* is the most widely-accepted system for standardizing assessment, determining treatment needs, placement, and utilization management.

- By organizing patient data into ASAM's 6 dimensions of assessment, providers can rapidly improve the quality of new patient intakes, speak in a consistent language of patient needs and strengths, streamline medical necessity presentations and negotiations, and upgrade treatment planning and outcomes measurement.

- The least intensive treatment should be used that safely and effectively can meet the patient's needs. Services should be used for WM, medications, co-occurring conditions, and support flexibly rather than in fixed placement configurations. One-size-fits-all placements and treatment plans, fixed bundles and durations of treatment, and fail-first medical necessity requirements should be avoided. Patients' needs should be served as they present, rather than requiring patients to meet the needs or expectations of treatment.

ACKNOWLEDGEMENTS

Supported by Grants # R01-DA08781 and K24-DA00427 to Dr. Gastfriend from the National Institute on Drug Abuse and the Norwegian Directorate of Health and the Drug and Alcohol Treatment in Central Norway Trust (Helsedirektoratet, Rusbehandling Midt-Norge).

DISCLOSURE

Dr D.R. Gastfriend is: President & CEO, RecoverySearch, Inc (royalties and consulting fees from ASAM, Inc, and FEi Systems, Inc). Co-founder & Chief Medical

Officer, DynamiCare Health, Inc (ownership, employment). Consultant, Farella Braun + Martel LLP for Federal District Court of No. District of California, Wit v. UBH Remedy Order (consulting fees). Scientific Advisory Board member, BioCorRx, Inc, IntentSolutions, Inc (options). Dr D. Mee-Lee is: Consultant, to The Change Companies (royalties and consulting fees)

REFERENCES

1. Mee-Lee D, Shulman GD, Fishman M, et al. The ASAM criteria: treatment for addictive, substance-related, and Co-occurring conditions. Third. Carson City, NV: The Change Companies; 2013.
2. Gastfriend DR, editor. Addiction treatment matching: research foundations of the American society of addiction medicine (ASAM) criteria. 1st edition. Binghampton, NY: Haworth Pr Inc; 2004.
3. ASAM-The American Society of Addiction Medicine. ASAM CONTINUUM. Available at: https://www.asam.org/asam-criteria/asam-criteria-software/asam-continuum. Accessed January 31, 2022.
4. Cohen C, Hernández-Delgado H, Robles-Fradet A. Medicaid section 1115 waivers for substance use disorders: a review. Washington, DC: National Health Law Program; 2021. p. 42.
5. Enos G. Ruling against UBH in class action resonates within treatment community. Alcohol Drug Abuse Weekly 2019. Available at: https://onlinelibrary.wiley.com/doi/abs/10.1002/adaw.32445. Accessed September 4, 2020.
6. American Association of Community Psychiatrists. LOCUS-level of care utilization system for psychiatric and addiction services. Vol Adult Version, 2010. Pittsburgh, PA: American Association of Community Psychiatrists; 2009.
7. Gastfriend DR, McLellan AT. Treatment matching. Theoretic basis and practical implications. Med Clin North Am 1997;81(4):945–66.
8. Hoffman NG, Halikas JA, Mee-Lee D. ASAM patient placement criteria for the treatment of psychoactive substance use disorders. American Society of Addiction Medicine; 1991.
9. Mee-Lee D. ASAM (American Society of Addiction Medicine) Patient placement criteria for the treatment of substance-related disorders. Chevy Chase, MD: American Society of Addiction Medicine; 1996.
10. Mee-Lee D. ASAM patient placement criteria for the treatment of substance-related disorders. Chevy Chase, MD: American Society of Addiction Medicine; 2001.
11. Turner WM, Turner KH, Reif S, et al. Feasibility of multidimensional substance abuse treatment matching: automating the ASAM Patient Placement Criteria. Drug and Alcohol Dependence 1999;55(1):35–43.
12. Kosanke N, Magura S, Staines G, et al. Feasibility of matching alcohol patients to ASAM levels of care. Am J Addict 2002;11(2):124–34.
13. Baker SL, Gastfriend DR. Reliability of multidimensional substance abuse treatment matching. J Addict Dis 2004;22(sup1):45–60.
14. Staines G, Kosanke N, Magura S, et al. Convergent validity of the ASAM Patient Placement Criteria using a standardized computer algorithm. J Addict Dis 2003; 22(Suppl 1):61–77.
15. Stallvik M, Nordahl HM. Convergent validity of the ASAM criteria in co-occurring disorders. J Dual Diagn 2014;10(2):68–78.
16. Sharon E, Krebs C, Turner W, et al. Predictive validity of the ASAM Patient Placement Criteria for hospital utilization. J Addict Dis 2003;22(Suppl 1):79–93.

17. Magura S, Staines G, Kosanke N, et al. Predictive Validity of the ASAM Patient Placement Criteria for Naturalistically Matched vs. Mismatched Alcoholism Patients. Am J Addict 2003;12(5):386–97.

18. Angarita GA, Reif S, Pirard S, et al. No-show for treatment in substance abuse patients with comorbid symptomatology: validity results from a controlled trial of the ASAM patient placement criteria. J Addict Med 2007;1(2):79–87.

19. Stallvik M, Gastfriend DR. Predictive and convergent validity of the ASAM criteria software in Norway. Addict Res Theor 2014;22(6):515–23.

20. Reggers J, Ansseau M, Gustin F. Adaptation and validation of the ASAM PPC-2R Criteria in french and dutch speaking belgian drug addicts. Presented at: The 65th Annual Meeting of the College on Problems of Drug Dependence; June 14, 2003; Bal Harbor, FL.

21. Hoopfer S, Ryan M, Lucena A, et al. ASAM PPC assessment software business plan. Boston, MA: Harvard Business School Volunteer Consulting Organization; 2011. p. 30.

22. American Society of Addiction Medicine. The ASAM Criteria Software National Demonstration Launch. Default. 2021. Available at: https://www.asam.org/blog-details/article/2021/08/09/the-asam-criteria-software-national-demonstration-launch. Accessed January 31, 2022.

23. Kolsky GD. Current state AOD agency practices regarding the use of patient placement criteria (PPC) |. NASADAD - The National Association of State Alcohol and Drug Abuse Directors; 2006. p. 17. Available at: https://nasadad.org/pageviewer/?target=resources/PPC_Report.pdf. Accessed January 25, 2022.

24. Wachino V. New service delivery opportunities for individuals with a substance use disorder. 2015. Available at: https://www.medicaid.gov/federal-policy-guidance/downloads/smd15003.pdf. Accessed November 30, 2016.

25. Richardson J, Cowell A, Villeneuve E, et al. Understanding substance use disorder (SUD)treatment needs using assessment data: final report. Washington, DC: Research Triangle Institute; 2020. Available at. https://aspe.hhs.gov/reports/understanding-substance-use-disorder-treatment-needs-using-assessment-data-final-report-0.

26. Guyer J, Traube A, Deshchenko O. *Speaking the Same Language: A Toolkit for Strengthening Patient-Centered Addiction Care in the United States.* American Society of Addiction Medicine. 2021. Available at: https://www.asam.org/docs/default-source/quality-science/final—asam-toolkit-speaking-same-language.pdf?sfvrsn=728c5fc2_2#page=13. Accessed November 9, 2021.

27. NIDA-The National Institute on Drug Abuse. Principles of drug addiction treatment: a research-based guide. Third Edition. National Institute on Drug Abuse; 2018. p. 60. Available at: https://www.drugabuse.gov/publications/principles-drug-addiction-treatment-research-based-guide-third-edition/preface. Accessed January 25, 2022.

28. Padwa H, Mark TL, Wondimu B. What's in an "ASAM-based Assessment?" Variations in Assessment and Level of Care Determination in Systems Required to Use ASAM Patient Placement Criteria. J Addict Med 2022;16(1):18–26.

29. Camilleri AC, Cacciola JS, Jenson MR. Comparison of two ASI-based standardized patient placement approaches. J Addict Dis 2012;31(2):118–29.

30. Kampman K, Jarvis M. American Society of Addiction Medicine (ASAM) National Practice Guideline for the Use of Medications in the Treatment of Addiction Involving Opioid Use. J Addict Med 2015;9(5):358–67.

31. The ASAM national practice guideline for the treatment of opioid use disorder: 2020 focused update. Rockville, MD: American Society of Addiction Medicine; 2020. p. 91.
32. Duncan BL, Miller SD, Sparks J. The heroic client: a revolutionary way to improve effectiveness through client-directed, outcome-informed Therapy. 2nd Edition. San Francisco: Jossey-Bass.; 2004.
33. Prochaska JO, DiClemente CC, Norcross JC. In search of how people change. Applications to addictive behaviors. Am Psychol 1992;47(9):1102–14.
34. Stallvik M, Gastfriend DR, Nordahl HM. Matching patients with substance use disorder to optimal level of care with the ASAM Criteria software. J Substance Use 2015;20(6):389–98.
35. Merrifield C. ASAM and CARF Launch Transformative Residential Addiction Treatment Certification Nationwide. 2020. Available at: http://carf.org/LOC-certification-launch/. Accessed January 28, 2022.
36. ASAM LOC Certification. Available at: http://www.carf.org/LOCcertification/. Accessed January 28, 2022.
37. Substance Abuse and Mental Health Services Administration. National survey of substance Abuse treatment services (N-SSATS): 2020, data on substance Abuse treatment facilities. CBHSQ Data; 2021. p. 313. Available at: https://www.samhsa.gov/data/report/national-survey-substance-abuse-treatment-services-n-ssats-2020-data-substance-abuse. Accessed February 8, 2022.
38. The Joint Commission. Enhanced substance use disorders standards for behavioral health organizations. Joint Comm 2019;7. Available at: https://www.google.com/search?q=SAMHSA+ASAM+Criteria+software&oq=SAMHSA+ASAM+Criteria+software&aqs=chrome..69i57j33i160.10264j0j7&sourceid=chrome&ie=UTF-8. Accessed January 31, 2022.
39. About the Addiction Treatment Needs Assessment. Available at: https://www.shatterproof.org/need-help/about-addiction-treatment-needs-assessment. Accessed January 31, 2022.
40. Boswell JF, Kraus DR, Miller SD, et al. Implementing routine outcome monitoring in clinical practice: benefits, challenges, and solutions. Psychother Res 2015; 25(1):6–19.
41. McLellan AT, McKay JR, Forman R, et al. Reconsidering the evaluation of addiction treatment: from retrospective follow-up to concurrent recovery monitoring. Addiction 2005;100(4):447–58.
42. Willenbring ML, Kivlahan D, Kenny M, et al. Beliefs about evidence-based practices in addiction treatment: A survey of Veterans Administration program leaders. J Subst Abuse Treat 2004;26(2):79–85.
43. Miller WR, Rollnick S. Motivational interviewing: Third Edition: helping people change. Guilford Press; 2012. Available at: https://www.guilford.com/books/Motivational-Interviewing/Miller-Rollnick/9781609182274. Accessed January 25, 2022.
44. Duncan B, Miller SD, Sparks J, et al. Preliminary Psychometric Properties of a "Working" Alliance Measure. 2004. Available at: https://www.semanticscholar.org/paper/The-Session-Rating-Scale%3A-Preliminary-Psychometric-Duncan-Psyd/385e71d09a5931a9eb3196f78951634a01c7c1f5. Accessed January 25, 2022.
45. Gormley MA, Pericot-Valverde I, Diaz L, et al. Effectiveness of peer recovery support services on stages of the opioid use disorder treatment cascade: a systematic review. Drug Alcohol Depend 2021;229(Pt B):109123.

46. Magill M, Ray L, Kiluk B, et al. A meta-analysis of cognitive-behavioral therapy for alcohol or other drug use disorders: treatment efficacy by contrast condition. J Consult Clin Psychol 2019;87(12):1093–105.

47. NIH - NIDA. Contingency management interventions/motivational incentives (alcohol, stimulants, opioids, marijuana, nicotine). National Institute on Drug Abuse; 2020. Available at: https://www.drugabuse.gov/publications/principles-drug-addiction-treatment-research-based-guide-third-edition/evidence-based-approaches-to-drug-addiction-treatment/behavioral-therapies/contingency-management-interventions-motivational-incentives. Accessed December 3, 2021.

48. Bolivar HA, Klemperer EM, Coleman SRM, et al. Contingency management for patients receiving medication for opioid use disorder: a systematic review and meta-analysis. JAMA Psychiatry 2021. https://doi.org/10.1001/jamapsychiatry.2021.1969.

49. Meyers RJ, Roozen HG, Smith JE. The Community Reinforcement Approach. Alcohol Res Health 2011;33(4):380–8.

50. Knopf A. CARF adds OBOT accreditation and ASAM certification. Alcohol Drug Abuse Weekly 2019;31(5):3–4.

51. McCorry F, Garnick DW, Bartlett J, et al. Developing performance measures for alcohol and other drug services in managed care plans. Joint Comm J Qual Improvement 2000;26(11):633–43.

52. Garnick DW, Lee MT, Horgan CM, et al. Adapting washington circle performance measures for public sector substance abuse treatment systems. J Subst Abuse Treat 2009;36(3):265–77.

53. Thomas CP, Garnick DW, Horgan CM, et al. Advancing performance measures for use of medications in substance abuse treatment. J Subst Abuse Treat 2011;40(1):35–43.

54. Cacciola JS, Alterman AI, DePhilippis D, et al. Development and initial evaluation of the Brief Addiction Monitor (BAM). J Subst Abuse Treat 2013;44(3):256–63.

55. Nelson KG, Young K, Chapman H. Examining the performance of the brief addiction monitor. J Subst Abuse Treat 2014;46(4):472–81.

56. Tai B, Volkow ND. Treatment for substance use disorder: opportunities and challenges under the affordable care act. Social Work Public Health 2013;28(3–4):165–74.

57. LaBelle CT, Han SC, Bergeron A, et al. Office-based opioid treatment with buprenorphine (OBOT-B): statewide implementation of the massachusetts collaborative care model in community health centers. J Subst Abuse Treat 2016;60:6–13.

58. Foster S, Lee K, Edwards C, et al. Providing incentive for emergency physician X-Waiver training: an evaluation of program success and postintervention buprenorphine prescribing. Ann Emerg Med 2020;76. https://doi.org/10.1016/j.annemergmed.2020.02.020.

59. Hollingsworth JM, Saint S, Hayward RA, et al. Specialty care and the patient-centered medical home. Med Care 2011;49(1):4–9.

60. Cohen JJ, Gabriel BA, Terrell C. The case for diversity in the health care workforce. Health Aff 2002;21(5):90–102.

61. NIDA. Principles of adolescent substance use disorder treatment: a research-based guide. National Institute on Drug Abuse; 2020. p. 42. Available at: https://www.drugabuse.gov/publications/principles-adolescent-substance-use-disorder-treatment-research-based-guide/evidence-based-approaches-to-treating-adolescent-substance-use-disorders/recovery-support-services. Accessed May 17, 2021.

62. Tanner-Smith EE, Steinka-Fry KT, Kettrey HH, et al. Adolescent substance use treatment effectiveness: a systematic review and meta-analysis. Nashville, TN: Peabody Research Institute, Vanderbilt University; 2016.
63. Coll KC, Freeman BJ, Juhnke GA, et al. Evaluating American Society of Addiction Medicine (ASAM) Dimension Assessment as an Outcome Measure: A Pilot Study with Substance Abusing Adolescents in Two Matched Residential Treatment Centers. 2015. Available at: https://www.counseling.org/knowledge-center/vistas/by-subject2/vistas-substance-abuse/docs/default-source/vistas/article_679b5a22f1 6116603abcacff0000bee5e7. Accessed January 26, 2022.
64. Gans J, Falco M, Shackman BR, et al. An in-depth survey of the screening and assessment practices of highly regarded adolescent substance abuse treatment programs. J Child Adolesc Subst Abuse 2010;19(1):33–47.
65. Heatherton B. Implementing the ASAM Criteria in community treatment centers in Illinois: opportunities and challenges. American Society of Addiction Medicine. J Addict Dis 2000;19(2):109–16.
66. Chuang E, Wells R, Alexander JA, et al. Factors associated with use of ASAM criteria and service provision in a national sample of outpatient substance abuse treatment units. J Addict Med 2009;3(3):139–50.
67. Fishman M, American Society of Addiction Medicine. ASAM patient placement criteria: supplement on pharmacotherapies for alcohol use disorders. Wolters Kluwer Health/Lippincott Williams & Wilkins; 2010. Available at: https://archive.org/details/asampatientplace0000unse. Accessed January 25, 2022.
68. American Society of Addiction Medicine. What is CO-Triage?. 2017. Available at: https://www.asamcontinuum.org/knowledgebase/what-is-continuum-triage-co-triage/. Accessed April 18, 2021.
69. Change Healthcare Partners with the American Society of Addiction Medicine to Transform Utilization Management for SUD. Recent News & Press Releases. Available at: https://newsroom.changehealthcare.com/press-releases/change-healthcare-partners-with-the-american-society-of-addictio. Accessed January 31, 2022.